D0886870

OXFORD MEDICAL PUBLICATIONS

Oxford Handbook of
Sports Medicine

Oxford University Press makes no representation, express or implied, that the drug dosages in this book are correct. Readers must therefore always check the product information and clinical procedures with the most up-to-date published product information and data sheets provided by the manufacturers and the most recent codes of conduct and safety regulations. The authors and the publishers do not accept responsibility or legal liability for any errors in the text or for the misuse or misapplication of material in this work.

Oxford Handbook of Sports Medicine

Editors
Eugene Sherry
Stephen F. Wilson

Assistant Editors
Lawrence Trieu
Sameer Viswanathan

KC
1211
.094
1998
Indiana University
Library
Northwest

Oxford   New York   Tokyo

OXFORD UNIVERSITY PRESS

1998

Oxford University Press, Great Clarendon Street, Oxford OX2 6DP

Oxford New York

*Athens Auckland Bangkok Bogota Bombay
Buenos Aires Calcutta Cape Town Dar es Salaam
Delhi Florence Hong Kong Istanbul Karachi
Kuala Lumpur Madras Madrid Melbourne
Mexico City Nairobi Paris Singapore
Taipei Tokyo Toronto Warsaw*

*and associated companies in
Berlin Ibadan*

Oxford is a trade mark of Oxford University Press

*Published in the United States
by Oxford University Press Inc., New York*

© *E. Sherry, S. Wilson, and the contributors listed on pxi, 1998*

*All rights reserved. No part of this publication may be
reproduced, stored in a retrieval system, or transmitted, in any
form or by any means, without the prior permission in writing of Oxford
University Press. Within the UK, exceptions are allowed in respect of any
fair dealing for the purpose of research or private study, or criticism or
review, as permitted under the Copyright, Designs and Patents Act, 1988, or
in the case of reprographic reproduction in accordance with the terms of
the licences issued by the Copyright Licensing Agency. Enquiries concerning
reproduction outside these terms and in other countries should be sent to
the Rights Department, Oxford University Press, at the address above*

*This book is sold subject to the condition that it shall not,
by way of trade or otherwise, be lent, re-sold, hired out, or otherwise
circulated without the publisher's prior consent in any form of binding
or cover other than that in which it is published and without a similar
condition including this condition being imposed
on the subsequent purchaser*

A catalogue record for this book is available from the British Library

Library of Congress Cataloging in Publication Data
*Oxford handbook of sports medicine / editors, Eugene Sherry, Stephen
F. Wilson; assistant editors, Lawrence Trieu, Sameer Viswanathan.
(Oxford medical publications)
Complements: Oxford textbook of sports medicine. 2nd ed.
Includes bibliographical references and index.
1. Sports medicine—Handbooks, manuals, etc. I. Sherry, Eugene.
II. Wilson, Stephen F. III. Oxford textbook of sports medicine.
IV. Series.
[DNLM: 1. Athletic Injuries handbooks. 2. Sports Medicine
handbooks. QT 29 098 1998]
RC1211.094 1998 617.1'027—dc21 98–11503
ISBN 0 19 262890 9*

NWST
1AKT1512

*Typeset by Joshua Associates Ltd., Oxford
Printed in Great Britain on acid-free paper by
The Bath Press, Avon*

Preface

Sports medicine is an exciting specialty charged with the care of sick and injured athletes. This includes performance parameters. In many countries this has become an independent specialty with its own colleges and associations; nevertheless its charge crosses the disciplines of orthopedics, rehabilitation medicine, nutrition, psychiatry, emergency medicine, pediatrics, geriatrics, gynecology, dermatology, and primary care. Perhaps this explains its appeal? It provides an opportunity to work with colleagues in an interdisciplinary way. Doctors can easily identify with their patients. Most are (or were) fit and highly motivated who want to get better (sometimes too soon).

The benefits of regular exercise are now well established for all groups in the community including the young, old, disabled, and the unwell. In some ways there is too much emphasis on sport with serious health problems, for example, eating disorders occurring in female athletes. We should never forget that we are primarily doctors and that may mean giving some unpopular advice to quit or delay sporting activity. This can best be done when armed with the facts.

Everyone has their idols. In the USA it seems to be Hollywood superstars, in the UK the aristocracy, with the Irish it is their writers, and in the Antipodes it is our sporting heroes. For the editors it is our teachers (ES—Ronald Huckstep, Bruce Shepherd, Geoff Cocker). ES learnt his craft as a general practitioner on the ski fields in the early 1980s where he treated over 10,000 skiing injuries before becoming an orthopedic surgeon. SFW developed his interest in sports medicine after competing in dinghy and yachting regattas from his teenage years until the present and went on to train in sports medicine at the London Hospital before returning to Sydney to practice rehabilitation medicine. He has been an honorary medical officer for Athletics NSW and more recently developed an interest as a national classifier for Swimmers with Disabilities. He was appointed a member of the NSW Government Sporting Injuries Committee and continues to research with a current interest in head and neck injuries in sport.

We are indebted to our contributors who bring their vast clinical experience and wisdom to this text (many of whom will be involved in the care of athletes in the Sydney 2000 Olympic Games); we are sure it will prove a useful practical guide to you as a medical student, primary care provider, sports medicine specialist, orthopedic surgeon, or rehabilitation physician.

A novel feature of this book is that the co-editors are available to answer your questions on Sports Medicine issues specifically related to this text by contacting us on our website, WorldOrtho (at http://www.worldortho.com). LT and SV have established this innovative website which is now the largest orthopedic and sports medicine site on the Internet. Our dedicated search engine (at http://www.orthosearch.com) can access further information for you. We invite you all to visit us on the web and in person at the Sydney 2000 Olympic Games.

ES
SFW
LT
SV

Sydney, 1998

Acknowledgments

We thank the publishers and authors of Greenwich Medical Media Ltd (GMM) for permission to reproduce figures and draw upon material from their text, *Sports medicine: Problems and practical management* (1997), Chap 4, Figs 4.4 and 4.5 are from Chap 5, Figs 9 and 12; Chap 23, Fig 23.1 is from Chap 17, Fig. 6; Chap 21, Figs 21.1 and 21.2, Table 21.2, Figs 21.3, 21.4, Tables 21.3, 21.4 and 21.5, Figs 21.5, 21.6, Tables 21.7 and 21.8 are from Chap 18, Figs 2, 11, 12.21, 26.27, 29, 32, 33.8 and 41 respectively. Table 4.3 is modified from Fig 1, p63.

We also thank William & Wilkins, Philadelphia, for permission to use Fig 2.1, p13, Chap 2 and Fig E-1, p290, Appendix E from ACSM's *Guidelines for exercise testing and prescription* (1995, 5th edn), W Larry Kenney (ed), Oxford University Press for permission to use Fig 1, p206, from the *Oxford textbook of sports medicine* by M Harries *et al* (1994); CRC Press for permission to use Tables 10–2, p83, for Table 4.1 and Tables 20.1 and 20.2 for Tables 22.2 and 22.3 from *Sports medicine for the primary care physicians* (1994, 2nd edn), RB Birrer (ed); and Hanley & Belfus, Philadelphia, (1944) for the use of the table from p431 in *Sports medicine secrets* (1994), MB Mellion (ed) for p94–5. We also thank the American Academy of Pediatrics for the use of their 1994 *Statement affecting sports participation* (Tables 1, 2, and 3, *Pediatrics* **49**, 5, 1994, p757–76) for. Tables 4.7 and 4.8. Figs 5.1, 19.14, 20.1, and 20.2 were supplied by Medical Illustrations, Royal North Shore Hospital, Sydney. Thanks also to the International Paralympic Committee for permission to use their logo.

Thanks are due to Professor John Thomson for providing editorial assistance, Vlasios Brakoulias (Bill) for the original illustrations, and to all the staff at Oxford University Press for all their help at all stages of production.

Contents

Dedicated to Conor, Declan, Tom (ES) and
inspired by a great sportsman—my father, Rupert (SFW)

Abbreviations and symbols

AAOS	American Academy of Orthopaedic Surgeons	ESR	erthrocycle sedimentation rate
ABC	**A**irway, **B**reathing, **C**irculation	EUC	electrolytes, urea, creatine
acetyl-CoA	acetyl-coenzyme A	FBC	full blood count
ACJ	acromioclavicular joint	FCR	flexor carpi radialis
ACL	anterior cruciate ligament	FDB	flexor digitorum brevis
ACSM	American College of Sports Medicine	FDL	flexor digitorum longis
		FDP	flexor digitorm profundis
ACTH	adrenocorticotropin hormone	FFA	free fatty acids
ADSA	Australian Drug Sports Agency	FHL	flexor hallucis longus
		FiO₂	partial pressure of oxygen in inspired air
ADT	anterior draw test	FPL	flexor pollicis longus
ADL	activities of daily living	FSH	follicle stimulating hormone
ADR	adverse drug reactions	FT	fast twitch
AO	(Weber's scheme)	FVC	forced vital capacity
AP	anterior–posterior (anterio-posterior)	GC/MS	gas chromatography/mass spectrometry
APL	abductor pollicis longus	GHJ	glenohumeral joint
ASDA	Australian Sports Drug Agency	GI	gastrointestinal
		GLUT4	glucose transporter proteins
ARDS	adult respiratory distress syndrome	GnRH	gonadotropin releasing hormone
ATFL	anterior talofibular ligament	GMM	Greenwich Medical Media
ATP–ADP	adenosine triphosphate–adenosine 5'-diphosphate	GSI	genuine stress incontinence
		HAPAD	transverse arch support
AVN	avascular necrosis	Hb	hemoglobin
BM	body mass	HBP	high blood pressure
BP	blood pressure	hCG	human chorionic gonadotropin
bpm	beats per minute		
CABG	coronary artery bypass graft	HCM	hypertrophic cardiomyopathy
CAD	coronary artery disease	HDL	high density lipoprotein
CHD	coronary heart disease	hGH	human growth hormone/somatropin
CHF	cardiac heart failure		
CHO	carbohydrate	HR	heart rate
CO	cardiac output	HRMS	high resolution mass spectrometer
CFS	cerebrospinal fluid		
CFL	calcaneofibular ligament	HRT	hormone replacement therapy
CMV	cytomegalovirus	HV	hallux vagus
CNS	cenral nervous system	Ig	immunoglobulin
CP	creatine phosphate	IGF-1	insulin-like growth factor
CPR	cardiopulmonary resuscitation	IHD	ischemic heart disease
CSF	cerebrospinal fluid	II	image intensifier
CT	computed tomography	IOC	International Olympic Committee
CV	cardiovascular		
CVS	cardiovascular system	IPJ	interphalangeal joint
CXR	chest x-ray	ISO	international sports organization
DCS	decompression sickness		
DEXA	dual energy x-ray absorptiometry	IUD	intrauterine device
		IV	intravenous
DI	detrusor instability	IVI	intravenous infusion
DIC	disseminated intravascular coagulation	K	potassium
		KOH	potassium hydroxide
DIPJ	distal interphalangeal joint	L	liter
DISI	dorsal intercalated segment instability	LB	loose body
		LDL	low density lipoprotein
DR	Danger Response	LCL	lateral collateral ligament
DRUJ	distal radioulnar joint	LFT	liver function test
DVT	deep venous thrombosis	LH	lutenizing hormone
EBV	Epstein–Barr virus	LLD	leg length difference
ECC	external cardiac depression	LV	left ventricle
ECG	electrocardiogram	LVH	left ventricular hypertrophy
ECRB	extensor carpi radialis brevis	MAST	military anti-shock trousers
ECRL	extensor carpi radialis longus	MCL	medial (ulnar) collateral ligament
ECU	extensor carpi ulnaris		
EF	ejection fraction	MET	metabolic equivalent unit
EMG	electromyogram	MDI	multidirectional instability
EPB	extensor pollicis brevis	mg	milligram
EPO	erythropoietin	MI	myocardial infarction

ml	milliliter	RBC	red blood cell count
MML	maximum MET level	RDI	recommended dietary intake
MPJ	metacarpophalangeal joint	rEPO	recombinant or synthetic EPO
MRI	magnetic resonance imaging	RICE	rest, ice, compression, elevation
MT	metatarsal	RM	repetition maximum
MTPJ	metatarsal joint	ROM	range of movement
MVA	motor vehicle accident	RTI	respiratory tract infection
Na	sodium	RTS	radial tunnel syndrome
ng	nanogram	RSD	reflex sympathetic dystrophy
NK	natural killer (cell)	RVH	right ventricular hypertrophy
NSAID	non-steroidal anti-inflammatory drug	SaO_2	arterial oxygen saturation
		SCD	sudden cardiac death
OA	osteoarthritis / osteoarthrosis	SCH	subconjunctival hemorrhage
OCD	osteochondritis dissecans	SCIWORA	spinal cord injury with-out radiographic abnormality
OCP	oral contraceptive pill		
OPG	orthopantomogram	SCJ	sternoclavicular joint
ORIF	open reduction and internal fixation	SIT	scaphoid impact test
		SLAP	superior labral anterior posterior
OTC	over-the-counter		
O_{2a-v}	arterial–venous oxygen difference	SOMI	sternal occipital mandibular immobilization
PA	posterior-anterior (postero-anterior)	ST	ST segment
		SUFE	slipped upper femoral capital epiphysis
PaO_2	partial pressure of oxygen in arterial blood		
		SV	stroke volume
PBT	pulmonary barotrauma	TA	tendon Achilles
PCL	posterior cruciate ligament	TCA	tricarboxylic acid cycle
PCR	polymerase chain reaction	TENS	transcutaneous electrical nerve stimulation
PCV	packed cell volume/pressure control ventilation		
		TFCC	triangular fibrocartilage complex
PE	pulmonary embolus		
PFT	pulmonary function tests	THC	tetrahydrocannabinol
PiO_2	partial pressure of oxygen in inspired air	TMJ	temporomandibular joint
		μg	microgram
PIPJ	proximal interphalangeal joint	U	unit
PMT	premenstrual tension	UCL	ulnar colateral ligament
PNF	proprioceptive neuromuscular facilitation	URTI	upper respiratory tract infection
POMS	Profile of Moods test	VF	venricular fibrillation
PR	per rectum	VISI	colar intercalated instability
PRE	progressive resistance exercise	VO_{2max}	maximum rate at which oxygen can be utilized
PTFL	posterior talofibular ligament		
RA	rheumatoid arthritis	VR	venous return
RAS	recticular activating system	WB	weight bearing

Contributors

Greg Bennett
Senior Director, Medical Division Nepean Health and President, NSW Branch, Australian Society of Geriatric Medicine, Sydney

Louise M Burke
Head of Sports Nutrition, Australian Institute of Sport, Canberra

John A Cartmill
Senior Lecturer in Surgery, University of Sydney and Staff Specialist Colorectal Surgeon, Nepean Hospital, Sydney

Donald John Chisholm
Head of Metabolic Research Program, Garvan Institute of Medical Research; Staff Specialist in Endocrinology, Sydney; Professor of Endocrinology, University of NSW

Manuel F Cusi
Visiting Fellow, School of Physiology and Pharmacology, University of NSW and Director of Sports Medicine, WorkSports Clinic, Pennant Hills, Sydney

Amitabha Das
Intern, Sydney

Carl Edmonds
Consultant in Diving Medicine, Sydney

John Estell
Rehabilitation Registrar, South Eastern Sydney Area Health Service, Sydney

Mark A Freeman
Intern, Sydney

Laurie Geffen
Professor of Psychiatry and Head, Cognitive Psychophysiology Laboratory, University of Queensland and Queensland Health Medical School, Herston, Queensland

Gina Geffen
Professor of Neuropsychology, Cognitive Psychophysiology Laboratory, University of Queensland and Queensland Health Medical School, Herston, Queensland

Saul Geffen
Registrar in Rehabilitation, Royal North Shore Hospital, Sydney

Jane A Gorman
Medical Student, University of Sydney

Tom Gwinn
Lecturer, School of Exercise and Sports Science, University of Sydney

Philippa Harvey-Sutton
Occupational Physician, Health Services Australia, Sydney

Anton D Hinton-Bayre
Postgraduate Scholar, Cognitive Psychophysiology Laboratory, University of Queensland and Queensland Health Medical School, Herston, Queensland

Simon R Hutabarat
Orthopaedic Registrar, Sydney

Barry Kirker
Clinical Psychologist, Sydney

Sue Ogle
Senior Staff Specialist Director, Department of Aged Care and Rehabilitation, Royal North Shore Hospital, Sydney

John Rooney
Orthopaedic Registrar, Sydney

Diana Rubel
Dermatology Registrar, Sydney

Jeni Saunders
Sports Medicine Specialist and Visiting Fellow, University of NSW, Sports Medicine Courses, Sydney

Eugene Sherry
Senior Lecturer in Orthopaedic Surgery, University of Sydney and Consultant Orthopaedic Surgeon, Nepean, Jamison, Hills Private and Sydney Adventist Hospitals

Diana E Thomas
Exercise Scientist, Sydney

Lawrence Trieu
Intern, Sydney

Sameer Viswanathan
Intern, Sydney

Stephen F Wilson
Senior Staff Specialist, Department of Aged Care and Rehabilitation Director Rehabilitation, Royal North Shore Hospital, Sydney

John D Yeo
Associate Professor of Surgery, University of Sydney and Senior Consultant to Spinal Injuries, Royal North Shore Hospital, Sydney

1 Sport and medicine: the human race—a philosophical aside

EUGENE SHERRY

Introduction

Sports medicine is concerned with the care and the potential performance of the athlete. It requires a comprehensive approach; unlike the fragmentation seen in technological medicine this century (today's medical students know more about T4 cell levels than a simple Colles' fracture). These principles of care were established by Herodicus of Selymbria (at the time of Socrates) and Claudius Galen (AD 131–201).[1] They emphasized training, diet, massage, and a medical approach to athletics.

Galen's contribution to scientific medicine was monumental. He placed the clinical instructions of Hippocrates on a sound experimental basis; for 1500 years his works dominated medical knowledge. He was a true sports medicine practitioner (the father of sports medicine). Pontifex Maximus made him physician to the gladiators in the Pergamon arena in Asia Minor (AD 158–161) and he published his methods of treatment (among his 500 known works). It is appropriate to set Galen's contribution among those of others.

1 RB Birrer 1994 *Sports medicine for the primary care physician* 2nd edn. CRC, Boca Raton.

When it happened

A history of significant sports medicine events is outlined:

Event	Significance
Bowling game (Egypt 5000 BC)	
Exercise with weights (Urina 3600 BC)	
Chariot races (Greece 1500 BC)	
Chinese book of Gung Fu (c.1000 BC)	Systematic teachings of exercise therapy
Text of the Hindu Atharva–Veda (c.1500 BC)	
Ancient Olympic Games (776 BC)	
Run of Pheidippedes (Marathon to Athens, 490 BC)	Heroism inspired Olympic ideals
Herodicus of Selymbria (time of Socrates 469–399 BC)	Emphasized medical gymnastics
Iccus of Tantrum (444 BC)	First treatise on athletic training
Claudius Galen (AD 131–201)	'Father of sports medicine'
Quintes of Sumer (c.4th century AD)	Described treatment of ankle sprains and boxing wounds
First rowing regatta (AD Venice 300)	Birth of the 'sacred' boat race (later cherished and idealized at Eton)
Avicenna (AD 979–1037)	'Father of Islamic medicine' Relevant writings during post Crusade period
First cricket game (UK 1250)	
Bergerius (1370–1440)	Regular exercises for children
Geronimo Mercuriali (1530–1606)	First illustrated book on sports medicine
Benjamin Franklin (1706–90)	Recommended resistance exercises
First Rugby Union game (Rugby School 1823)	
Oxford–Cambridge Boat Race (1829)	
Edward Hitchcock MD (1854)	America's first college team physician
John Morgan's paper on longevity of elderly oarsmen (mid 19th century)	Benefits of exercise scrutinized
Modern Olympic Games (1896)	Greek doctors in attendance at marathon
Death of Lazaro, a Portuguese runner, from heat stroke after Stockholm marathon (1912)	Physical examinations subsequently required for marathoners
Paris Olympic Games (1924)	First US team doctor in attendance
International Federation of Sports Medicine (FIMS) founded by Sr. Moritz (1928)	
Berlin Olympic Games (1936)	Nazi political perversion of Games
First Paraplegic Games (1948)	Sport for all
First Asian Games (1951)	Reflecting improved standards of nutrition and health
American College of Sports Medicine founded (1954)	
R.G. Bannister, 4-minute mile (1954)	'Physiological barrier' broken (3min 59.4sec), 'glimpse of the greatest freedom that a man can ever know'
President's Council (Eisenhower 1956) on youth and fitness	US Governmental efforts to promote physical fitness through sport
American Academy of Orthopaedic Surgeons establish Committee on Sports Medicine (1962)	Formalization of orthopedic surgeons' long-term involvement with care of athletes

Event	Significance
Terrorism at Munich Games (1972)	Terrorism at the Games
Black Boycott, Montreal Games (1976)	Politics at the Games
Olympic competitors keep sponsorship money (1981)	End of amateurism
Ben Johnson, 100-metre sprint, banned for steroid use (1988)	'End' of use of drugs for performance enhancement
'Unified Team' at Barcelona (1992)	'End' of communist domination of Games
'Coca-Cola' Games in Atlanta (1996)	'Beginning' of corporate control of sports (? started in Los Angeles 1984)

Today, sports medicine has evolved into a respected discipline with dedicated associations, colleges, institutes, and literature in most countries.

Why it happened

Modern man seems obsessed by sport (both as spectator and participant). 25–30% regularly compete in sports.[1] This is not surprising. The health benefits of regular exercise are well documented (decreased: coronary artery disease, high blood pressure, non-insulin dependent diabetes, colon cancer, anxiety, depression, death rates) and all responsible medical practitioners promote it as 'the easiest way to preserve health'.[2] However, there is concern that we are not doing enough participant sport (<50% of children aged 10–17 years regularly exercise, only 10–20% of adults aged 18–65 years vigorously exercise, and <80% over age 65 years exercise).[1] In developing countries, people's lack of exercise, together with tobacco and alcohol consumption, seem likely to create a health catastrophe by the year 2020.[3]

Although sporting fitness/prowess is important, we are perhaps creating modern nations of fit but godless morons (note declining church attendance and literary levels in developed countries). The downtown city gym is the cathedral of this modern age. The appeal and realism of 'Beavis and Butthead', two illiterate adolescent US movie characters, is worrisome. US educators have already sounded the alarm bells about the lack of competitiveness from lack of education in a knowledge-based global economy.[4] Certainly, sporting events can serve other needs. The Roman emperors staged elaborate and costly gladiatorial spectacles (264 BC—AD 325) to entertain and appease the masses so that they could maintain political control. The Circus Maximus in Rome (1st century BC) held up to 150,000 spectators; 2,000 gladiators and 230 wild animals were billed to die in one such show. During this century, the Nazis (Berlin 1936) and Communist regimes (1956—88) used the Olympic Games as spectacles to showcase and legitimize their systems of social control. More recently, the corporate sector is using the Games for financial advantage (Los Angeles 1984, Atlanta 1996). It is thought that the Sydney 2000 Games will be the 'Green Games'—promoting an 'ecological' approach to progress.

Although Baron Pierre de Coubertin's statement that 'the Olympic movement tends to bring together in a radiant union of all the qualities which guide mankind to perfection' appears naïve and idealistic it is not unreasonable to want to use sport to improve the 'human lot' and make it more 'bearable' for all. But why use sport as this vehicle? We need to look further back (in fact, to 4600 billion years ago).

1 J Bloomfield *et al* 1995 *Science and medicine in sport.* 2nd edn p xiii. Blackwell Science 2 RB Birrer 1994 *Sports medicine for the primary care physician.* 2nd edn. p v. CRC, Boca Raton 3 CJL Murray, AD Lopez 1996 *Evidence-based health policy—Lessons from the Global Burden of Disease Study.* Science **274** 740–3 4 *Years of promise: A comprehensive learning strategy for America's children.* Carnegie Corp, New York, Sept. 1996.

How it happened

Man evolved this way.[1] Planet Earth is 4600 million years old. Initially, there was no oxygen. Ultraviolet radiation, which was not blocked by an ozone barrier, stimulated photosynthesis to produce *organic molecules* from water, carbon monoxide, and ammonia.

- Anaerobic metabolism developed 3500 million years ago.
- These original organisms released oxygen into the atmosphere and anaerobic metabolism developed (2000 million years ago). Nucleated unicellular organisms (the eukaryote with the ATP–ADP energy system) arrived 1500 million years ago.
- Large animals appeared 700 million years ago; the first primate, 60–70 million years after the dinosaurs disappeared; mammals, flowering plants, and birds appeared.
- Hominids arrived 5–20 million years ago; *Australopithecus* 4 million years ago. Upright posture with bipedal gait freed the hands to allow the use of tools (and so the brain expanded). Thus followed *Homo habilis*, *H. erectus* (hunters and food gatherers who used fire), *H. sapiens Neanderthalensis* (formed tribes and used common language) and modern man (*H. Sapiens sapiens* 50000 years ago). Modern man's success is due to bipedal gait (sea to land), upright posture (head to sky), use of tools (with opposition of the thumb), and the brain and speech (with universal interests). The orthopaedic markers of this progress are the foot, spine, and thumb/hand (precision grip).
- The above steps (evolution) occurred according to modified Darwinian theory, which states that the gradual accumulation of genetic variants (from mutations and chromosomal rearrangements) allows nature to select the 'best' variants.

It is clear that outdoor activities of hunting and food gathering have been an essential part of our development for millions of years and so constitute an important part of even modern man's emotional, social, and intellectual well-being. The urbanized sophisticate may sit with laptop computer on knee, mobile phone by ear, dictaphone in hand, cable TV on view but yearns for the open sport's field to fulfil a primitive biological need (the Wild Wild Web, the Internet, cannot meet all our needs) to hunt (deer stalking, fishing), to fight (bull as in bull fighting, man as in boxing, environment as in mountaineering) and to use tools (Formula 1 car racing, snow skiing)—that is, *to compete/confront.*[2]

Organized sport

Organized sporting competition can be shown to have three major milestones:

    1 *The Ancient Calendar* with: Egyptian (exercises 5000 BC, running rituals at Meriphis 3800 BC), Chinese (Emperors encouraged subjects to exercise daily, 3600 BC), Indian (text of Hindu Atharva-Veda) and Islamic (Avicenna's writings) events.

    2 *The Olympic Games*—the Greco-Roman tradition with the

1 P Astrard 1994 Introduction—Man as an athlete. In M Harries *et al* (ed) *Oxford textbook of sports medicine* p1–10. OUP   **2** Ernest Hemingway said he only lived to fight, write and to make love. From AE Hotchner 1986 *Papa Hemingway*. William Morrow, New York

Ancient Games (776 BC) and the Modern Games (1896). Olympic competition introduced idealism (dedicated to the Glory of Zeus—the mind, body and spirit of man) with a celebration of the mind and body (by the Greeks) and the need to rise above politics (the Modern Games). Sport functioned to elevate man to a plane of idealistic behaviour above our biological needs.

3 *The Great English Public Schools* recognized (before Baron Pierre de Coubertin) the civilizing influence of organized sport. It served to subvert the energies of their school pupils (the future masters of the British Empire and the Western World) into enterprises of co-operation and heroism on the football field (Eton Wall Game) and the water (rowing). The same schoolboys went up to University (Oxford–Cambridge Boat Race, 1829) and out to the Colonies (where sporting powers developed to maintain status and successful competition with mother England—US football, NZ rugby champions, West Indies cricket, Australian swimming and tennis). All schools and universities eventually established athletic events as an important part of their curriculum.

What will happen

Sport will play a critical part in our future. The scientific endeavours of this century have been directed at military conquest (nuclear bombs), wealth accumulation (commerce) and medicine (disease treatment and prevention). 'All research leads to biomedical advances'.[1] Sports medicine will showcase the achievements of medical science. The health problems of the world (the Global Burden of Disease)[2] are currently respiratory infections, diarrhoea, perinatal problems, depression, and heart disease. The risk factors for these problems are no food, no water, no sanitation, no exercise, no safe sex, too much tobacco and alcohol use, high blood pressure, drug use, and air pollution. By the year 2020 the health problems (from older populations and the rise of the developing regions) will be: heart disease, depression, road accidents, strokes, lung disease; all largely attributable to occupation, alcohol, and tobacco use. Many of these problems can be related to the destruction of our environment (rapid population and industrial growth) in the following way:[2]

- Urban air pollution (oxides)
- Water pollution (waste products)
- Food contamination
- Nuclear weapons (pollution)
- Wars (destroyed ecosystems)
- Loss of ozone in atmosphere (ultraviolet radiation)
- Global rewarming (vector-borne diseases, such as malaria, droughts, floods, starvation)
- Deforestation (with infectious disease epidemics)
- Failure of the modern city (urban homelessness, poverty, underclass, collapse of public health infrastructure). Tuberculosis is at the highest rate in history. The benefits of our civilization are only bestowed on the privileged few, with an urban underclass and the developing world as sick as the Irish city-dwellers of the 1830s, and not much better off than the hunter/food gatherers of the Stone Age.[3]

We need to see some order to see our way forward. Today there are basically two classes of countries—The Developed (wealthy western-styled democracies existing on national debts and cable TV) and the Developing (with widening wealth gap, either few or outrageous prospects and either courted by the multi-glomerates or dependent on the World Bank). The citizens of these countries fall into four groups—can't stop (the super achievers, names found in *Encyclopaedia Britannica*), can cope (solid citizens who uphold the system and pay tax), won't cope (criminal groups) and can't cope (mentally and physically handicapped who need help). 'Can't stop' will plan and 'can cope' will carry out an answer to these problems.

We must protect our environment otherwise our children will be playing sport in a planetary junkyard. Sport may help us. It can modify risk factors (i.e. protect the body) by allowing and encouraging us to:

- reduce alcohol and tobacco use
- avoid physical inactivity

1 J Daie, R Wyse 1996 *Editorial Science* **274** 701   2 CJL Murray, AD Lopez 1996 *Evidence-based health policy—Lessons for the Global Burden of Disease Study. Science* **274** 740–3.   3 MN Cohen 1989 *Health and the rise of civilization.* Yale University Press, New Haven, CT

- avoid the need for illicit drug use
- prevent hypertension and depression (documented)

In fact, the benefits of sport may be taken further to protect the environment. If the purpose of sport is to enhance our health then it is irrational and dangerous to exercise in a polluted environment (the environment is the main determinant of our health—food, water, clean air). Urban runners have been found to have elevated blood lead levels ($>2.51\mu mol/L$), despite decreased levels for the average American from the use of lead-free petrol.[1]

Urban athletes inhale above-average levels of air pollutants (respiratory minute volume increases up to 20 times) which bypasses the nose filter with an open mouth.[2] These pollutants are either a reducing or oxidant form of smog. The reducing forms (carbon fuels) consist of smoke particulate, Sulfur di- or trioxide, and may cause bronchospasm with respiratory infection, viral myocarditis (especially in children in big cities). The oxidant forms (vehicle exhausts with sunlight) are carbon monoxide (can be lethal in the elderly and possibly the young in competition, swimming times are slower when levels exceed 30 parts per million), hydrocarbons, ozone, and nitrogen oxides (these impair the respiratory system, and this is seen in competitive cyclists on open roads). Skaters have developed chemical pneumonitis from the nitrogen oxides given off by propane fuel-propelled resurfacing machines. Swimmers can have exposure-dependent chloroform blood levels (from chlorination, a suspected carcinogen). Team doctors have been needed to monitor and advise on levels (the danger level of nitrogen oxide is 58 parts per billion; obtain the air pollution index from the weather bureau; cancel events when necessary; move to air-conditioned venues; check ventilation facilities).

Athletic events should only be staged in cities and countries with a commitment to safe and clean environments. The culture of sport may need to develop a new creed: *Protect my body and my environment.* There should be an awareness of the need of ecological compatibility of athletic performance with the environment in which the event is held. The Sydney 2000 Olympic Games plan to use this approach. A 'Medic-O-Games' could go further to provide a forum for medical doctors to discuss the health and environmental problems facing us and to participate in Olympic sporting events themselves.

The sporting events of the future will be called on to serve these greater human needs and in increasingly spectacular ways. I predict that the 'circus masters' of the future (political leaders, corporate bosses, media moguls, cable TV proprietors) will stage these shows (Olympics and gladiatorial shows) and accomplish it by these methods:

- Sports medicine will be used to showcase the advancements of medical science.
- World records (the ultimate goal of competition) will continue to be broken by improved training techniques, tactics, equipment, and nutrition.

1 W O Roberts 1996 Environmental concerns. In *ACSM's Handbook for the team physician. Williams and Williams* p185–7 Williams & Wilkins, Baltimore

- The athletic 'machine' will be trained in environmental cocoons to avoid the adverse effects of pollutants on performance. Genetic bioengineers will develop techniques to extend anaerobic and aerobic potentials. The Human Genome Project is already underway decoding the genetics of disease and soon the genetics of deviant behaviors and human enhancement may also be understood.

- Peripheral brains (biocomputers) will be implanted to alter personality and psychological barriers and to enhance neuromuscular and cardiorespiratory performance. *The Internet* is already coding and expanding our current knowledge database; it will facilitate scientific inquiry and invention. *Fractal geometry* will be the powerful mathematical tool for the scientists of the next century along with quantum computers.

- Design engineers will improve sporting equipment and facilities to better performance and lessen injuries (faster cycles, safer helmets, better splints, spring-loaded basketball courts to minimize impact problems).

- Athletes may undergo biomechanical alterations to their bodies to enhance performance (lengthen femurs, create metatarsus adductus, 'pigeon toes').

- Human beings may be cloned and developed for sporting spectacles. Already the All Blacks (NZ Rugby) are in effect pre-selecting a genetic prototype for successful outcomes (large players of Polynesian extraction).[1]

Our philosophical acceptance of these things will depend on whether we consider that such ventures improve the 'human lot'. We are entering a daring age in which NASA has established the 'Origins' program to tackle, scientifically, the major questions of life (origins of life and structure in the universe/life beyond Earth).[2]

Sports medicine faces a new millennium with great expectations and on an ambitious scientific foundation.

---

[1] Although the superb performance of All Black C Cullen in the All Black-Wallabies game in Melbourne on 26 July 1997 in Melbourne would suggest otherwise [2] EJ Chaisson 1997 NASA's new science vision editorial *Science* 275 735

1 Sport and medicine: the human race

What will happen

Part I
Fundamentals

2 Epidemiology of sporting injuries

EUGENE SHERRY

16

Introduction

Epidemiology is the medical discipline which deals with the occurrence, causes, and prevention of disease. Its methodology, used in public health to study outbreaks of disease and to design preventive measures, is widely applied in sports medicine to injury rather than illness or disease. The epidemiological approach contributes much to better understanding of the incidence and causes of injuries and allows planning of prevention programs and the proper allocation of medical resources.

An understanding of the implications of assumptions inherent in the statistical methods underlying epidemiological methods is necessary if some common pitfalls are to be avoided (e.g. no clear hypothesis under test, poor definition of injury type, inappropriate controls, population under study not defined, overgeneralization of results).

Snow skiing injuries have been extensively studied as has American football (because of the high incidence of head and spinal injuries). Interventional studies now being published examine the role of knee and ankle braces in injury prevention. With time, more multi-centre studies will be planned to gather data on the effects of interventional measures.

Investigating sports injuries

Epidemiological approaches to sports injuries may be *descriptive* or *analytical* (**1,2**). Descriptive studies define the problem in terms of *incidence* and *prevalence*. Analytical studies seek to identify risk factors with the goal of doing something about the injury rate, or to evaluate the effectiveness of treatment regimes.

Incidence and prevalence

Incidence (rate) of injury is the number of cases per unit time. The rate of injury is measured as the number of injuries or injured athletes (note the significance of the distinction in relation to multiple injuries which may be of different type) over a specified period, and may be expressed in absolute or relative terms (e.g. 3 skiing injuries per 1000 skier days). The *risk of injury* (the probability that an individual will be injured) is measured in the exposed population as a cumulative incidence giving the proportion injured, by actuarial methods (difficult), or from incidence densities. These two parameters provide the basis for most studies of sports injuries.

Risk factors

Identification of risk factors provides a means for doing something about the sports injury problem. Both the observational and experimental approaches of analytical epidemiology are used (**3**).

Observational study designs are of three main types:

1 *Case–control* (Fig. 2.1)—the injured group is compared with a non-injured group in relation to a potential risk factor. Such studies are *retrospective*, easy to conduct and commonly used, but careful matching of controls is important. The possible sources of bias, role of sampling vagaries, and confounding variables must be carefully assessed.

2 *Cohort* (Fig. 2.2)—similar design, but *prospective* in that groups exposed or not exposed to a potential risk factor are recognized before injury and then followed through time. This approach is less susceptible to information bias (see below). Data collection takes longer and the method is more expensive to implement. Variations include *surveillance designs* (continuous monitoring of a group of athletes as under the National Athlete Injury/Illness Reporting System in the USA or NEISS). In survival designs, survival curve analysis is used to follow the reduction in proportion of uninjured/injured over the study period (as in follow-up of orthopedic joint replacement).

3 *Cross-sectional* (Fig. 2.3)—documents injuries and risk factors at one point in time, describing prevalence and injury patterns. This approach is of limited value where rehabilitation times after injury are long.

Experimental study designs are interventional. Subjects are assigned randomly to treatment or control groups (e.g. prophylactic wearing of ankle splints in basketball). Ethical problems may arise in relation to allocation/withholding of potentially useful treatment.

Effectiveness of treatment

The effectiveness of treatment is best studied in *randomized clinical trials* (Fig. 2.4) which should be double-blinded as compliance with protocol is otherwise difficult to achieve. The study plan covers selection of patients (inclusion and exclusion criteria must be clearly defined), random allocation of treatments, treatment, and analysis.

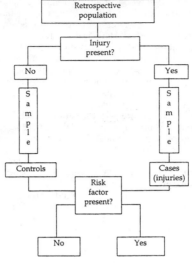

Fig. 2.1 Structure of case–control study

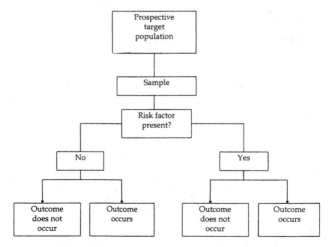

Fig. 2.2 Structure of cohort study

Steps in study design and implementation

Appropriate study design may at first appear daunting to the sports medicine doctor. It is good practice to enlist collaboration with an epidemiologist or statistician before embarking on an investigation to avoid the frustration of having your work rejected on the grounds of unsound design, incorrect statistical analysis, or simply failure to prove an hypothesis (hindsight often shows that this would have been possible with proper planning to ensure adequate statistical power, see below). Plan the investigation with definite objectives in view by formulating test(s) of a working hypothesis (see discussion of null hypotheses below). Know what questions you are asking and why they are relevant in the context of treatment or prevention. Data crunching of large amounts of information 'dredging' for statistically significant relationships of no particular medical significance may be ridiculous and perhaps unethical. Key stages in planning research on sports injuries include:

Definition of injury: specification of the particular injury type(s) to be considered will start the investigation. Usually injury is defined as being serious enough to need medical attention from a doctor.

Diagnostic tests needed for the study should be assessed for *accuracy* or *predictive value* (ability to detect the condition). This depends on: (1) *sensitivity*, measured as the fraction of people with the condition who are actually identified as positives by the test; and (2) *Specificity*, measured as the fraction of people without the condition who are identified as negatives by the test. Predictive value should ideally be near 100% (achieved when both sensitivity and specificity are near 100%). The *kappa coefficient* estimates interobserver reliability (two or more observers using the same test get the same result). Intraobserver error is a measure of the consistency of one observer over multiple tests.

Injury recording requires a numerator (the number of injuries) and denominator (the population at risk, e.g. the number of persons skiing during a specified time period). The population time is the number of participants at risk by the time exposed to potential injury (usually 1000 player games). In skiing the unit is 1000 skier-days (1000 persons skiing for 1 day). These units provide a basis for comparisons between studies and between sports.

Controls must be similar to the study group, using the same inclusion and exclusion criteria (apart from injury).

Bias is systematic error (usually unintentional) resulting in inaccuracy which must be minimized. Such errors may arise from the way that subjects or controls are chosen (*selection bias*) or measured (*information bias*), or from confounding variables. Common sources are *recall bias* (in case–control studies arising from retrospective recall of risk factors), *follow-up bias* (in cohort studies where players leaving the study differ from those remaining), and *historical bias* (where 'historical controls' in sequential periods are not aware of other changes).

Confounders (confounding variables) are systematic factors associated with the study variable (e.g. risk factor) and the occurrence of injury in such a way as to obscure the true relationship between study variable and injury. The confounder may itself be another risk factor. Features of experimental design may help to mitigate difficulties caused by confounding variables. For instance, in *stratified trials*, subjects are divided according to one or more of the variables

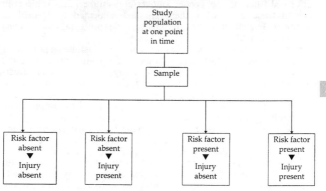

Fig. 2.3 Structure of cross-section study

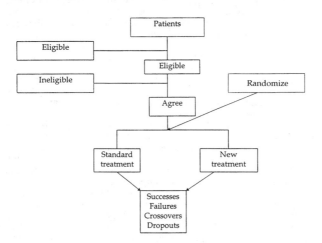

Fig. 2.4 Randomized clinical trial

concerned (such as age, gender, smoker/non-smoker) and subjects in each of these groups are then randomly allocated to control or treatment. The effect of the grouping variable (potential confounder) is thus eliminated.

Informed consent of participating patients must be arranged as appropriate in relation to the nature of the investigation before the study can be commenced. This is especially important where treatment alternatives are planned. Where the study may identify particular persons or ethnic/cultural groups, especially in publications dealing with the results, approval of the project by the appropriate community leaders may be required (usually monitored by the research/ethics committees of the researcher's institution). Many journals now require evidence that such approvals were obtained before considering the results of such studies for publication.

Pilot studies (small-scale preliminary investigations) are often helpful or even essential. Commencement of a definitive study will typically require approval or award of peer-reviewed competitive funding as well as research/ethics committee approval from the sponsoring institution. Both will ordinarily necessitate assessment of the statistical power (see below) of the proposed investigation. Such calculations require estimation of the expected magnitude and variance of the differences between the groups being compared, and hence the scale of the anticipated response to treatment. Preliminary evaluation of possible confounding factors may also be necessary. A pilot study is often the only way of providing this information where the proposed research breaks new ground. Further, a pilot study may also be helpful in testing and justifying proposed inclusion and exclusion criteria for study subjects, and in providing evidence that proposed recruitment rates are realistic in relation to the proposed time frame of the investigation.

Statistical power and the calculation of required sample size. Does the observed difference between two groups being compared reflect a real difference between them or is it merely a reflection of chance sampling effects? Statistical tests enable calculation of the probability (P) that a difference as large or larger than observed would arise from random sampling effects alone. If sampling effects would account for differences of the observed magnitude only rarely, we may judge it unlikely that chance alone accounts for the difference and conclude that other systematic factors are involved. But just when do we regard the differences as sufficiently likely to involve factors other than chance sampling effects that we call them 'statistically significant'? Where we set the cut-off between 'significant' and 'non-significant' is entirely arbitrary. We can set the *significance level*, denoted as alpha, to any P-value that we consider appropriate for a particular situation. However, by common usage to the point of it having become conventional in biomedical studies, the critical threshold value of P is generally set at 0.05 (i.e. alpha = 0.05). At this threshold, if there is 1 chance in 20 or less ($\leqslant 5\%$ probability) that random sampling effects could account for a difference at least as great as that observed, we regard the difference as significant, i.e. likely to arise from systematic causes such as the effects of treatment. Other significance levels, such as alpha = 0.02 or 0.01 may of course be chosen according to circumstances, but the criterion to be applied in an investigation should be decided before the analysis is commenced.

Formally, the use of probability in this way is based on testing the validity of the *null hypothesis* (H0) that there is no difference between the populations of which the groups being studied represent random samples in relation to the attributes being compared (mean, variance, proportion, survival curve). For each null hypothesis an *alternative hypothesis* (H1) exists, here that the populations represented by the study samples are in fact different. In the specific context of risk factor analysis a null hypothesis may be phrased to state that there is no association between the dependent variable (risk factor) and the independent variable (injury).

Once the null hypothesis has been formulated and an appropriate statistical test has been selected (Table 2.1), *P* can be calculated and statistical significance judged according to where alpha was set.

Statistical errors of two kinds, known as *type I and type II errors*, relate to the null hypothesis as follows:

Null hypothesis accepted	*Null hypothesis rejected*	
True	Correct	Type I error
False	Type II error	Correct

A type I error arises if the null hypothesis is rejected (because the calculated value of *P* is less than alpha) even though the null hypothesis is in fact true. A type I error is equivalent to the mistake made if a verdict of guilty is brought in when the accused is innocent. The probability of making a type I error is alpha which was set by the investigator. The lower the alpha is set, the fewer the type I errors, but the higher the chance of type II errors. A type II error arises when the null hypothesis is accepted even though it is false (i.e. the alternative hypothesis, H1, is true). A type II error is equivalent to the mistake made by a verdict of not guilty when the accused is in fact guilty. The probability (beta) of making a type II error depends on the size of the difference specified by the alternative hypothesis (H1), and this reflected a decision on the part of the investigator as to the minimum difference regarded as of practical value or clinical significance. Simultaneously reducing the chances of making type I and II errors means increasing sample size. Whether this is feasible will depend on practical considerations (e.g. recruitment rates) and cost/benefit considerations.

Statistical power and the calculation of sample size. The *power* of a statistical test is defined as (1-beta) where beta is the probability of making a type II error (see above). Statistical power is the probability of finding a significant difference when the difference between the populations sampled is delta. The larger the sample size the greater the power of the test. Methods for calculating sample size (**4,5**) appropriate for studies of different kinds are provided in most statistical packages (see below). Remember to include an adequate allowance for likely drop-outs during the study. Long-term studies are particularly susceptible to drop-out losses and poor follow-up rates (few have been successfully completed in the field of sports injuries).

Confidence intervals. In many circumstances, the arbitrary decision significant/not significant may advantageously be replaced or supplemented by specifying confidence intervals (CI, set to any level, but typically 95%) within which population values or differences estimated from the study sample(s) must lie (**5**).

Outliers. Once data are collected, occasional values may be seen to fall outside the range of the main body of data points. These must all be accounted for and must not be arbitrarily discarded as erroneous without investigation. Some will turn out to be due to clerical or instrumental (e.g. calibration shift) errors, unrecognized pathology in the subject, missed exclusion criteria, etc. Residual exceptions for which no explanation is found at the time may in future yield new insights.

What statistical tests should be used for the analysis? This depends on the objectives of the study and on the kind of data, whether measures of variables with underlying Gaussian (normal) distributions, rank or score data, binomial (two outcome) data or survival curves (Table 2.1) (**5,6,7**). For large-scale or complex investigations it is generally prudent to recruit professional statistical collaboration at the planning stage of the project. It may be too late to achieve the full potential of an investigation if this is delayed until after data collection.

Implementation of data analysis will typically involve use of a computer software package. Amongst the more widely used professional level packages for independent desktop use are:

Package	Company
SYSTAT V	Systat Inc, Evanston, IL, USA
STATISTICA	StatSoft Inc.
SPSS/PC+	SPSS Inc, Chicago, IL, USA
SAS	SAS Institute Inc, Cary, NC, USA
MINITAB	Minitab Inc, State College, PA, USA
STATGRAPHICS Plus	STSC International Ltd., Windsor, Berks, UK

Authoritative but less comprehensive (and less expensive) although adequate for many smaller scale projects are:

Package	Company
INSTAT and PRISM	GraphPad Software Inc, San Diego, CA, USA
STATVIEW	Abacus Concepts Inc

What conclusions should be drawn from the study? If the research project was properly planned with clearly formulated objectives based on well-stated hypotheses, the analysis will necessarily provide the basis for statistical (mathematical) findings. But statistical significance does *not* carry an inference of clinical importance (an observed effect in the real world). Some statistical findings are medically meaningless and sometimes statistics may not detect an important relationship from a given data set (chance, statistical power too low).

In summary:

- Shape the investigation by formulation of one or more testable hypotheses
- Estimate the necessary sample sizes; allow for drop-outs; check that proposed recruitment rates are realistic in relation to the available subject pool
- Obtain necessary ethics approvals and informed consent of parties and individuals concerned
- Use eligible subjects; apply inclusion and exclusion criteria rigorously
- Collect accurate information
- Watch for, and avoid, bias
- Eliminate or control confounding variables
- Practice good management procedures through all phases of the study

Table 2.1 Selection of appropriate statistical tests according to study objective and type of data

Objective	Type of data to be analysed			
	Mesurements of continuous variable (Gaussian distribution)	Ranks, scores, or measurements of variable (non-Gaussian distribution)	Binomial categorization (2 alternative outcomes)	Duration of survival
Description of study group	Mean, SD	Median, interquartile range	Frequency, proportion	Kaplan–Meier survival curve
Comparison of study group and reference value	t-test	Wilcoxon	*Chi*-square binomial	
Comparison of 2 groups, unpaired subjects	Unpaired t-test	Mann–Whitney	Fischer's exact, *Chi*-square	Log rank, Mantel–Haenszel
Comparison of 2 groups, paired subjects	Paired t-test	Wilcoxon	McNemar	Conditional PHR*
Comparison of ≥3 groups, unmatched subjects	One-way ANOVA	Kruskal–Wallis	*Chi*-square	Cox PHR*
Comparison of ≥3 groups, matched subjects	Repeated-measures ANOVA	Friedman	Cochrane Q	Conditional PHR*
Measure association between 2 variables	Pearson correlation	Spearman correlation	Contingency coefficients	
Predict value of 1 variable from another	Simple linear, non-linear regressions	Non-parametric regression	Simple logistic regression	Cox PHR*
Predict value of 1 variable from ≥2 others	Multiple linear and non-linear regressions		Multiple logistic regression	Cox PHR*

* PHR, proportional hazard regression
From Motulsky 1995 *Intuitive biostatistics* OUP

- Evaluate data (examine outliers, check for breakdown of recruitment, or blinding criteria)
- Choose statistical tools appropriate in relation to data type and study objectives
- Draw conclusions cautiously, with emphasis on medical (rather than mathematical) importance.

Example: trends in skiing injuries in Australia

Downhill snow skiing injuries lend themselves to epidemiological study; large numbers of injuries in one place over a short time period make it possible to collect many data quickly. Trends in skiing injury type and rates in Australia were established from a review of 22,261 injuries over 27 years (**8**).

Type of study	Observational, care series, retrospective
Definition of injury	Injury requiring medical attention
Rate of injury	3.22 injuries per 1000 skier days in (1988)
Risk of injury	Not relevant here
Size of sample	All injuries within acceptance criteria for duration of study
Analyses	computer-based statistics package was used to generate descriptive statistics and for characterization of changes in the pattern and rates of injury over the study period. F-statistics were used for the overall injury rate analysis as this data exhibited non-Gaussian distribution. Injury classes (upper body, thumb, knee, tibial fracture, ankle fracture, lacerations) were examined by contingency analysis. The threshold for significance was set at alpha = 0.5. Statistically significant trends were demonstrated in 4 of the 6 injury types.
Conclusions	Data on rate and type of injury were presented. Recommendations were made in regard to upper body protection, thumb safety, binding function, organization of ski slopes, and instruction.

2 Epidemiology of sporting injuries
Example: trends in skiing injuries in Australia

Overview of sports injury rates

There is little doubt that sporting injuries are on the increase and being seen more frequently in emergency rooms around the world. In Sweden (where comprehensive injury statistics are collected by national registration) the proportion of patients presenting with sports trauma rose from 1.4% of all injuries in 1955 to 10% in 1988 (**9**). The number of participants has increased with 25% to 30% of the population of most Western countries involved in sport (over 100 million in North America).

In general, the cause of injuries can be grouped into *personal factors* (age, gender, experience—the last often not a major contributor), *sports factors* (contact, high-velocity, indoor, activities with high jump rates are more dangerous), and *environmental factors* (usually greater in good weather due to increased exposure) (**10**).

The relative risks of injury in different sports is reasonably well documented. Insurance data from Sweden (Folksam Insurance Survey covering 27,000 injuries from 1976 to 1983) (**11**) showed that ice-hockey had the highest injury rate with basketball the lowest, with many only minor. The Swiss organization Youth and Sports (**12**) involves 350000 young people annually: ice-hockey, handball and soccer had the highest injury rates with athletics and gymnastics the lowest (Table 2.2). Overall females were at greater risk of injury. Studies of extensive series of injuries reveal that most are minor (65% are contusions or sprains and contusions) and the overall incidence of injury is low (0.8%) (**13**). The lower extremity (foot and ankle) is the most common site of injury (**14**).

MacLeod has reviewed rugby football injuries. Of these, 30% affected face and neck, 20–35% were severe (necessitated missing 2 weeks play), 5–22% suffered concussion (not graded, higher in school boys), catastrophic injury (quadriplegia) occurred sporadically (true incidence not known) (**15**). Football injuries in the USA have also been closely studied (**16**). Some 50% of all National Football League (NFL) players are injured each season; 5% of the injuries involve concussion.

Severity of injury is more important than **incidence** in relation to permanent disability, spinal injury or death. Sherry found those most at risk of severe skiing injury to be males, children (<14 years), experienced skiers, in collisions, using steep slopes, at high speed, on slushy or deep snow, using long skis, without head protection and without operative binding releases. Severe injuries (<5%) were considered to be life- or limb-threatening and to require hospital care or cause long-term morbidity (**17**).

The Swedish Folksam study (**11**) found a 2.5% permanent disability from soccer, mainly involving a motor vehicle accident (MVA) en route to/from games, or knee injuries (an element of over-reporting was noted).

The relative risks of spinal injuries are outlined in Table 2.3. Diving shows the highest incidence with downhill snow skiing (including specialist aerial maneuvers) surprisingly low (see Chapter 7). The incidence of spinal cord injury in Rugby Union in New South Wales (Australia) is 0.53 per 10,000 registered participants per year (0.18 for Rugby League) (**18**).

Rule changes help. A dramatic reduction in lethal cervical spine injuries in American football occurred between 1975 and 1984 after

Table 2.2 The relative incidence of injury of different sports

Sport	No. of injuries	%	No. of particip.	Hours of exposure	Incidence rates	95% CI of IR*
Ice-hockey	1,570	12.1	29,911	1,824,535	8.6	8.2/9.0
Handball	1,052	8.1	30,876	1,452,907	7.2	6.8/7.7
Soccer	7,264	55.8	192,690	10,973,085	6.6	6.5/6.8
Wrestling	105	0.8	4,927	167,085	6.3	5.1/7.5
Hiking	821	6.3	76,149	2,308,797	3.6	3.3/3.8
Basketball	243	1.9	15,094	693,952	3.5	3.1/3.9
Volleyball	152	1.2	13,739	500,631	3.0	2.6/3.5
Alpine skiing	502	3.9	58,960	1,667,207	3.0	2.8/3.3
Alpinism	126	1.0	21,398	434,133	2.9	2.4/3.4
Judo	102	0.8	17,837	442,361	2.3	1.9/2.8
Fitness training	296	2.3	57,068	1,726,600	1.7	1.5/1.9
Athletics	268	2.1	43,448	1,646,962	1.6	1.4/1.8
Apparatus gymn.	90	0.7	12,441	602,524	1.5	1.2/1.8
Other sports	425	3.3	114,836	3,986,578	1.1	1.0/1.2
Total	13,016	100.3	689,374	28,427,357	4.6	4.5/4.7

* CI, confidence interval; IR, incidence rates
From M de Loes 1995 *International Journal of Sports Medicine* **16** 135

Table 2.3 Spine fractures and neurological deficits related to sports

Sport/Recreation	Absolute frequency	%	% with neurological deficit for particular sport	
			Absolute frequency	%
Diving	34	25	24	71
Snowmobile	16	12	7	44
Equestrian	16	12	4	25
Parachute/skydiving [a]	14	10	3	21
All-terrain vehicles [b]	12	9	4	33
Toboggan	11	8	1	10
Bicycle	4	4	1	25
Rugby	4	4	1	25
Ice hockey	3	2	1	33
Downhill skiing	3	2	1	33
Surfing	3	2	1	33
Football	2	1	0	0
Mountaineering	2	1	1	50
Other [c]	10	8	4	40
Total	134	100	53	?

[a] Includes hand-gluding and ultralite plane. [b] Includes only 1 case of trampoline injury. [c] Includes motocross racing, dirtbike, and all-terrain (3-wheel) vehicles each with 4 cases.
Reproduced with permission from *Oxford textbook of sports medicine* OUP. 1994

law changes in 1976 outlawed contact with helmet/face mask (**19**). The likelihood of death from sport is important. Downhill snow skiing, for instance, has 0.87 fatalities per 1 million skier days (subdivided into traumatic 0.24; cardiovascular, 0.45; environmental/hypothermia, 0.18) (20). Other sports have significantly higher death rates (e.g. water sports, 2.8; firearm sports, 1.3; football, 2.0/ 100,000, respectively) (**21**). There is a greater likelihood of dying from car accidents to/from sporting events than from participation (in one ski season in the Perisher region, Australia, 12 car deaths occurred whereas there were 29 ski deaths over the previous 32 years).

The cost of injuries from sport has been estimated in Sweden to amount on average to US$330 per case when treated in the emergency room, but US $4178 if admitted. Note that the cost to society of treating osteoporosis at this time was 100 times the total cost of sporting injuries.

References

(1) M Schootman *et al* 1994 Statistics in sports injury research. In JC DeLee, D Drez (ed) *Orthopaedic sports medicine* p160–83. Saunders, Philadelphia

(2) J Ryan, A Pearl 1994 Epidemiological concepts in sports medicine. A brief review. *Update in Sports Medicine* AAOS 3–16

(3) RL Lieber 1994 Experimental design and statistical analysis. In SR Simon (ed) *Orthopaedic basic science* p626–59. AAOS, IL

(4) DG Altman 1991 *Practical statistics for medical research*. Chapman & Hall, London

(5) H Motulsky 1995 *Intuitive biostatistics*. OUP

(6) HA Kahn, CT Sempos 1989 *Statistical methods in epidemiology*. OUP, New York

(7) WL Hays 1988 *Statistics*. 4th edn. Harcourt Brace Jovanovich, Orlando, FL

(8) E Sherry, L Fenelon 1991 Trends in skiing injury type and rates in Australia *MJA* **155** 513–15

(9) E Ericksson 1994 An introduction and brief review. *Oxford textbook of sports medicine*, p341–2. OUP

(10) FJG Backx *et al* 1991 Injuries in high-risk persons and high risk sports. *Am J Sports Med* **19** 124–30

(11) *Folksam sports injuries, 1976–83*. A report from Folksam, Stockholm, 1985

(12) M de Loes 1995 Epidemiology of sports injuries in the Swiss organization 'Youth and Sports', 1987–1989. *Int J Sports Med* **16** 134; 135

(13) ER Larkowski *et al* 1995 Medical coverage for multievent sports competition. *Mayo Clin Proc* **70** 549–55

(14) EM Tenvergert *et al* 1992 *J Sp Med Phys Fitness* **32** 214–20

(15) DAD MacLeod 1993 In GR McLatchie, CME Lennox (ed). *The Soft tissues. Trauma and sports* p372–81. Butterworth, Guildford, UK

(16) KN Waninger, JA Lombardo 1993 In MB Mellion (ed) *Sports Medicine Secrets* p343. Hanley & Belfus, Philadelphia

(17) E Sherry 1986 Factors determining the severity of skiing trauma. MPH thesis, Univ Sydney

(18) SF Wilson *et al* 1996 Spinal cord injuries have fallen in Rugby Union players in NSW. *BMJ* **313** 1550

(19) JS Torg, B Sennet 1987 *Clinics in Sports Medicine* **6** 61–72

(20) E Sherry, L Clout 1988 Death from skiing in Australia. *MJA* **149** 615–18

(21) JE Sheahy 1983 Death in downhill snow skiing. *Ski Trauma and safety* p349–57. ASTM, Philadelphia

3 Basic sports medicine science

DIANA E THOMAS, JANE A GORMAN,
JOHN ROONEY, SIMON HUTABARAT

Section I Exercise metabolism

Diana E Thomas

Introduction

Knowledge of the biochemistry and physiology of exercise is essential for interpreting the complex reactions involved in physical exertion. This knowledge can be applied to improve not only the performance of athletes, but also to monitor the health of the exercising public and to improve some medical conditions. Exercise has beneficial metabolic effects relevant to many areas of medicine, such as in diabetes, in the prevention of atherosclerosis and obesity, and in the management of stress. Regular exercise lowers: the resting heart rate, blood pressure, diabetic insulin requirements, LDL (low density lipoprotein) and triglycerides, while it increases: HDL (high density lipoprotein) and lean body mass. With appropriate exercise, the cardiovascular capacity overall improves and the cardiovascular risk is lowered. In some medical conditions fatigue occurs after mild exertion (e.g. peripheral vascular disease). From information based on the metabolism of exercise and the ensuing fatigue, assessment and treatment can be implemented through strategies such as suitable nutrition and training programs.

In general, genetic reproduction, adaptive capability, and metabolism maintain the human condition. You walk (if intelligent, rather than run) to kill your prey in the jungle or boardroom with spear or pen, carry it home, and then write a letter to your mother (historical record = civilization) about it. There are 65 billion body cells, about 50% are muscle cells which require the delivery of nutrients and the removal of waste products (increased demand with exercise). This is met by the cardiovascular and pulmonary systems.

Cardiovascular response to exercise[1]

During exercise, the cardiac output increases, enabling the cardiovascular system to increase the transport of oxygen to the working muscles and to remove the metabolic heat produced by transferring it to the skin surface for evaporation, while still maintaining the blood pressure to supply blood to the brain.

Maximum exercise capacity is determined by increased oxygen delivery from increased cardiac stroke volume (SV) and so cardiac output (CO = SV × HR), vasodilatation, and to a much lesser extent increased mitochondrial volume. Such capacity decreases with age from ↓max HR and ↓SV, although exercise may maintain it. (See Chapter 4 p128–31.)

1 E Sherry 1997 Basic sports medicine science In E Sherry, D Bokor (ed) *Sports medicine Problems and practical management* p19–20 GMM, London

Pulmonary response to exercise

During exercise, the pulmonary ventilation also increases in order to augment oxygen supplies to the exercising muscles and remove waste carbon dioxide from the increased oxidative metabolism. Exercise improves the efficiency of the respiratory muscles and increases the total lung capacity by reducing the residual volume. The vital capacity is increased and élite athletes have a very large vital capacity. The maximum minute volume is also increased by athletic training and endurance athletes are able to process large volumes of air during competition (from 6L/min at rest up to 120L/min during exercise) (1).

In fact, the athletes pulmonary capacity may determine full metabolic potential and who becomes a champion (i.e. those with the largest 'vital capacities').

Quantifying exercise capacity

Exercise capacity can be measured in a variety of ways. As a general measure of fitness, the measurement of aerobic capacity is the most useful indicator.

1 Anaerobic capacity can be quantified using the Wingate test, where the subject cycles maximally for 30sec on a cycle ergometer weighted at 75g kg body mass. The peak power output and the time to reach it, the rate at which fatigue occurs and the average power output over the period can then be calculated.

2 Aerobic capacity can be quantified by measuring the maximal oxygen uptake (VO_{2max}), the maximum rate at which oxygen can be utilized. It is CO (HR $\times$ SV) $\times$ O_{2a-v} (the arterial–venous oxygen difference) and is genetically determined. This encompasses the capacity of both the cardiovascular and respiratory systems to supply oxygen to the muscles, as well as the potential of the muscles to utilize it. VO_{2max} is assessed by the exercise intensity on a cycle ergometer being gradually increased by a standard protocol until the maximal oxygen consumption is reached. As heart rates (HRs) can increase in direct correlation, VO_{2max} can be closely approximated by monitoring heart rates, then converting to the relative VO_{2max}. VO_{2max} values for sedentary subjects are about 30ml/kg/min, while those for trained athletes can be up to 85ml/kg/min (**2**). VO_{2max} can be increased by 5% in the fit and up to 25% in the unfit over 8–12 weeks.

Skeletal muscles

Up to 45% of the total body mass may be skeletal muscles, which are composed of muscle fibers, classified as either type I and slow twitch (ST), or type II and fast twitch (FT, subdivided into FTa and FTb). There are well-defined differences between fibers in the type II group, which is the reason why FT fibers have been differentiated further into FTa fibers (relatively higher oxidative potential) or FTb fibers (relatively higher glycolic potential), making at least three categories of discernible muscle fibers. Although muscle fiber types are mainly genetically determined, it appears that small changes are possible and training has been shown to alter the nature of some fibers (**3**). The type I fibers have slow contraction times, are red in color, have a high potential for oxidative metabolism, have more triglycerides and mitochondria, and are recruited more for endurance activities. They are the first to atrophy with disuse (more vascularized, appear red in color—and so remember as 'slow red ox'). The type II fibers are white in color, have a higher glycolytic capacity, and are employed more for sprinting (**4**) and fine motor skills. Hence, élite endurance athletes tend to have a majority of type I muscle fibers, while élite sprinters and weight lifters generally have high percentages of type II. Some characteristics of muscle fibers are outlined in Table 3.1.

Table 3.1 Comparison of muscle fiber types

	Slow Twitch	FTa	Fast twitch FTb
Contraction time	Slow	Fast	Fast
Colour	Red	Pink	White
Blood supply	Good	Medium	Low
Mitochondrial content	High	Medium	Low
Oxidative potential	High	Medium	Low
Glycolytic potential	Low	Medium	High

Systems of the provision of energy during exercise

There are several systems in the body that enable the increased energy requirements for exercise to be met. At exercise onset, the initial requirement for instant energy is met by the very small stores of adenosine triphosphate (ATP) already in the cell and then by synthesis of further ATP using creatine phosphate (CP) cell stores. However, these processes can only sustain the first few seconds of exercise. To sustain prolonged, strenuous exercise, energy then needs to be supplied aerobically.

Instant energy: ATP and creatine phosphate

ATP is the compound that supplies the energy to the exercising muscles, but it cannot be transported into the muscle cells, and so must be resynthesized within them.

$$ATP^{4-} + H_2O \rightarrow ADP^{3-} + P_i^{2-} + H^+$$

While a marathon runner would consume about 75kg of ATP in one race, only about 100g ATP are stored in the muscle cells, so to provide fuel for exercise, ATP must be continuously resynthesized from ADP (adenosine diphosphate) within each cell (**1**).

$$ADP^{3-} + phosphocreatine_i^{2-} + H^+ \rightarrow ATP^{4-} + creatine$$

Energy from the small quantities of creatine phosphate already present in the cell can fuel this rapid anaerobic synthesis of ATP for a few seconds. For exercise of longer duration, the energy for phosphorylation must be generated by the metabolism of ingested carbohydrates, fats, and to a lesser extent, proteins.

Short-term energy: glycolysis

Glycolysis can provide, anaerobically, a rapid energy source for the resynthesis of the high-energy phosphates required for the exercise after the first few seconds. Carbohydrate (CHO) is especially important in exercise metabolism, since it is the only fuel that can be used anaerobically to generate ATP. Hence, stored glycogen and plasma glucose are the principal sources of energy in the early minutes of exercise while the oxygen supply is limited (**5**). The process of *anaerobic glycolysis* may be summarized as:

$$glucose \rightarrow 2\ lactate^- + 2H^+$$

Further energy may be obtained by the conversion of lactate to glucose in the liver and its recycling back to the muscles (the Cori cycle). *Anaerobic*:

$$1\ molecule\ CHO \rightarrow 2ATP$$

As anaerobic metabolism only resynthesizes a net of 2ATP per mole of CHO. However, strenuous exercise for longer than 2–3 minutes requires energy to be more efficiently supplied and this is achieved through aerobic metabolism.

Long-term energy: aerobic metabolism

Hence, for prolonged strenuous exercise, energy for ATP regeneration must be supplied aerobically during the oxidation of glycogen and triglycerides (intramuscular fuels) and glucose and free fatty acids (plasma substances). In this second stage CHO breakdown, pyruvate is converted to acetyl-coenzyme A (CoA), which is then metabolized in the tricarboxylic acid cycle (TCA). Hydrogen ions released are oxidized via the respiratory chain and the energy generated is coupled to phosphorylation. From the metabolizing of 1 mole of CHO, a net 36 ATP molecules are formed, about one-third being conserved in the ATP bonds and two-thirds dissipated as heat (5). *Aerobic*:

$$1 \text{ molecule CHO} \rightarrow 36\text{ATP}$$

Fuel substrates for exercise

The major fuels for exercise are carbohydrates (CHO: muscle glycogen, liver glycogen, and blood glucose) and free fatty acids (FFA). While the body can theoretically store FFA supplies in vast quantities, it can only store about 500g CHO, the fuel essential for strenuous exercise, of which about 350–400g is muscle glycogen, 90–110g is liver glycogen and 15–20g is blood glucose (6). These energy supplies, if used individually, would fuel exercise for quite different periods of time. If one fuel could be used exclusively, a marathon runner could run over 4000min using free fatty acids, but only for 71min using muscle glycogen, for 18min using liver glycogen, and for 4min using blood glucose (7). However, this does not occur and a combination of fuels must be used, depending on the type of exercise. Research has centered on increasing the CHO supplies, since this is the limiting fuel. These CHO stores can be augmented by nutrition strategies in the days prior to the exercise to increase glycogen stores, or through ingestion of drinks or foods before or during the exercise to increase the blood glucose supply.

Muscle glycogen

Is the storage form of glucose in the muscles, is an essential fuel for exercise, but can only be used as an energy source in the muscle where it is stored, since muscles lack glucose-6-phosphatase, the enzyme essential for the transport of glucose across membranes (6). The rate of muscle glucagon utilization during prolonged exercise depends on the intensity and duration of the exercise and intense exercise performed to fatigue can deplete the muscle glycogen stores (8). Modified CHO-loading techniques can increase the stores to about 500g and in extreme conditions, some élite athletes may be able to store more (9).

Liver glucose and gluconeogenesis

In the non-exercising state, the liver is another of the body's limited glycogen storage sites, derived from CHO from ingested food. Following an overnight fast, these stores decrease to about 75–90g. CHO from ingested food can then increase these hepatic glycogen stores during the absorptive phase after a meal, when dietary glucose is released into the bloodstream and taken up by the liver and muscles. Post-absorptivity (3–6h after meal), hepatic glycogenolysis and gluconeogenesis are the only sources of glucose for essential organs such as the brain. Hepatic glycogen is utilized at only about 0.1g/min supplying about 75% of the glucose (10).

However, when exercise commences and there are large increases in glucose uptake by working muscles, hepatic glycogenolysis increases rapidly to provide a glucose supply to maintain plasma glucose levels, and about 18–20g hepatic glycogen is mobilized during the first 40min (11). As the liver glycogen supplies are utilized, hepatic gluconeogenesis increases, continuing to replenish the blood glucose at a rate similar to that of glucose utilization by the working muscles. During exercise, the increase in hepatic glucose production and the relative contribution from glycogenolysis or gluconeogenesis depends on exercise intensity and duration (12).

Blood glucose

In the non-exercising state, blood glucose is only a minor energy for muscle oxidative metabolism, and plasma glucose and insulin concentrations control the glucose uptake by muscles. Glucose transport across the cell membranes is a major rate-limiting step in glucose utilization and an important site of muscle metabolic regulation. As the plasma glucose concentration increases, the rate of glucose entry into the muscle approaches the maximum (13). Once inside the cell, glucose is metabolized either oxidatively, by glycolysis, the TCA cycle and oxidative phosphorylation to produce ATP, or non-oxidatively, when glycogen or lactate may be formed (7).

During strenuous exercise (>60% VO_{2max}), as muscle glycogen stores deplete, there is a gradual increase in glucose uptake by the muscles to minimize the CHO oxidation, peaking at 90–120min and after 40min of strenuous exercise, blood glucose provides about one-third of the energy. Hence, CHO ingested either before or during the exercise can provide an important source of blood glucose to be utilized as fuel. CHO foods of a differing glycemic index consumed before exercise have been investigated as well as CHO-containing drinks (14, 15). There is increased muscle glucose uptake after pre-exercise glucose feedings, as the sudden rise in plasma glucose concentration stimulates insulin to clear the blood of excess glucose (16). A large percentage of the glucose fed to glycogen-depleted subjects either 15min before or during strenuous exercise was found to be metabolized during exercise (17). Glucose can also be supplied to the blood by CHO-containing drinks during exercise and CHO ingested during exercise at 50–70% VO_{2max} has been shown to supply up to two-thirds of blood glucose (18, 19).

Free fatty acids

During exercise, muscle uptake of FFA is proportional to the plasma FFA concentration. As exercise continues any glycogen reserves deplete, FFA must supply a greater percentage of the energy and during prolonged exercise, FFA may supply nearly 80% of the total energy (20). As plasma glucose and insulin levels decrease, the plasma glucagon concentration increases, reducing the CHO metabolism and stimulating the release of FFA. However, even though there is an enormous supply of potential energy from stored lipids, CHO fuel is still an essential requirement to maintain strenuous exercise, and when CHO is depleted, the FFA cannot maintain the strenuous exercise at an equivalent level.

Fuel regulation during exercise

The fuel mixture during exercise depends on the intensity and duration of the exercise and the availability of substances, as well as the nutritional state and degree of training (**21, 22**). While CHO is essential for exercise, the proportion of the fuel mixture it comprises varies. At rest or during mild exercise levels (30% VO_{2max}), CHO contributes only about 25% of the fuel, with the larger percentage being supplied by FFA (**23**). As the exercise intensity increases, the requisite percentage of CHO in the fuel mixture increases (**6**). Hence, at moderate exercise levels (50% VO_{2max}), the fuel mixture is approximately 50% CHO and 50% FFA, while at higher exercise intensities (>60% VO_{2max}), CHO is the predominant fuel.

At the onset of exercise there is a sudden increase in glucose uptake by muscle, resulting in increased hepatic glycogenolysis and then increased gluconeogenesis. Early in submaximal exercise, about 40–50% of the requisite energy is supplied by hepatic glycogen and glycogen in the exercising muscles. Changes in hormonal secretion and metabolism increase the mobilization of fuels from both the extra-and intramuscular stores. There is increased glucagon, cortisol, and growth hormone. Although the plasma insulin concentrations fall, insulin sensitivity is increased and, during exercise, the role of insulin is more complex than in the non-exercising state. Exercise stimulates the secretion of catecholamines, which increase the glycogenolysis in both the liver and the muscle, and stimulate hepatic gluconeogenesis (**24**). Adrenaline enhances the breakdown of muscle glycogen during both low and high intensity exercise.

Muscle glycogen and blood glucose are the main energy source during high-intensity exercise (**6**). At the onset of exercise, the muscle uptake of blood glucose increases rapidly and continues to do so as exercise continues. Muscle glucose utilization may be controlled by the rate of glucose transported into the cells intracellularly. The increase in muscle glycogen breakdown causes glucose-6-phosphate concentrations to increase, which, by inhibiting hexokinase, may limit the increased glucose uptake caused by the exercise. During prolonged exercise, glycogen stores becomes depleted and glucose-6-phosphate production declines, resulting in greater rates of glucose transport into the muscle sell. Hence, the blood glucose contribution to energy metabolism increases as exercise progresses (**23**). After 40min of exercise, the glucose uptake rises 7–20 times the uptake at rest, depending on the intensity of the exercise, and in prolonged strenuous exercise may even increase by up to 40 times.

As exercise continues and the oxygen stores become reduced, an increasingly greater percentage of the energy is supplied through FFA metabolism. The stimulation of lipolysis results on raised FFA levels. Eventually, liver glucose output decreases compared to its use by muscles, and blood glucose concentration may decrease (**25**). Blood glucose levels may even fall to hypoglycemic levels after 90min of continuous exercise.

Regulation of body temperature

During prolonged, strenuous exercise, the body's ability to regulate temperature, in addition to its capacity to exercise and its potential peak performance, is decreased by dehydration, so it is important for an athlete to drink sufficiently to maintain the correct fluid balance. Dehydration post exercise is also important. Most of the heat from metabolic reactions during exercise is lost in sweat evaporation at the rate of about 1–2l/h or up to 3l/h in very hot conditions (**26, 27**).

There is an increased possibility of hyperthermia during heavy exercise in the heat, however, in addition to drinking fluids, heat acclimatization can lessen the risk. When conditions for athletic events are predicted to be extremely hot, the athlete should acclimatize to the heat prior to the competition by training in hot conditions. This can induce adaptations for exercise in the heat such as increasing the volumes of both plasma and sweat, and reducing heart rate and body temperature. The sweating can commence earlier and be more dilute. Exercise during hot conditions may induce increased rates of muscle glycogenolysis; however, heat acclimatization may also reduce this (**28**).

Training

Can improve athletic performance through changes in metabolism, muscle, and psychological approach. Weight training can increase the size of the individual muscle fibers. Endurance training can improve athletic performance by increasing the reliance on FFA as a fuel and by decreasing the total CHO oxidation (**29**, **30**). In trained muscle, FFA uptake increases linearly with FFA delivery, whereas in untrained muscle, uptake becomes saturated with time, partly explaining the increase in lipid oxidation in trained subjects and indicating that muscle training adaptations are involved in FFA utilization during prolonged exercise (**31**).

Training has several effects on the heart. After training, the heart rate at rest or for a particular level of exercise is lower than that before training. During exercise in trained subjects, the increase in stroke volume with more blood leaving the heart for each contraction, causes an increased cardiac output. Training also increases the heart size and reports indicate that Paavo Hurmi, who won 9 Olympic gold medals for distance running, had a heart three times the normal size (**7**). Training also has hormonal effects. After training, less insulin is required to clear excess glucose from the circulation, because exercise training improves insulin sensitivity. Endurance-trained athletes have a lower plasma concentration of catecholamines than untrained at the same absolute workload (**25**).

Training strategies to improve aerobic capacity should include several basic elements. They should exercise large muscle groups and be performed at intensities between 40% and 85% VO_{2max}. The intensity should gradually be increased as the subject becomes fitter. There should be 3–5 sessions per week, each of 15–60min in duration.

Strength (weight) training

Strength is achieved by a variation of intensity (the load or resistance lifted per repetition), volume (weight lifted), frequency (every other day), and the use of rest periods (<60s is best). It is beneficial (if supervised) for young athletes (prevents injury, aids rehabilitation, betters self-esteem). It should include a warm-up (of 15–20min calisthenics or stretching), a lifting session and a cool-down period (as for warm-up).

55

Fatigue

Muscle fatigue may be defined as an inability of the muscles to maintain a particular power output (**32**). While fatigue has often been assumed to be due to hypoglycemia or depletion of muscle glycogen, there are other possible causes some of which have been identified and others which are still being investigated. Proton accumulation with the resultant drop in pH in the muscle is one of the most likely reason for fatigue in sprinters:

$$\text{glucose} \rightarrow 2 \text{ lactate}^- + 2H^+$$

During short, high intensity exercise, acidosis can result from the production rate of these protons exceeding their utilization whereas under non-exercising conditions, the protons produced are utilized in other reactions. The depletion of muscle phosphocreatine is another contribution to fatigue occurring in sprinters (**1**).

Fatigue may have many causes. There are numerous points in the process of skeletal muscle activation where fatigue could occur:

1 Mental state
2 Brain
3 Spinal cord
4 Peripheral nerve
5 Neuromuscular junction
6 Muscle fiber membrane
7 Sarcoplasmic reticulum
8 Ca^{2+} ions
9 Actin and myosin interaction

In prolonged strenuous exercise, fatigue could be caused by not only CHO depletion, but also possibly by a decrease in Ca^{2+} available for release from the sarcoplasmic reticulum, or by changes in the plasma concentration of some amino acids, as well as by physical factors such as hyperthermia (**33**).

Exercise science

Research into the biochemistry and physiology of exercise is ongoing and as new discoveries are made, they are applied, where possible to athletes, enabling the frontiers of human achievement to be pushed a little further. Even one minor discovery, if it can be translated into a biomechanical or metabolic improvement in the athletic field, can make the difference between record-breaking performances and mediocrity.

References

(1) EA Newsholme, AR Leech 1994 *Keep on running*. Chichester, John Wiley and Sons.

(2) PO Astrand, K Rodahl 1970 *Textbook of work physiology*. McGraw-Hill, New York

(3) E Jansson *et al* 1978 Effect of diet on the utilisation of blood-borne and intramuscular substrates during exercise in man. *Acta Physiol Scand* **104** 235–7

(4) B Saltin *et al* 1977 Fibre types and metabolic potentials of skeletal muscles in sedentary man and endurance runners. *Annal NY Acad Sci* **301** 3–20

(5) WD McArdle *et al* 1991 *Exercise physiology; energy, nutrition and human performance*. Lea & Febiger, Philadelphia

(6) P Felig, J Wahren 1975 Fuel homeostasis in exercise. *Ann NY Acad Sci* **301** 30–44

(7) EA Newsholme, AR Leech 1983 *Biochemistry for the medical sciences*. Wiley, Chichester, UK

(8) L Hermansen *et al* (1967) Muscle glycogen during prolonged severe exercise. *Acta Physiol Scand* **71** 129–39

(9) KJ Acheson *et al* 1988 Glycogen storage capacity and de novo lipogenesis during massive carbohydrate overfeeding in man. *Am J Clin Nutr* **48** 240-247

(10) H Hers 1990 Mechanisms of blood glucose homeostasis. *J Inherited Metabolic Disorders* **13** 395–410

(11) E Hultman 1978 Liver as a glucose supplying source during rest and exercise, with special reference to diet. In *Nutrition, physical fitness and health*. University Park Press, Baltimore

(12) JP Wahren *et al* 1971 Glucose metabolism during leg exercise in man. *J Clin Invest* **50** 2715-25

(13) JO Holloszy *et al* 1986 Activation of glucose transport in muscle by exercise. *Diabetes/Metab Rev* **1** 409–23

(14) DE Thomas *et al* 1991 Carbohydrate feeding before exercise: effect of glycemic index. *Int J Sports Med* **12(2)** 180–86

(15) G Ahlborg, O Bjorkman 1987 Carbohydrate utilization by exercising muscle following pre-exercise glucose ingestion. *Clin Physio* **7** 181–95

(16) G Ahlborg, P Felig 1977 Substrate utilization during prolonged exercise preceded by ingestion of glucose. *Am J Physiol* **233** E188-94

(17) A Bonen *et al* 1981 Glucose ingestion before and during intense exercise. *J Appl Physiol* **50** 766–71

(18) P Van Handel *et al* 1980 Fate of C-14—glucose ingested during prolonged exercise. *Int J Sports Med* **1** 127

(19) EF Coyle 1992 Carbohydrate supplementation during exercise [Review]. *Nutrition* **122**(3 Suppl) 788–95

(20) PD Gollnick *et al* 1981 Availability of glycogen and plasma FFA for substrate utilization in leg muscle of man during exercise. *Clin Physiol* **1** 27–42

(21) HG Ahlborg *et al*, 1974 Substrate turnover during prolonged exercise in man. *J Clin Invest* **53** 1080–90

(22) E Jansson, L Kaijser 1982 Effect of diet on the utilisation of blood-borne and intramuscular substrates during exercise in man. *Acta Physiol Scand* **115** 19–30

(23) B Essen 1977 Intramuscular substrate utilization during prolonged exercise. *Ann NY Acad Sci* **301** 30–44

(24) H Galbo 1983 *Hormonal and metabolic adaptation to exercise*. Thieme, Stuttgart

(25) G Ahlborg, P Felig 1982 Lactate and glucose exchange across the forearm, legs, and splanchnic bed during and after prolonged leg exercise. *J Clin Invest* **69** 45–54

(26) JR Brotherhood 1984 Nutrition and sports performance. *Sports Med* **1** 350–89

(27) S Fortney, NB Vroman 1985 Exercise, performance and temperature control: temperature regulation during exercise and implications for sports performance and training. *Sports Med* **2** 8–20

(28) LE Armstrong, CM Maresh 1991 The induction and decay of heat. acclimatisation in trained athletes. *Sports Med* **12** 302–12

(29) E Hultman, J Bergstrom 1973 Local energy-supplying substrates as limiting factors in different types of leg muscle work in normal man. In *Limiting factors of physical performance* p113–25. Thieme, Stuttgart

(30) J Karlsson, *et al* 1974 Muscle glycogen utilization during exercise after training. *Acta Physiol Scand* **90** 210–17

(31) L Turcotte *et al* 1992 Increased plasma FFA uptake and oxidation during

prolonged exercise in trained vs. untrained humans. *Am J Physiol* **262**(6 Pt 1) E791–9

(32) RHT Edwards 1981 Human muscle function and fatigue. *Ciba Found. Symp.* **82** 1–18

(33) N Vollestad 1988 Biochemical correlates of fatigue. *Eur J Appl Physiol* **57** 336–47

Section II

Jane A Gorman, John Rooney, Simon Hutabarat

Bone

Forms the mobile structural framework of the body and serves to protect vital internal organs (brain, lungs, heart, viscera). Bone also plays a critical role in regulating calcium and phosphate metabolism, and maintains a stable calcium gradient across the extracellular and intracellular compartments. Bone is self-repairing and continuously remodels throughout life in response to mechanical demands (Wolff's law). It is a well-organized, lightweight tissue with tensile strength almost that of cast iron. It consists of:

Macroscopically: two types (Fig. 3.1).

1 *Cortical* (also called dense or compact) bone has four times the mass of cancellous bone, but one-eighth of the metabolic turnover. Cortical bone has a smaller surface area, and comprises the outer envelope of bones and the diaphysis of long bones. It is subject to bending, torque, and compression loads. (Fig. 3.2).

2 *Cancellous* (also called spongy or trabecular) bone is found in the epiphysis, metaphysis, and vertebrae. It is composed of a 3-dimensional branching lattice aligned along stress lines, and is mainly exposed to compression loads.

Microscopically: several types—(Fig. 3.2)

3 *Woven*: immature, primitive bone, found in the embryo and neonate, in fracture callus, metaphyseal bone, in tumors, pagetoid bone, and osteogenesis imperfecta. It is coarse-fibered with no uniform arrangement of its collagen, and randomly placed cells. Woven bone has isotropic mechanical properties.

4 *Lamellar*: present in mature bone, from remodeling of woven bone (complete by 4 years of age). Has anisotropic mechanical properties, so the greatest strength is parallel to the longitudinal axis of its collagen fibers.

5 *Plexiform*: found in large animals, as a result of rapid growth, where layers of lamellar and woven bone sandwich vascular channels.

6 *Haversian (cortical)*: complex structure, composed of osteons made by sheets of lamellar bone around vascular channels, forming canals oriented to the long axis. They are the major structural unit of cortical bone, which also features interstitial lamellae between the osteons and circumferential lamellae around the bone surface.

Bone is surrounded by periosteum, composed of an outer fibrous layer, continuous with joint capsules; and an inner loose layer, highly vascularized and osteogenic. Periosteum is more highly developed in children.

Cell types in bone (Fig. 3.3).

- *Osteoblasts*[1] form bone, synthesize, and secrete matrix to form collagen.
- *Osteocytes*: 90% of bone cells in the mature person, maintains bone. They develop from osteoblasts trapped in matrix, and help control extracellular Ca^{2+} and PO_4^{3-}.
- *Osteoclasts*: giant cells that resorb bone rapidly in Howship's lacunae, which is coupled to formation. They also produce H^+ to increase the solubility of hydroxyapatite, then the organic matrix is removed by proteolytic digestion.

1 The gene responsible for turning precursors into osteoblasts has been identified. It is CBFA-1. S Dickman 1997 *Science* **276** 1502

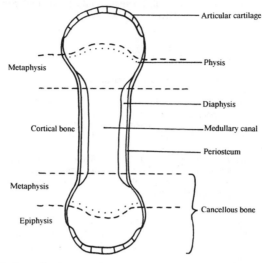

Fig. 3.1 Regions of an immature bone

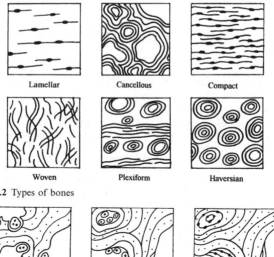

Fig. 3.2 Types of bones

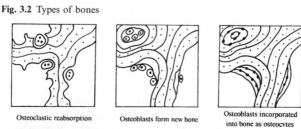

Osteoclastic reabsorption   Osteoblasts form new bone   Osteoblasts incorporated into bone as osteocytes

Fig. 3.3 Bone remodeling

Bone (*cont*)

- *Osteoprogenitor* cells: line canals, endosteum and periosteum. These cells are the osteoblast precursors.

Bone matrix

- *40% organic*
  - 90% collagen (type 1) with cross-linking to increase tensile strength
  - proteoglycans—have compressive strength, inhibit mineralization
  - matrix protein—promotes mineralization and bone formation (e.g. osteocalcin), attracts osteoclasts, and is related to the regulation of bone density, osteonectin regulates Ca^{2+} and mineral organization
- *60% inorganic (mineral)*:
  - calcium hydroxyapatite ($Ca_{10}(PO_4)_6(OH)_2$), provides compressive strength. Mineralization occurs primarily in gaps in the collagen, then in the periphery
  - osteocalcium phosphate

Circulation (Fig. 3.4)

5–10% of cardiac output is delivered to bone via:

- Nutrient artery—goes through the diaphyseal cortex to the medullary canal, supplies inner two-thirds of diaphyseal cortex. High pressure system.
- Metaphyseal/epiphyseal system—from periarticular vascular plexuses (e.g. geniculate arteries).
- Periosteal system—supplies outer one-third of diaphyseal cortex. Low pressure system, flows from internally to externally.
- Venous blood flows from the cortex to venous sinusoids to internal nutrient (or emissary) veins.

In fractures, initially there is a reduction in blood flow by disruption, followed by an increase in blood flow which peaks at 2 weeks and returns to normal in 3–5 months. Vascular supply is the major determinant of fracture healing.

Bone formation in the fetus[1-5]

- *Endochondral ossification*—occurs at extremities and in weight-bearing bones. A cartilage model is made of the bone, which is vascularized, then osteoblasts infiltrate to form a sleeve of periosteal bone by 8 weeks gestation (primary ossification). The marrow space develops by central resorption and invasion by myeloid precursor cells. Secondary ossification at the ends of the bone occurs at cartilaginous epiphyseal centers (growth plates), to produce longitudinal growth.
- Growth plates consist of:
  - *reserve zone* of chondrocytes
  - *proliferative zone*—involves cell proliferation and matrix production. Has high proteoglycan, resulting in low calcification

1 RMH McMinn 1995 *Last's anatomy: Regional and applied.* Churchill Livingstone, Edinburgh 2 MD Miller 1996 *Review of orthopaedics* Saunders, Philadelphia 3 AW Rogers 1992 *Textbook of anatomy.* Churchill Livingstone, Edinburgh 4 MH Ross *et al* 1989 *Histology: A text and atlas.* Williams & Wilkins, Baltimore 5 SR Simon 1994 *Orthopaedic basic science.* American Academy of Orthopaedic Surgeons, Columbus, OH

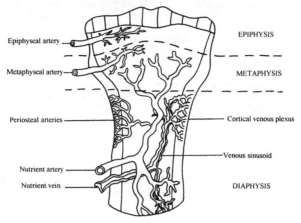

Fig. 3.4 Blood supply of a mature long bone

Bone (*cont*)

- *hypertrophic zone*—involves maturation and degeneration of cells, and provisional calcification. This zone is most likely to fracture and undergo slippage. New osteoblasts use cartilage as a scaffold for bone formation
- The metaphysis removes mineralized cartilaginous matrix, forms bone and remodels cancellous trabeculae. (Fig. 3.5)
- Intramembranous ossification—occurs in flat bones and the clavicle, and is responsible for increase in **width** of long bones (appositional growth) by subperiosteal bone formation. Involves mesenchymal cells aggregating to the periosteal membrane, then differentiating to osteoblasts which form directly in the collagenous matrix.

66

Aging (Fig. 3.6)

Bone resorption increases with aging, particularly in females after the menopause when the protective effect of estrogen is lost. Available estrogen is further reduced by smoking and minimal body fat. Bone density is reduced, resulting in fewer, thinner trabeculae subjected to a greater strain. Loss of trabeculae is irreversible and very damaging because new bone needs a scaffold on which to develop.

Bone injury and repair

Bone fails under breaking loads (fracture) or submaximal forces (stress fractures). Fractures heal by orderly phases:

Process	Result	Time
Inflammation	1 Haematoma	Immediate
	2 Granulation tissue	Hours/days
Repair	3 Immature callus	Weeks
	4 Mature bone (cortical or cancellous)	Months
Remodel	5 Remodeling according to stresses (Wolff's law)	Up to 7 years

Callus formation is reduced with solid immobilization (as in open reduction with internal fixation), leading to primary healing of the cortex. Closed reduction (allowing some movement of the fracture) leads to enchondral healing with periosteal callus.

Growth of bone occurs at the growth plates (the physis and the epiphysis) and under the periosteum. Fractures in children often involved these growth plates and may disturb subsequent growth arrests with shortening and angulation: Salter–Harris classification 1-6, see also Fig. 21.4).[1]

1 Basic sports medicine science In E Sherry, D Bokor (ed) 1997 *Manual of sports medicine*, Ch10, p125–44. GMM, London

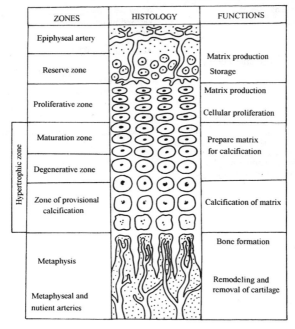

67

ZONES	HISTOLOGY	FUNCTIONS
Epiphyseal artery		Matrix production
Reserve zone		Storage
Proliferative zone		Matrix production
		Cellular proliferation
Maturation zone		Prepare matrix for calcification
Degenerative zone		
Zone of provisional calcification		Calcification of matrix
Metaphysis		Bone formation
Metaphyseal and nutient arteries		Remodeling and removal of cartilage

Hypertrophic zone (bracketing Maturation zone, Degenerative zone, and Zone of provisional calcification)

Fig. 3.5 Histology and function of the growth plate

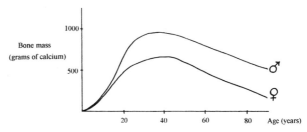

Fig. 3.6 Change in bone mass with age

Complications of fractures include:

Disruption	Result
Healing	Delayed union
	Non-union
	Mal-union
Blood supply	Avascular necrosis
Infection (seen after ORIF)	Osteomyelitis
Soft tissue	Skin (fracture blisters/pressure ulcers/RSD)
	Tendon entrapment
	Ligament rupture
Artery entrapment	
Compartment syndrome	
Nerve injuries	Growth plate disruption (in children)
Growth arrest with shortening and angulation	General
ARDS, fat embolism, DVT	Late
Secondary osteoarthritis	

Joints

Are of three types (Fig. 3.7):

1 *Fibrous* (synarthrosial)—bones are joined by fibrous tissue, as in skull sutures (which gradually ossify with age) and the distal tibulo-fibular joint. Movement is negligible.

2 *Cartilaginous* (amphiarthrodial)—articular surfaces are covered by hyaline cartilage and joined by fibrocartilage (a network of type I collagen, proteoglycan, glycoprotein, and fibrochondrocytes) as in the symphysis pubis or intervertebral disks (in which the fibrocartilage is filled with gel). Limited movement is possible.

3 *Synovial* (diarthrodial)—articular surfaces are covered with hyaline cartilage, surrounded by a capsule and reinforced with ligaments, and lined with a synovial membrane. All limb joints are synovial. The synovium regulates the composition of synovial fluid (an ultrafiltrate), which nourishes hyaline cartilage by diffusion, and provides lubrication. Synovial joints may contain intraarticular fibrocartilage (such as the knee menisci) which deepen the articular surface and so play a role in load distribution and shock absorption.

The knee meniscus is composed of fibrocartilage (a network which is 75% type 1 collagen fibers arranged radially and longitudinally, dissipates the hoop stresses).The meniscus expands under compressive loads to increase contact area. Only the outer quarter of the meniscus has a blood supply and so is capable of healing.

Fatty pads are present in the hip and talocalcaneonavicular joint to spread synovial fluid. Hyaline cartilage (Fig. 3.8) is composed of:
- 65% water
- 10–20% type II collagen for tensile strength
- 10–15% proteoglycan for compressive strength
- 5% chondrocytes
- other proteins (e.g. fibronectin)

Aging of cartilage, exacerbated by immobilization, results in fewer chondrocytes, less proteoglycan and water, increased protein, and stiffening. Joints may be damaged by osteoarthritis (OA) (especially after a fracture), rheumatoid arthritis, avascular necrosis (secondary to steroids or disrupted blood supply), infection, or hemorrhage. Cartilage heals superficially by chondrocyte proliferation, and deeply by fibrocartilaginous scarring (aided by continuous passive motion).

Sports and intense physical activity wear out joints (in fact, intensive sporting activity results in a 4.5 times increased incidence of OA of the so-called skier's hip, which may go up to 8.5 times when combined with occupational exposure).[1]

1 E Vingaard *et al* 1993 *Am J Sports Med* **21** 195–200

Fibrous joint

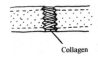

Collagen

Cartilaginous joint

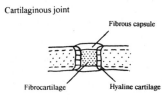

Fibrous capsule

Fibrocartilage   Hyaline cartilage

Synovial joint

Fibrous capsule   Hyaline cartilage

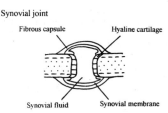

Synovial fluid   Synovial membrane

Fig. 3.7 Classification of joints

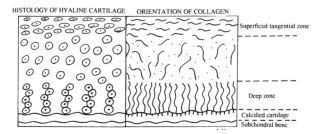

HISTOLOGY OF HYALINE CARTILAGE   ORIENTATION OF COLLAGEN

Superficial tangential zone

Deep zone

Calcified cartilage
Subchondral bone

Fig. 3.8 Histology of hyaline cartilage

Skeletal muscle

Is composed of muscle fibers (the basic unit of contraction), surrounded by endomysium, then arranged in fascicles which are in turn surrounded by perimysium (Fig. 3.9). The whole muscle is surrounded by epimysium. Each muscle fiber is composed of myofibrils ($1-3\mu m$ in diameter and $1-2cm$ long), made up of numerous sarcomeres of thick (myosin) and thin (actin) filaments which slide by each other, resulting in muscle contraction. The signal to contract is delivered to the muscle unit (of 10–1000 muscle fibers, depending on the precision required of the unit) via an α-motor neurone. The signal is then mediated by Ca^{2+} stored in the intracellular sarcoplasmic reticulum and released via T-tubules to each myofibril, to stimulate contraction.

Types of muscle contraction:

1 *Isotonic* (dynamic)—allows constant tension during concentric contractions (muscle shortening) or eccentric contractions (muscle lengthening). Variable resistance refers to a changing external load during weight lifting.

2 *Isometric* (static)—tension is generated but there is no muscle shortening. This exercise causes muscle hypertrophy, which increases cross-sectional area so allowing greater force production, but has no benefit to endurance. When the muscle is stretched in isometric contraction, generated tension increases up to a point at which the muscle is overstretched and damaged (see Fig. 3.10).

3 *Isokinetic* (dynamic)—involves maximal tension generation in a muscle contracting at constant speed over the full range of motion.

4 *Functional*—dynamic exercises which allow rapid rehabilitation (e.g. jump ropes).

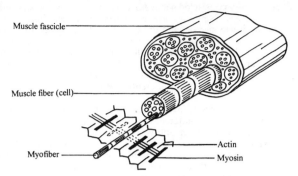

Fig. 3.9 Structure of muscle

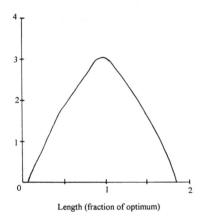

Length (fraction of optimum)

Fig. 3.10 Isometric tension-length curve of skeletal muscle

Nerves

Peripheral nerves consist of nerve fibers (axons), blood vessels and connective tissues. Neurones are composed of a cell body with dendrites to receive signals, and an axon to deliver signals to other cells via synapses. Axons may be surrounded by myelin to facilitate conduction of electrical signals. Myelin is formed by Schwann cells, which wrap around segments of axon, with spaces (nodes of Ranvier) between them (Fig. 3.11). Nerves may be afferent (sensory) going to the central nervous system, or efferent (motor) delivering signals to muscle.

Spinal reflexes usually involve the sudden stretching of a tendon, which sends a signal in an afferent nerve to the spinal cord, where the nerve synapses to an efferent nerve via one or more interneurones (most human reflexes are polysynaptic). The efferent signal to the muscle stimulates it to contract briefly in response to the initial stretch. Reflexes may therefore be used to assess peripheral nerves and the spinal cord at a certain level.

The blood supply to a nerve may be extrinsic (vessels travel in connective tissue around the peripheral nerve) or intrinsic (interconnected vascular plexuses in connective tissue sheaths within the nerve). Peripheral nerves may be damaged in three ways:

1 *Neuropraxia*—transient denervation (1–2 months) due to mild nerve injury such as compression.

2 *Axonotmesis*—complete denervation, in which the distal axon dies and Wallerian degeneration of myelin occurs. Axonal regeneration occurs slowly (2.5cm per month), and is influenced by guidance from remaining Schwann cells, and neurotrophic (growth) factors.

3 *Neuronotmesis*—complete denervation, occurring when the axons and the myelin sheaths are transected. Recovery is poor, even with nerve repair.

Note: there is little valid evidence that suggests exercise influences the function of motor neurones.

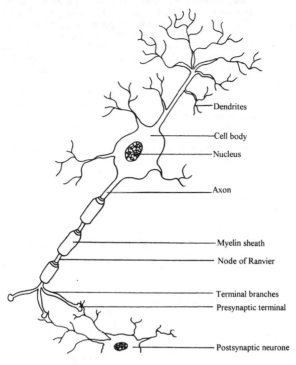

Fig. 3.11 Structure of a neurone

Tendons

Are dense, regular connective tissues that attach muscle to bone via Sharpey's fibers (transitional, calcified fibrocartilage which incorporates into the bone). Tendons are composed of proteoglycans and parallel bundles of type I collagen (85% of tendon) produced by fibroblasts which lie in fascicles surrounded by loose areolar tissue. The collagen bundles are separated by endotenon, surrounded by epitenon, and the whole tendon is enclosed in paratenon (the tendon sheath).

Tendons are nourished by blood vessels, synovial folds, and periosteal attachments. After damage (acutely or by tensile overload/overuse), tendons repair by the action of fibroblasts and macrophages, with maximal weakness at 7–10 days and maximum strength 6 months post injury. Early mobilization increases the range of movement but decreases the strength of the tendon repair.

Sports Tendon Overload

Site	Sport
Tendo achilles/ECRB	Tennis
Iliotibial band/patellofemoral/patellar tendon/plantar fasciitis/ shin splints	Running
EPB/APL	Rowing

Injuries occur at the muscle–tendon junction and in muscles crossing two joints (the hamstrings and the Achilles tendon). Most of these involve the lower limb (look for a cause), and do not overlook other overuse injuries, such as stress fractures/chronic compartment syndrome/shin splints. Causes include training errors (sudden increase in mileage such as >64km/week; inadequate stretching; wrong scheduling), anatomical factors (varus knee, pronated foot), training surfaces (hills, irregular tracks, too hard, too soft, too much friction), weather/altitude, and running shoe problems (worn out, wrong size, poor maintenance).[1] Rehabilitation is critical (acute phase—rest, NSAIDs, protected ROM, isometrics, isotonics; recovery-careful loading, ROM, resistive and functional exercises).

1 E Sherry 1997 Basic sports medicine science In E Sherry, D Bokor (ed) *Manual of sports medicine* Ch10, p125–44. GMM, London

Ligaments

Help stabilize joints, and usually insert into bone indirectly, with fibers inserting into periosteum at an acute angle. Direct insertion involves deep fibers attaching at 90°, with a transition from ligament to fibrocartilage, to mineralized fibrocartilage, to bone; and superficial fibers joining the periosteum directly. Avulsion injuries usually occur between the unmineralized and mineralized fibrocartilage layers. Ligaments are composed of type I collagen (70% of ligament tissue) with variable fibers and a high elastin content, and have mechanoreceptors to assist with joint stabilization.

The blood supply to ligaments enters at the insertion into bone. Extraarticular ligaments heal by hemorrhage, then inflammation, and finally type III collagen (later maturing to type I collagen) is formed by fibroblasts. Intraarticular ligament healing is halted by the presence of synovial fluid. Immobilization causes stiffness and reduces the strength of repair.

4 Medical problems of athletes

EUGENE SHERRY, SAMEER VISWANATHAN,
LAWRENCE TRIEU, DONALD JOHN CHISHOLM,
AMITABHA DAS

Section I The environment and sport

Introduction

Athletes do battle with themselves, their competitors, and the environment. The results may be glory, injury, or illness. In this chapter we describe the medical and environmental problems facing athletes. Many are potentially serious but can often prevented by proper preparation and education.

Heat

It is important to understand thermoregulatory factors. Thermoregulation results from reflex responses from the various temperature receptors in the skin, central vessels, viscera, and (preoptic area) anterior hypothalamus, signaling sympathetic shunting of blood and sweat gland stimulation when the temperature exceeds 37 °C (Benzinger reflex (Fig. 4.1). The body maintains a core temperature between the normal range of 36.1–37.8 °C by balancing heat production/gain and heat loss. Heat is produced by metabolic functions (65–85kcal/h at rest) and work done by muscles (both smooth and skeletal; muscular contraction produces 300–700 kcal/h). Heat is gained by radiant energy from the sun (100–200 kcal/h). Fever can add, at a rate of about 8%, a rise per degree Celsius of fever.[1]

Heat is lost to the environment in the following ways:

- Radiation (65% heat loss, only works when body temperature is greater than ambient temperature).
- Evaporation (sweating, air–skin interface), the latent heat of evaporation is the amount of heat passed to the environment by vaporization (0.6kcal of heat/ml sweat), it is the major physiological defense against overheating as the ambient temperature rises, reduced by high humidity as the ambient vapour pressure approximates moist skin).[2]
- Convection (needs air movement: 12–15%)
- Conduction (direct contact).
- Reflected radiation (from nearby surfaces).

1 MD Bracker 1992 *Clin Sports Med* 11 419–36   2 M J Leski 1994 Thermoregulation and safe exercise in the heat. In MB Mellion (ed) *Sports medicine secrets* p77–82. Hanley & Belfus, Philadelphia

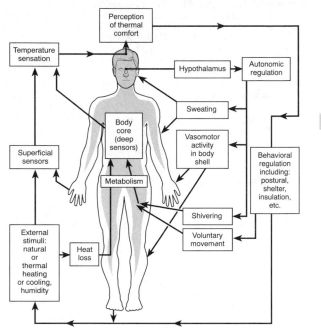

Fig. 4.1 Temperature regulation in the body.

Wet bulb globe temperature (WBGT)

It is important to evaluate all aspects of the exercise environment, i.e. temperature, humidity, air movement (if outdoors) and solar radiation. This is done by the WBGT (Fig. 4.2), which is a single temperature and is dependent on air temperature, solar and ground radiation, humidity, and wind velocity. It thus represents a sum of the impact of the environment on the athlete.[1] It can be measured with inexpensive simple instrumentation or calculated with data from the weather bureau (either degrees F or C).The WBGT calculation uses three measurements: (1) natural wet-bulb temp (place a wet wick over the thermometer bulb): (2) air temp; and (3) globe temp (temp inside a copper globe painted matt black). WBGT is calculated as follows:

Indoor WBGT = $(0.7 \times$ natural wet-bulb temp$) + (0.3 \times$ globe temp$)$
Outdoor WBGT = $(0.7 \times$ natural wet-bulb temp$) + (0.2 \times$ globe temp$) + (0.1 \times$ air temp$)$

Whether to or how to exercise in hot environments can be decided by considering the two criteria: Recommended alert limit (RAL), above which action should be taken to reduce heat stress: and Ceiling limit (CL), above which exercise should not be undertaken without changing the environment). Figure 4.3[2] shows limits based on exercise intensity (energy expenditure per hour) and WBGT. When the temperature is between C and RAL exercise is possible, but has risks. Therefore:

Change the environment (fans or air conditioning) or move to area where WBGT is within acceptable limits.

- For the exercise session, decrease the intensity of the exercise (slow the pace and/or add rest periods).Useful guide is the *target heart rate* (unchanged from cool conditions). Exercise heart rate is increased 1 beat/minute (bpm) for every degree centigrade above 25C and 2bpm for every mmHG above 20mmHg water vapour pressure. Maintain to a fixed heart rate.

Marron and Tucker have provided a useful guide for exercise in the heat (Table 4.1).[3]

It is important to acclimatize to exercise in a hot environment: 25% of the thought-to-be healthy population may be heat intolerant if unacclimatized (but will decrease to 2% with proper preparation with aerobic exercise starting with a 10–15min and over a 10–14-day period). Especially for those >60 years (as thirst becomes less useful guide to hydration). The following conditions predispose to heat stress:

- high blood pressure (alters control of skin blood flow)[4]
- diabetes (because of neuropathy)
- drugs (diuretics, beta-blockers, α agonists, vasodilators, opiates, salicylates, thyroxine, CNS stimulants, parasympatholytic, or anticholinergics)

1 W Kennedy *et al* 1995 Eds *ACSMs guidelines for exercise testing and prescription* 5th edn p288–93. Williams & Wilkins, Philadelphia   2 National Institute for Occupational Safety and Health 1986 *Criteria for a recommended standard . . . occupational exposure to hot environments.* DHHS NIOSH Publ No 86–113. US Dept Health and Human Services, Washington, DC   3 JT Marron, JB Tucker 1994 Environmental factors In RB Birres (ed) *Sports medicine for the primary care physician* ch10. CRC, Boca Raton   4 WL Kenney, E Kamon 1984 *Eur J Appl Physiol* **52** 196–201

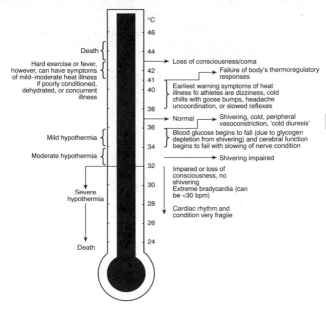

Fig. 4.2 Temperature effects on the body

Wet bulb globe temperature (WBGT) (*cont*)

- alcohol
- obesity
- prior heat tolerance problems

In 1984, the American College of Sports Medicine (ACSM) recommended that it was unsafe to proceed with endurance events if the WBGT >28 °C.

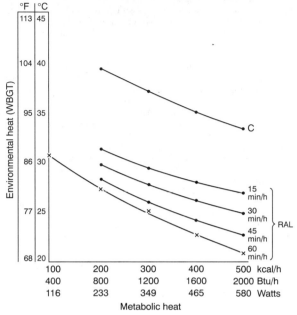

Assumes 70kg (154lb) body weight and 1.8m² (19.4ft²) body surface

Fig. 4.3 Recommended heat stress alert (RAL) and ceiling (C) limits.

Table 4.1 Exercise in the high temperatures

WBGT reading (°C)	Recommendations
Football practice	
15.5	Go ahead
16–19	Watch for >3% water loss
19.5–22	Have water available
22.5–25	Change schedule (30min work/rest periods
25.5	Cancel
Running	
>28	Cancel
23–28 red flag	High risk, postpone until after 4pm or before 9am, not for those at risk
18–28 amber flag	Moderate risk
10–18 green flag	Minimal risk
<10 white flag	Risk of hypothermia, especially slow runners in the cold over long distances

Heat problems

These are a group of clinical presentations due to increased core temperatures that are generally classified into mild, moderate, or severe. There is an increased risk in children, female athletes (where prolonged exercise in the luteal phase), and older athletes.[1]

Mild

Presents as heat fatigue, (heat) cramps, or syncope. Symptoms include weakness, fatigue and muscle cramps which occur during exercise, whereas fainting or dizziness usually occurs at the end of exercise (when venous blood pools). Usually of short duration but may be excruciating. Signs are muscle tightness or cramps. **Treatment** is rest, ice, and massage of cramps. Oral fluids. Lie in cool area and elevate legs if syncope. Remove excess clothing.

Note other terms used: heat edema (self-limiting swelling of hands/feet, resolves with acclimatization); heat tetany-carpopedal spasm; miliaria (prickly heat); rubramaculopapular rash from keratin plugs (over clothed areas, better hygiene needed).

Moderate

Also known as heat exhaustion. There is headache, weakness, exhaustion, nausea, vomiting, ataxia, and mild confusion. Examination reveals increased sweating, hypotension (especially postural), and tachycardia. Raised core temperature is present but its significance is doubtful since well marathon runners can have temperatures up to 41 °C. Rectal temperature should be measured to monitor true temperature status and to exclude heat stroke. **Treatment:** measures as for *mild*, as well as ice packs to groin and axillae, and possibly intravenous fluids.

Severe (heat stroke)

Core temp >41 °C. There is collapse with impaired consciousness from exercise.

Note: Clinical picture may be masked by presence of hot, dry skin or cold and sweaty skin, therefore always take rectal temperature.

Classic heat stroke

Occurs in those at risk (old, homeless, poor, ill, obese, drunk, drugged); whereas exertional heat stroke occurs in summer in those exercising. **Treatment**: Initiate ABC of resuscitation. Start rapid cooling (cool packs over neck/groin/axillae; atomized spray of warm air with fanning with warm air—Mecca Cooling Unit) and intravenous fluids (1–2L of dextrose–saline solution). Transfer to hospital as this is a medical emergency with potentially life-threatening multiorgan failure with DIC (with similarities to septic shock).

Pathophysiology and complications

In *severe heat* problems, the following chain of events occurs:

- *Heat injury* → gut ischemia → endotoxins enter portal circulation → hepatic clearance overwhelmed → cytokine release

1 JR Sutton 1994 In M. Harries *et al* (ed) *Oxford textbook of sports medicine* Ch2.4. OUP

- *Dehydration and cytokines* both contribute to hypotension and other complications. Complications of *severe heat problems* include:
- *Cardiac*   Postural hypotension, conduction disturbances, myocardial infarct, and cardiac failure.
- *Neurological* Convulsions, cerebrovascular events, and coma.
- *Abdominal*   Gastrointestinal bleeding, liver damage, and renal failure.
- *Other*   Rhabdomyolysis or breakdown of skeletal muscle membrane. This results in toxic metabolites, such as myoglobin, which may lead to renal failure. Presents with myoglobinuria (brown urine) and raised serum phosphokinase and potassium. An associated disseminated intravascular coagulation may also develop.

Prevention of heat problems

The following is a summary of the guidelines introduced since the 1971 City-to-City race, Sydney, Australia:[1]

- Wear appropriate cool, light-colored clothing.
- Stay well hydrated before, during, and after exercise (2 cups cold water 15–20min prior exercise, 1 cup every 15min of exercise, and more than thirst demands afterwards).
- Adequate physical fitness preparation for sport/event/conditions is essential. This may include heat acclimatization. The physiological adjustments in increased blood volume, venous tone, and especially sweating, seen during acclimatization usually requires 2 weeks to take effect (although this is variable).
- Avoid exercise in extreme heat (and humidity). At-risk events and sports should have guidelines with medical advice.
- Do not exercise with intercurrent illness (such as fever, URTI, or gastroenteritis).
- Proper planning with fluids, sunscreen, and medical /or first aid cover.
- Obtain informtion on the early signs of heat illnesses.
- Run within one's capabilities

Note: *One victim of heat stress means others are at risk in the group.*

Hyponatremia

This can cause collapse associated with exercise in heat and is commonly mistaken for heat stroke. Only seen in ultra-endurance events (>34h), under extreme conditions, there is profuse sweating, no acclimatization. Thought to be caused by fluid overload from hypotonic drinks.

1 D Richards *et al* 1979 *Med J Austral* **2** 457–61

Cold problems

Although less of an immediate worry than heat stress, need to consider frostbite, exposure (hypothermia), and masking of angina (cold air and/or cold peripheries may mask the onset of angina, lower the threshold or cause angina at rest).[1] Those involved in snow, water, and mountaineering sports are at risk as well as endurance events in cold temperatures.[2] The wind chill factor accelerates temp loss through convection and radiation.[3] Hypothermia (defined as physiological state where core temp falls below 35 °C) can be mild, moderate, or severe and clinical features vary accordingly:

- **Mild:** core temp (34–36°C). Athlete usually displays cold extremities, shivering, tachycardia, tachypnoea, urinary urgency, and slight incoordination. Patient is aware of this temperature loss.
- **Moderate:** core temp (32–34°C). Blood sugars begin to fall and cerebral function begins to fail at 35 °C, with unsteadiness, muscle weakness, cramps, and increased incoordination. If warmth, shelter, and food are found at this stage, recovery is rapid. If exposure to the cold continues, **a failure of shivering** (the critical difference between *mild* and *moderate* as when shivering stops patient can no longer rewarm spontaneously and external heat is necessary) and a loss of vasoconstrictor tone results in an accelerating loss of temperature control, speech becomes slurred, fatigue, dehydration, amnesia, poor judgment, drowsiness, anxiety, and irritability takes place.
- **Severe:** core temp (<32 °C). Significant mortality with total loss of shivering, inappropriate behavior, impaired or loss of consciousness (coma), muscle rigidity, hypotension, pulmonary edema, extreme bradycardia, and cardiac arrhythmias (especially ventricular fibrillation, VF).

Treatment: measure rectal temperature to assess the severity of hypothermia and to monitor treatment (the diagnostic dilemma of unexpected confusion and agitation in the snow is solved by measuring the rectal temp). Principles of treatment include basic life support measures (e.g. fluids, nutrition, and cardiac support), minimizing further heat loss, rewarming in a controlled manner, treatment of other injuries, and transportation. It is a fallacy that voluntary activity increases body heat (in fact, movement increases peripheral blood flow and so increases body surface area exposure to the surrounding elements, resulting in increased heat loss and body heat requirements). Use full cardiac and oximetric monitoring, establish an IV line, start CPR, if necessary. **Remember that a cold patient is not pronounced as dead until he/she is 'warm and pink'.** CPR may need to be continued for well over an hour until you are convinced there are no sustainable signs of life in the rewarmed patient. This can be a difficult decision—if possible talk to a more senior colleague. In a severely hypothermic and pulseless patient (suspended animation) start CPR, at half standard rates, should only be started if full warming can be done. **Treatment**: establish airway (may need to intubate). Then institute rewarming maneuvers. Rewarming can be:

1 W Larry Kennedy *et al* 1995 (ed) *ACSMs guidelines for exercise testing and prescription* 5th edn 294. Williams & Wilkins, Philadelphia 2 E Sherry D Richards 1986 *Med J Austral* **144** 457–61 3 See *US Air Force survival manual* 64–3

- **Passive**—insulation from wet, wind, and cold. Removal of wet clothing and drying the body (even in dry snow!). Allowing the body to gradually rewarm by its **own** metabolic heat.
- **External active**—hot packs and baths, heated aerosols, electric blankets, another body these measures are adequate for mild or moderate hypothermia). Caution should be exercised in severe cases where shift of already reduced fluid volume to a warmed periphery may cause hypotension and a cardiac event.
- **Internal active**—warm drinks or food are reasonably simple measures. Most effective is venous-to-venous hemodialysis (raise temp $\frac{1}{2}$ –1°C/h).Otherwise use nasogastric tube, urinary catheter, peritoneal catheter, and enema tube with warm fluids. The rough handling of the patient can precipitate irreversible ventricular fibrillation.

Frostbite

Is a local destruction of superficial tissues caused by cold exposure (commonly toes, fingers, ears), subdivided into:

- *Frost nip* Incipient frostbite with sudden blanching of skin and is painless.
- *Superficial* Skin place, waxy and firm but not frozen.
- *Deep frostbite* Cold, pale, solid, fragile tissue.

Treatment is local rewarming, analgesia, protection (with blanket, cottonwool), and gentle handling. Avoid rubbing area or applying snow, and watch for secondary vascular occlusion by edema, gangrene, and infection. Possible use of calcium channel blockers (peripheral vasodilatation) and NSAIDs (protect against prostaglandin effects).

Cold urticaria

Some patients exposed to cold develop urticarial eruptions which may evolve into angioedema. Severe cases may develop hypotension and syncope. Urticaria is mast cell-mediated, IgE-dependent disorder, although cryoglobulins and cold agglutinins may be recognized in the blood. Urticaria may only affect the exposed limb. Previous asymptomatic exposure to cold stimuli does not exclude cold urticaria. **Treatment** is rewarming, antihistamines, and sympatheticomimetic agents if severe.

Prevention of cold problems

- *Adequate preparation* (clothing, communication, equipment, weather forecasts).
- *Stay* well hydrated and nourished (chocolate bar in pack). Caution with alcohol.
- *Do not* exercise to exhaustion.
- *Adequate* fitness level for required activity including cold and altitude acclimatization if indicated.

Note: cold acclimatization is less effective than heat acclimatization.
Note: death in snow avalanche is from suffocation, injury, hypothermia (in that order).

Altitude problems

Distinct medical problems are encountered in sport at high attitudes and are made worse with rapid ascent. Performances at high altitude are helped by reduced wind resistance and gravity, and worsened by the reduced oxygen pressure (FiO_2 remains constant but ↓ barometric pressure and so ↓ PiO_2 and possibly ↓ PaO_2 and ↓ SaO_2) and by the dropping temperatures (temperatures reduce by about $2\,°C$ for every additional 300m above sea level). Changes with physical activity (acclimatization) at high altitude include:

- ↑ pulmonary ventilation (with breathlessness), variable, may not become apparent for several days, leads to mild respiratory alkalosis (to counter the ↓ PaO2).
- ↑ HR in order to ↑ CO and offset the ↓ SaO_2 (to maintain oxygenation), this ↑ HR is transient (returns to N after 2–3 days but HR_{max} may remain below sea level value). **Note** target HR guidelines developed at lower altitudes are still useful guide in presence of high heat and humidity.
- ↓ Vo_{2max} (by 5% at 1200m; 4000 feet) with ↓ physical work capacity, (and greater above 1200m; 4000 feet).
- ↑ RBC (to ↑ oxygen-carrying capacity blood) with shift of oxyhemoglobin curve over days to weeks.
- ↑ capillary and ↑ mitochondrial density over weeks.

Note: myocardial ischemia may occur where CAD, because of relative hypoxia.

A resolution was made at the 20th World Congress of Sports Medicine (Melbourne 1974) urging extreme caution at altitudes of more than 2600m (8700ft) and an absolute prohibition of contests above 3000m (10,000ft). Various adaptations occur over varying time frames at altitude, including a reduction in bicarbonate, an increase in hemoglobin levels, a restoration of blood volume, and an increase in various tissue enzymes. Problems encountered at altitudes include the following.

Acute mountain sickness: AMS (> 2400m; 8000ft)

With non-specific symptoms such as headache, dizziness, nausea, vomiting, irritability, and insomnia from hyperventilation and associated acid-base disturbances. It is usually a temporary condition affecting the first 2–3 days of a rapid ascent over 2000m (6650ft). There is mild tachycardia and peripheral edema. **Symptomatic treatment** is usually adequate (rest, hydration, analgesics), in severe cases return to lower altitudes is advisable and the use of acetazolamide[1] (125mg, twice daily) may help (beware diuretic effect on plasma volume).

High altitude pulmonary edema: HAPE[2] (> 3000m; 10,000ft)

A life-threatening (non-cardiac) condition occurring in the first few days of an ascent and manifests with symptoms dyspnea, blood-stained (pink) frothy sputum, coughing, and chest diskomfort/pain. Signs of tachycardia and tachypnea, low grade fever, and cyanosis. It is more common in the presence of intercurrent cardiorespiratory conditions. O2 desaturation (moderate to severe) with relative hypoventilation. **Treatment** immediate on descent, oxygen, nifedipine

---

1 Acetazolamide is banned from Olympic competition 2 RB Schoene 1994 In MB Mellion (ed) *Sports medicine secrets*, p430–4. Hanley & Belfus, Phildelphia, with permission

(20mg slow release 8-hourly) and dexamethasone (4mg, 6-hourly).[1]
(*Note*: both these drugs thought to be useful but not proven.)
Hyperbaric therapy (if descent not possible).

High altitude cerebral edema: HACE (>3600m; 12,000ft)

A rare condition with severe headache, confusion, hallucination,
impaired consciousness, or coma. Signs of ataxia, focal neurologi-
cal/visual signs, retinal hemorrhage. Usually associated with rapid
ascents above 4000m (13,300ft). Moderate oxygen desaturation.
Treatment is urgent return to low altitude, oxygen and intravenous
corticosteroids (dexamethasone 8mg bolus then 4mg, q6h), hyperbaric oxygen bag (if descent not possible).

Chronic mountain sickness: CMS (>3000m; 10,000ft)

Takes months/years to develop. There is lethargy and reduced exercise
capacity. Signs of plethora, peripheral edema, and conjunctival
injection.[1] Polycythemia, hypercapnia, (relative), and oxygen desaturation. **Treatment** is descent, oxygen, and respiratory stimulants
(acetazolamide, progesterone, phlebotomy). **Prevention** is possible
and essential:

- Avoid rapid ascents
- Altitude acclimatization. Approximately 3 weeks at a moderate
  altitude (2500–3000m; 8300–10,000ft).
- Appropriate medical screening (patients with pulmonary hyperten-
  sion, uncompensated CHF, unstable angina, recent MI or severe
  anemia are at greater risk when travelling to higher altitudes).[2]
- Education of participants about early symptoms, signs, and man-
  agement of altitude illnesses.
- Susceptible patients (often young and healthy) need a slow gradual
  ascent with prophylactic use of nifedipine
- Consider carrying a portable hyperbaric bag. (In the USA, the
  Gamow Bag is available from Chinook Medical Products, Boulder,
  CO.)

Retinal pathology

These small retinal hemorrhages are mainly benign and occur above
altitudes of 4000m (13,300ft). Visual impairment can occur with
central scotomata and impaired color vision.

1 PP Bartsch *et al* 1991 *N Engl J Med* **325** 1284–89   **2** R W Squires 1985 *J Cardiopulmon Rehab* **5** 421–6

Section II Acute management of the sick and injured athlete

Introduction

Regardless of particular medical expertise in medicine all doctors need to know how to resuscitate and handle a life-threatening injury. Especially in sports medicine where the athlete is 'young' and salvageable. The number of such situations that are life-threatening is probably low. The author has found that <5% of snow skiing injuries require immediate hospital treatment.[1] The risk of these injuries or illness amongst athletes depends on the type and level of sport (amateur vs professional), previous illness or injury, and the level of fitness. The profile of skiers with serious injury is male, under 14 years, experienced skier, colliding with rocks, on steep slopes, at high speed, slushy snow, long skis, no head protection, and bindings did release.[2]

A **simple approach** is essential in any case of potential life-threatening injury (Table 4.2) or illness.

1 E Sherry 1984 *Med J Austral* **140** 530–1 **2** E Sherry 1986 MPH thesis University of Sydney

Table 4.2 On field approach to Injury

Injuries can be:		Action
Minor	Cuts/abrasions/sprains/ cramps	Return to game
Moderate	Sprains (swelling, pain, ↓ ROM)	Treat on site/later refer
Severe	Severe pain, swelling, deformity (sprains, fractures, dislocations)	Expert medical care
Life threatening	Stroke, head/neck injury, heart attack	Resuscitate

Sick and injured athlete[1]

Resuscitating a patient falls into two basic groups: (1) non-trauma (dehydration, heat stress, cardiac—start basic life support and medical therapy); and (2) trauma (injury, IV start, stop bleeding, splint, transport). Various treatment algorithms have been designed for each group (Australian Resuscitation Council, American Heart Association, Early Management of Severe Trauma, Advanced Trauma Life Support). For athletes requiring resuscitation it is essential to determine from *the onset of first aid, if there has been any trauma* present. If there is uncertainty about the presence or absence of trauma, *assume trauma is involved and treat accordingly* (Table 4.3).

Use:
A airway
B breathing
C circulation

History: brief talk to athlete or witness/details of accident/extent pain/ assess severity. **Examination:** check for: swelling/deformity/tenderness/ROM, and classify (as above). **Treat**

1 S Stapleton 1997 In E Sherry, D Bokor (ed) *Sports Medicine*, Ch5, p61–71. GMM, London.

Table 4.3 Are they conscious?

NO	YES
Call for help (Dial emergency number) Trauma-related?	STOP Stop, talk, observe, prevent

NO	YES
Assess: **A B C** Initiate CPR Remove from further danger Assist emergency medical services Ensure rapid transport to definitive care	Secure airway with neck immobilization Assess breathing Assess circulation Control external bleeding Remove from further danger Assist emergency medical services Ensure rapid transport to definitive care

Care of the collapsed or seriously ill athlete

The basic principles of the resuscitation of the collapsed or seriously ill patient are the Chain of Survival:

- *Early access* to emergency medical services. This 'call for help' allows the rapid delivery of care in the field by ambulance services to commence early stabilization and delivery of the patient to a hospital for definitive care.
- *Early commencing of bystander cardiopulmonary resuscitation (CPR)*, when required. This will buy time for the arrival of ambulance personnel, particularly where cardiac arrest, where early defibrillation is the most important factor determining survival.
- *Early defibrillation* is the most important factor in determining survival in cardiac arrest due to either ventricular fibrillation or pulseless ventricular tachycardia.
- *Early advanced care* implies the rapid delivery of the seriously ill patient to hospital. In the non trauma-related illness this allows the early administration of advanced medical care.
- *Early access to emergency medical services*: emergency medical services achieves two major goals:

1 the early resuscitation and stabilization of the seriously ill patient
2 the rapid delivery of the patient to definitive care.

This is best achieved when bystanders 'call for help' as the initial step in the caring for the seriously ill patient. If 2 or more bystanders are present, one person should dial the Emergency telephone number, whilst the other commences CPR. Relate clear information regarding the location of the patient, and any other information requested by the operator.

- *For the infant or child,* in arrest, the most likely cause is an airway problem. Here it is best to commence CPR, then call for help.
- *'Call for help'* also implies gaining assistance at the scene, before the ambulance arrives. Even for people experienced in resuscitation, CPR is always easier with 2 or more people lending help. *Do not hesitate in seeking help.*

Commencing early CPR

The window of opportunity for survival from cardiac arrest is small. As such, the aim of bystander CPR is to increase the time before death occurs, allowing emergency medical services the opportunity to deliver early defibrillation, and other advanced care techniques. After assessing the person's responsiveness, the steps in bystander CPR or basic life support for the collapsed patient are:

- **Secure the airway.** *First clear the airway, and then open the airway.* Clear the airway means removing any foreign bodies from the airway including dentures, broken teeth, food, vomit, or blood. This is done by the finger sweep, although care must be taken not to dislodge any loose teeth, especially in young children. If available a suction device should be used. After clearing the airway, it may need to be opened by a combination of extending the head, chin lift and jaw thrust (not neck extension as this may damage the cervical spine). An oropharyngeal airway (Geudel's airway) should be used.
- **Assess and ensure breathing** (*rescue breathing or expired air resuscitation*). To assess the presence/ absence of breathing look for movement of the chest with inhalation and exhalation, feel for chest movement and listen for the air movement. *If there is no evidence of breathing*, rescue breathing should be commenced immediately. This is commenced with 2 slow breaths, by the mouth-to-mouth technique, ensuring that the chest rises (Fig. 4.4). If possible use a mouth-to-mask device to reduce the risk of infection.

The rates and ratios of external cardiac compression and rescue breathing are: *Ventilation*: 15 breaths/min. *Chest compressions*: 80–100 compressions/min and a ratio of 15 breaths/2 compressions (when one rescuer) and 5/1 (when two).

- **Assess and maintain circulation** (*external cardiac compression, ECC*). To assess the circulation feel for the carotid pulse in the neck at the angle of the jaw. *If the pulse is present,* but the patient is not breathing spontaneously, continue rescue breathing at a rate of 15 breaths/min, until either help arrives or spontaneous breathing commences.
- **If there is no detectable carotid pulse,** commence ECC immediately. The hands are placed on the lower third of the sternum, with the arms locked at the elbows and the rescuer kneeling over the patient (Fig. 4.5). Compressions are approximately 5cm deep in the adult, at a rate of between 80 to 100 compressions/min. Tiring work (if needed over a prolonged period), so do not delay in getting help from bystanders (change every few minutes). *To determine the adequacy of ECC*, feel for the carotid pulse, and after every 2min of full CPR, check whether there is spontaneous breathing and circulation. Continue full CPR until either help arrives, or there is return of spontaneous circulation.
- **Stabilization and transport**. When pulse and breathing have returned place in the coma position until help arrives (patient semi-prone, hands under head, upper knee bent forward in front of lower). Check airway patency, breathing and circulation frequently, and respond to any deterioration. Then transport.

Assess the adequacy of rescue breathing by watching the
chest move while maintaining an open airway

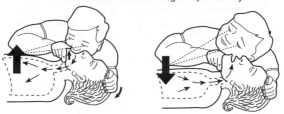

Fig. 4.4 Rescue (mouth-to-mouth) breathing. Watch the chest move as you
maintain the airway.

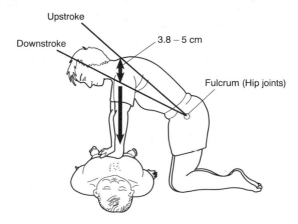

Fig. 4.5 Technique of CPR. Hands over lower one-third of sternum, elbows
locked, rescuer kneeling over patient.

Seriously injured athlete

Care is similar to that of the seriously ill athlete, with several points of note. The system taught in Advanced Trauma Life Support and the Early Management of Severe Trauma courses, is easy to remember (Table 4.4). **Remember the following**:

- *Remove from danger,* in order to prevent further injury. While doing so it is essential to protect the patient's neck, to prevent any trauma to the cervical spine and spinal cord (hold the neck firmly without any movement as when removing a football helmet).

- *Airway management includes care of the cervical spine.* In the non-injured patient, one of the first airway opening maneuvers is to extend the neck. This should not done in the injured patient, especially if unconscious, as it may damage the cervical spine. All airway-clearing maneuvers must be accompanied by in-line cervical immobilization. The neck should be immobilized with a rigid cervical collar.

- *In controlling the circulation, control blood loss. Use direct pressure. Do not use limb tourniquets* (may cause arterial or nerve damage). Immobilize long bone fractures, especially of the femur (Donway splint) to reduce blood loss and control pain.

- *In the unconscious, injured athlete always consider severe head injury.* These patients need rapid stabilization and transfer to a hospital for life-threatening intracranial bleeding (urgent operation).

Table 4.4: The approach to the severely injured athlete.
(*At the scene,* it is important to prevent further injury by removing the patient from any danger. It is *essential to care for the patient's neck whilst doing so.*)

Primary Survey

- Airway and cervical spine immobilization
  - Immobilize head and neck with in-line stabilization
  - Clear airway
  - Open airway, remember not to extend neck

- Assess and ensure adequate breathing/ventilation
  - Commence rescue breathing

- Control bleeding and control circulation
  - Apply pressure to external bleeding
  - Commence external chest compressions, if **no** pulse

- Assess disability (neuro loss)
  - If unconscious, assume major head injury and transport to hospital **asap**
  - If unable to move arms or legs, assume spinal injury (**do not move** until further help arrives)

- Control environment
  - Remove from danger
  - Prevent excessive heat loss if injured
  - Gather information about series of causative events

Resuscitation

- Fix any immediate life-threatening problems from primary survey

Secondary Survey

- Done in hospital
- Head to toe, front to back
- examination looking for injuries
- Includes x-rays and blood tests

- Examine all systems
  - good history
  - allergies
  - medications
  - last tetanus
  - last ate
  - events of injury

Stabilization and transport

- Reassess ABC, before moving
- Splint any limb injuries

- Transport to hospital **asap**

Exercise testing and prescription

The purpose of an exercise prescription is to enhance physical fitness, reduce risk factors and ensure safety during exercise. In regard to intensity of exercise consider level of fitness, current medications, risk or cardiovascular or orthopedic injury, individual's preference, and objectives. Can use target heart rate range as guide (Target HR range = [(HR max–HR rest) × 0.5 and 0.85] + HR rest). METS are a useful concept of judging the energy costs of various sports (Table 4.5) for fit athletes. **Note**: METs × 3.5 × bodyweight(kg)/200 = kcal/min

- **Exercise duration**: 20–60min continuous aerobic activity (American College of Sports medicine, ACSM, recommendation)
- **Exercise frequency**: Where functional capacity <3METs then multiple short daily sessions; 3–5 METs use 1–2 sessions/day; >5METs use 3–5 sessions/week.
- **Progression of exercise**: Initial (weeks 1–5) at 60–70% VO_{2max} for 12–20min duration: *Improvement* (weeks 6–27) at 70–80% VO_{2max} for 20–30min duration; and *Maintenance* (after 28 weeks) at 70–85% VO_{2max} for 30–45min.
- **Muscular flexibility guidelines**: *Frequency*: 3 sessions/week; *Intensity*: to mild discomfort; *Duration*: 10–30s each stretch; *Repetitions*: 3–5 each stretch; Type: static.
- **Muscular fitness (resistance training)**. Gain strength with weights near max, gain endurance with greater number of repetitions. Dynamic exercises are better for adults. For a fit adult: 8–10 exercises for major muscle groups, set of 8–12 repetitions and 2 days per week.
- **Supervised** where athlete has >2 CAD risk factors or functional capacity <8METs.

The benefits of regular physical activity are now well established:[1]
- improved cardiorespiratory function (↑max O_2 uptake, myocardial oxygen cost for a given task, ↓HR and BP for a task, ↑exercise threshold for accumulation of lactate, ↑threshold for onset of disease, e.g. angina)
- reduction in CAD risk factors (↓HBP both systolic and diastolic, ↑serum HDL cholesterol, ↓serum triglycerides, ↓body fat, ↓insulin needs with better glucose tolerance)
- decreased mortality and morbidity (primary prevention as lower fitness is associated with ↑CAD, secondary prevention showing ↑longevity and postMI have ↓cardiovascular mortality)
- other (anxiety, ↑well-being, ↑performance at work/recreation/sport)

In general, it is a matter of 'getting more people to do more activity more of the time'. Exercise will also lessen the impact of many chronic diseases (all cause mortality, CAD, HBP, obesity, stroke, cancer colon, Non-insulin diabetes, osteoporosis).[2]

Health screening prior to sport

This important for safe participation in sport, as it:
- Identifies individuals at risk
- Defines a need for supervision of sport
- Clarifies special needs

1 RA Hahn *et al* 1990 *JAMA* 264 2654–9 **2** In WL Kennedy *et al* (ed) *ACSMs guidelines for exercise testing and prescription* 5th edn Chs 1 to 3 1995 p1–48. Williams & Wilkins, Philadelphia

Table 4.5 METS for various sports (metabolic equivalent unit; the amount of energy expended per 1min of rest, and equals the VO_2 at rest, 3–5ml/kg/min)

Sport	Range
Archery	3-4
Backpacking	5-11
Basketball	7-12
Cricket	4-8
Field hockey	8 (mean)
Golf	4-7 (walking)
Running	16.3 (6min/mile)
Skiing	5-8 (downhill)
Soccer	5-12
Tennis	4-9

Data from Table 7-3 p164 In W Larry (ed) 1990 *ACSMs guidelines for exercise testing and prescription* 5th edn. Williams & Wilkins, Phildelphia

It must be cost and time effective (the PAR-Q from the ACSM is reproduced in the Appendix). Risk stratification is possible (into *apparently healthy*—healthy with no more than one coronary risk factor; *increased risk*—possible cardiopulmonary disease or metabolic disease and/or two or more; *known disease*—known cardiac, pulmonary, or metabolic problems).[1] *Cardiac patients* should be further stratified into low-, moderate-, or high-risk groups. Use either the American College of Physicians or the American College of Cardiovascular and Pulmonary Rehabilitation systems (Table 4.6).[2,3]

Pre-test evaluation

08

Performed prior to exercise testing:

- History (standard and include exercise and work history)
- Physical examination (standard)
- Blood tests (cholesterol, fasting glucose, blood chemistry)
- Other (ECG, CXR, PFT, other tests as indicated).

No exercise test when recent ECG change, recent MI, unstable angina, ventricular or atrial arrhythmia, third degree hear block without pacemaker, acute CHF, severe aortic stenosis, dissecting aneurysm, myocarditis, pericarditis, thromphlebitis, thrombi, PE, acute infections, emotional stress

Relative contraindications are BP at rest >200/115,valvular heart disease, electrolyte problems, fixed pacemaker infrequent ventricular ectopic, ventricular aneurysm, uncontrolled metabolic disease, chronic infectious disease, advanced/complicated pregnancy, musculoskeletal disease aggravated by exercise

Physical fitness testing

Wear comfortable clothing, be rested/hydrated and fed beforehand. No coffee, food, alcohol, for 3h prior. *Measure body composition* (hydrostatic weighing, skinfold measures, height, weight, girth). *Measure* VO_{2max} (open circuit spirometry) using maximum-effort (for the fit) and submaximum for most using a cycle ergometer (use the ACSM Health/Fitness Instructor (sm) examination). *Other methods* are the submaximal treadmill tests (Bruce and Balke protocol), 3min step tests (YMCA protocol), and field tests (Cooper 12min test and the 1.5 mile, 2.4km, test for time).

Stop test when angina, drop in systolic BP >20mm or does not rise with exercise, BP rises >260/115, poor perfusion, change heart rhythm, wants to stop, severe fatigue, failure of equipment.

Muscular fitness

Muscular strength (in Newtons) can be measured in static mode (cable tensiometers, handgrip dynamometers) or in dynamic mode (1-RM ≡ the heaviest load that can be lifted once; warm-up permitted, use bench press or military press or for lower limbleg press). Isokinetic testing uses equipment which allows control of the speed of joint rotation (measure torque).

1 CAD risk factors are Age(M > 45, F > 55); Family History (MI or sudden death before 55 of male or 65 for female relative);Cigarette smoker; HBP(> 140/90); ↑chol (> 200 mg/dl); Diabetes mellitus (IDDM > 30 years or NIDDM > 35 years); Sedentary **2** Health and Policy Committee. Am Coll Physicians, Cardiac Rehab Service 1988 *Ann Int Med* **15** 671–3 **3** Am Assoc of Cardiovascular and Pulm Rehab 1994 *Guidelines for cardiac rehab programs* 2nd edn. Human Kinetics, IL

Table 4.6 Risk Stratification for cardiac patients

Low risk

- Uncomplicated MI, CABG, angioplasty, atherectomy
- Functional capacity > or = 8METS 3weeks after event
- No (resting or exercise-induced) ischemia/left ventricular dysfunction (EF >50%)/ complex arrhythmias
- Asymptomatic at rest with exercise tolerance satisfactory for most requirements

Moderate risk

- Functional capacity <METS 3 weeks after event
- Shock or CHF during recent MI (<6 months) or EF <31 to 49%.
- Failure to comply with exercise advice
- Exercise-induced ST-segment depression <1–2mm or reversible ischaemic defects

High risk

- Severely depressed LV function (EF <30%)
- Resting complex ventricular arrhythmias (low grade IV or V) or with exercise
- PVCs with exercise
- Exertional hypotension (↓systolic by >15mm Hg with exercise or failure to rise with exercise)
- Recent MI (<6 months) complicated by serious ventricular arrhythmias/ CHF/shock
- Exercise-induced ST-segment depression >2mm
- Survivor of cardiac arrest

Muscular endurance

The measure of a muscle group to perform repeated contractions over a set time to cause fatigue. Use the 60s sit-up test or the maximum number of push-ups performed without rest. Can also use resistance training and isokinetic equipment (e.g. YMCA bench press test with 30 repetitions/min and 80lb (36kg) barbell for men and 35lb (16kg) for women).

Flexibility (ability to move a joint through ROM)

Measure with goniometer, Leighton flexometer, the shoulder elevation test, ankle flexibility test, trunk flexion (sit-and-reach) test and trunk extension test.[1] Use ACSM fitness book for list of good stretches.

Prescription for cardiac and pulmonary patients

This is beyond the realm of this text, refer to the ACSM's *Guidlelines for exercise testing and prescription* (Williams & Wilkins, PA 1995).

Conditions limiting sports participation

Firstly classify sports into contact v non-contact (see Table 4.7).

Guidelines for particular sports (Table 4.8)

[1] Actual tests described in: *et al* (ed) 1989 *Y's way to physical fitness* 3rd edn. Human Kinetics, Publishers, IL

Table 4.7 Contact versus non-contact

Contact		Non-contact		
Collision	*Limited*	*Strenuous*	*Somewhat Strenuous*	*Non-strenuous*
Boxing	Baseball	Aerobics	Badminton	Archery
Field hockey	Basketball	Crew	Curling	Golf
Football	Cycling	Fencing	Table tennis	Shooting
Ice hockey	Diving	Track and field (discus, shot put)		
Martial arts	Track and field (high jump)	Running on track		
Rodeo	Gymnastics	Swimming		
Soccer	Horseback riding	Tennis		
	Skiing	Weight lifting		
	Softball			
	Squash			

Table 4.8 Medical conditions and sports participation

This table is designed to be understood by medical and nonmedical personnel. In the 'Explanation' section below, 'needs evaluation' means that a physician with appropriate knowledge and experience will need to assess the safety of a given sport for an athlete with the listed medical condition. Unless otherwise noted, this is because of the variability of the severity of the disease or of the risk of injury among the specific sports in Table 1, or both.

Condition	May participate?
Atlantoaxial instability (instability of the joint between cervical vertebrae 1 and 2)	Qualified Yes
Explanation: Athlete needs evaluation to assess risk of spinal cord injury during sports participation.	
Bleeding disorder	Qualified Yes
Explanation: Athlete needs evaluation.	
Cardiovascular diseases	
Carditis (inflammation of the heart)	No
Explanation: Carditis may result in sudden death with exertion.	
Hypertension (high blood pressure)	Qualified Yes
Explanation: Those with significant essential (unexplained) hypertension should avoid weight and power lifting, body building, and strength training. Those with secondary hypertension (hypertension caused by a previously identified disease), or severe essential hypertension, need evaluation. Reference 4 defines significant and severe hypertension.	
Congenital heart disease (structural heart defects present at birth)	Qualified Yes
Explanation: Those with mild forms may participate fully; those with moderate or severe forms, or who have undergone surgery, need evaluation. Reference 3 defines mild, moderate, and severe disease for the common cardiac lesions.	
Dysrhythmia (irregular heart rhythm)	Qualified Yes
Explanation: Athlete needs evaluation because some types require therapy or make certain sports dangerous, or both.[3]	
Mitral valve prolapse (abnormal heart valve)	Qualified Yes
Explanation: Those with symptoms (chest pain, symptoms of possible dysrhythmia) or evidence of mitral regurgitation (leaking) on physical examination need evaluation. All others may participate fully.[3]	
Heart murmur	Qualified Yes
Explanation: If the murmur is innocent (does not indicate heart disease), full participation is permitted. Otherwise the athlete needs evaluation (see congenital heart disease and mitral valve prolapse above).	
Cerebral palsy	Qualified Yes
Explanation: Athlete needs evaluation.	

Condition		May participate
Diabetes mellitus		Yes
Explanation:	All sports can be played with proper attention to diet, hydration, and insulin therapy. Particular attention is needed for activities that last 30 minutes or more.	
Diarrhoea		Qualified No
Explanation:	Unless disease is mild, no participation is permitted, because diarrhoea may increase the risk of dehydration and heat illness. See 'Fever' below.	
Eating disorders		Qualified Yes
Anorexia nervosa		
Bulimia nervosa		
Explanation:	These patients need both medical and psychiatric assessment before participation.	
Eyes		Qualified Yes
Functionally one-eyed athlete		
Loss of an eye		
Detached retina		
Previous eye surgery or serious eye injury		
Explanation:	A functionally one-eyed athlete has a best corrected visual acuity of <20/40 in the worse eye. These athletes would suffer significant disability if the better eye was seriously injured as would those with loss of an eye. Some athletes who have previously undergone eye surgery or had a serious eye injury may have an increased risk of injury because of weakened eye tissue. Availability of eye guards approved by the American Society for Testing Materials (ASTM) and other protective equipment may allow participation in most sports, but this must be judged on an individual basis.[9,10]	
Fever		No
Explanation:	Fever can increase cardiopulmonary effort, reduce maximum exercise capacity, make heat illness more likely, and increase orthostatic hypotension during exercise. Fever may rarely accompany myocarditis or other infections that may make exercise dangerous.	
Heat illness, history of		Qualified Yes
Explanation:	Because of the increased likelihood of recurrence, the athlete needs individual assessment to determine the presence of predisposing conditions and to arrange a prevention strategy.	

Table 4.8

Condition		May participate?
HIV infection		Yes
Explanation:	Because of the apparent minimal risk to others, all sports may be played at that the state of health allows. In all athletes, skin lesions should be properly covered, and athletic personnel should use universal precautions when handling blood or body fluids with visible blood.	
Kidney: absence of one		Qualified Yes
Explanation:	Athlete needs individual assessment for contact/collision and limited contact sports.	
Liver: enlarged		Qualified Yes
Explanation:	If the liver is acutely enlarged, participation should be avoided because of risk of rupture. If the liver is chronically enlarged, individual assessment is needed before collision/contact or limited contact sports are played.	
Malignancy		Qualified Yes
Explanation:	Athlete needs individual assessment.	
Musculoskeletal disorders		Qualified Yes
Explanation:	Athlete needs individual assessment.	
Neurologic		Qualified Yes
History of serious head or spine trauma, severe or repeated concussions or craniotomy.		
Explanation:	Athlete needs individual assessment for collision/contact or limited contact sports, and also for noncontact sports if there are deficits in judgment or cognition. Recent research supports a conservative approach to management of concussion.	
Convulsive disorder, well controlled		Yes
Explanation:	Risk of convulsion during participation is minimal.	
Convulsive disorder, poorly controlled		Qualified Yes
Explanation:	Athlete needs individual assessment for collision/contact or limited contact sports. Avoid the following noncontact sports: archery, riflery, swimming, weight or power lifting, strength training, or sports involving heights. In these sports, occurrence of a convulsion may be a risk to self or others.	
Obesity		Qualified Yes
Explanation:	Because of the risk of heat illness, obese persons need careful acclimatization and hydration.	

Organ transplant recipient
Explanation: Athlete needs individual assessment.

Ovary: absence of one
Explanation: Risk of severe injury to the remaining ovary is minimal

Respiratory
Pulmonary compromise including cystic fibrosis
Explanation: Athlete needs individual assessment, but generally all sports may be played if oxygenation remains satisfactory during a graded exercise test. Patients with cystic fibrosis need acclimatization and good hydration to reduce the risk of heat illness.

Asthma
Explanation: With proper medication and education, only athletes with the most severe asthma will have to modify their participation.

Acute upper respiratory infection
Explanation: Upper respiratory obstruction may affect pulmonary function. Athlete needs individual assessment for all but mild disease. See 'Fever' above.

Sickle cell disease
Explanation: Athlete needs individual assessment. In general, if status of the illness permits, all but high exertion, collision/contact sports may be played. Overheating, dehydration, and chilling must be avoided.

Sickle cell trait
Explanation: It is unlikely that individuals with sickle cell trait (AS) have an increased risk of sudden death or other medical problems during athletic participation except under the most extreme conditions of heat, humidity, and possibly increased altitude. These individuals, like all athletes, should be carefully conditioned, acclimatized, and hydrated to reduce any possible risk.

Skin: boils, herpes simplex, impetigo, scabies, molluscum contagiosum
Explanation: While the patient is contagious, participation in gymnastics with mats, martial arts, wrestling, or other collision/contact or limited contact sports is not allowed. Herpes simplex virus probably is not transmitted via mats.

Spleen, enlarged
Explanation: Patients with acutely enlarged spleens should avoid all sports because of risk of rupture. Those with chronically enlarged spleens need individual assessment before playing collision/contact or limited contact sports.

Testicle: absent or undescended
Explanation: Certain sports may require a protective cup.

	Qualified Yes
	Yes
	Qualified Yes
	Yes
	Qualified Yes
	Qualified Yes
	Yes
	Qualified Yes
	Qualified Yes
	Yes

115

116

Physical Activity Readiness
Questionnaire - PAR-Q
(revised 1994)

PAR - Q & YOU

(A Questionnaire for people Aged 15 to 69)

Regular physical activity is fun and healthy, and increasingly more people are starting to become more active every day. Being more active is very safe for most people. However, some people should check with their doctor before they start becoming much more physically active.

If you are planning to become much more physically active than you are now, start by answering the seven questions in the box below. If you are between the ages of 15 and 69, the PAR-Q will tell you if you should check with your doctor before you start. If you are over 69 years of age, and you are not used to being very active, check with your doctor.

Common sense is your best guide when you answer these questions. Please read the questions carefully and answer each one honestly: check YES or NO.

YES	NO		
☐	☐	1.	Has your doctor ever said that you have a heart condition *and* that you should only do physical activity recommended by a doctor?
☐	☐	2.	Do you feel pain in your chest when you do physical activity?
☐	☐	3.	In the past month, have you had chest pain when you are not doing physical activity?
☐	☐	4.	Do you lose your balance because of dizziness or do you ever lose consciousness?
☐	☐	5.	Do you have a bone or joint problem that could be made worse by a change in your physical activity?
☐	☐	6.	Is you doctor currently prescribing drugs (for example, water pills) for your blood pressure or heart condition?
☐	☐	7.	Do you know of *any other reason* why you should not do physical activity?

Continued on Next Page

Reprinted with permission from Reference 7.

YES to one or more questions

If you answered

Talk with your doctor by phone or in person BEFORE you start becoming much more physically active or BEFORE you have a fitness appraisal. Tell your doctor about the PAR-Q and which questions you answered YES.

- You may be able to do any activity you want—as long as you start slowly and build up gradually. Or, you may need to restrict your activities to those which are safe for you. Talk with your doctor about the kinds of activities you wish to participate in and follow his/her advice.
- Find out which community programs are safe and helpful for you.

DELAY BECOMING MUCH MORE ACTIVE:

- if you are not feeling well because of a temporary illness such as a cold or fever—wait until you feel better; or
- if you are or may be pregnant—talk to your doctor before you start becoming more active.

NO to all questions

If you answered NO honestly to all PAR-Q questions, you can be reasonably sure that you can:

- start becoming much more physically active—begin slowly and build up gradually. This is the safest and easiest way to go.
- take part in a fitness appraisal—this is an excellent way to determine your basic fitness so that you can plan the best way for you to live actively.

You are encouraged to copy the PAR-Q but only if you use the entire form

Informed Use of the PAR-Q: The Canadian Society for Exercise Physiology, Health Canada, and their agents assume no liability for persons who undertake physical activity, and if in doubt after completing this questionnaire, consult your doctor prior to physical activity.

Note: If the PAR-Q is being given to a person before he or she participates in a physical activity program or a fitness appraisal, this section may be used for legal or administrative purposes.

I have read, understood and completed this questionnaire. Any questions I had were answered to my full satisfaction.

NAME _____

SIGNATURE _____ DATE _____

SIGNATURE OF PARENT _____ WITNESS _____
or GUARDIAN (for participants under the age of majority)

©*Canadian Society for Exercise Physiology* *Supported by:* Health Canada Santé Canada
Société canadienne de physiologie de l'exercice

Continued

Section III Medical problems in sport

Donald John Chisholm

Diabetes mellitus

When considering sport and diabetes it is important to keep in mind that there are different types of diabetes that represent different disease procesIses and often require different approaches to therapy (**1**).

Type 1 diabetes (insulin dependent, juvenile onset) usually occurs in childhood or young adult life, requires insulin injections throughout life and is associated, within a few years of onset, with a total lack of endogenous insulin production. People with this type of diabetes are prone to substantial blood glucose fluctuations and considerable attention is needed to diet, insulin doses, and exercise to maintain satisfactory blood glucose control.

Type II diabetes (non-insulin dependent, maturity onset) accounts for 85–90% of diabetes in the community in Australia and most developed countries—and the percentage is even higher in many developing countries. It usually has its onset in middle aged or older people; it can generally be treated with diet and exercise with or without oral hypoglycemic agents. However, with time insulin therapy is sometimes necessary, but even when the patient requires insulin therapy he/she will still have some endogenous insulin and is not prone to the degree of blood glucose fluctuation that occurs in type I, nor to ketoacidosis.

Other types of diabetes. About 2–3% of people with diabetes have a specific cause such as Cushing's syndrome, steroid therapy, hemochromatosis, pancreatitis, etc. Most people with these unusual causes of diabetes behave similarly to people with type II diabetes.

Benefits of sport or exercise

- *Increased insulin sensitivity* is a well-demonstrated response to regular physical activity in either non-diabetic or diabetic people (**2–4**). As type II diabetes is in large part due to insulin resistance, exercise has a specific therapeutic benefit in combating insulin resistance and is therefore a recommended component of therapy. It is also proven to be useful in prevention of type II diabetes. Enhanced insulin sensitivity with exercise appears to involve increased muscle capillarity, an increase in oxidative enzymes, increased production of glucose transporter proteins (GLUT4), and a reduction in abdominal (visceral) fat mass (**3,5**). The GLUT4 glucose transporter is responsible for insulin induced glucose transport into muscle as insulin translocates this protein from the cell cytoplasm to the cell wall, thus generating increased glucose transport. Visceral fat is highly correlated with, and is probably a major causative factor in, insulin resistance (**6**)—apparently by supplying fatty acids through the portal vein to the liver, and also increasing general systemic supply of fatty acids to muscle. Increased fatty acid supply to the liver opposes insulin action at the liver and increases hepatic glucose output. Increased fatty acid availability in muscle inhibits both glycolysis and glycogen synthesis.
- Regular physical activity also improves insulin sensitivity in type I diabetes and often leads to a reduced insulin dose requirement—but does not usually result in better blood glucose control.
- *A reduction in cardiovascular risk* appears to result from regular

exercise in the non-diabetic population. People with diabetes have an approximately 3 times increased risk of coronary artery disease and 10 times increased risk of peripheral vascular disease. There is a strong belief that regular physical activity will reduce risk of cardiovascular disease to a similar degree in the diabetic population as in non-diabetic subjects (7). However, it must be stated that there has been no adequate controlled trial or substantial epidemiological study to prove this. On the other hand the improvement in cardiovascular risk factors seen in non-diabetes with regular exercise seems in general to hold true for people with diabetes (i.e. increase in HDL cholesterol, reduction of triglycerides, lowered blood pressure, and reduced platelet aggregability).

- *Weight reduction* is benefited by exercise (**8**), and there is specific loss of central abdominal fat. Many subjects with type II diabetes are overweight and have excess abdominal fat; regular physical activity may be very helpful in their management.
- *The improvement in general well-being and psychological parameters* can be helpful in the diabetic as in the non-diabetic population (**9**),

Problems and risks of sporting activity in the diabetic population

People with diabetes are prone to all the usual risks of sporting activity which apply to the general population—but are probably somewhat more liable to problems such as hyperthermia, hypothermia, dehydration, etc. Such problems represent a greater upset, and carry increased risk for the diabetic as compared to the non-diabetic athlete. However, the particular risks which are most important in people with diabetes undertaking sporting activity—and which must be the subject of education and preventative measures are:

- *Hypoglycemia.* This is a major potential problem in people with type I diabetes (**10**) but may also occur in people with type II diabetes who are on insulin therapy or sulphonylureas.
- *Hyperglycemia or ketoacidosis* may occur if a person with type I diabetes has an intercurrent illness at the time they undertake exercise or if they make too great a reduction in their insulin doses in preparation for exercise. It should be noted that when type I diabetic subjects exercise at a time when they are hyperglycemic and insulin-deficient, there is an additional rise in blood glucose and ketone levels with exercise (**10**).
- *Foot lesions*—especially in older people or those who have neuropathy or peripheral vascular disease (**11**).

Approach to metabolic control in athletes with diabetes

1 *Finger prick blood glucose monitoring.* Self-blood glucose monitoring is an invaluable tool in the hands of a person with diabetes and their doctor. A finger prick blood glucose should be done at any time when there is a question of hypo- or hyperglycemia, and should be used frequently when undertaking new or different sporting activities, or altering the time schedule of activities. In general, it is likely that a similar blood glucose response will occur to the same physical activity done at the same time on different days (**12**), so regular blood glucose monitoring when the person commences a new activity can be used to predict the metabolic response on future occasions.

2 *Diet* (**10**). For relatively short-term physical activity (less than an hour) the major issue is adjustment of carbohydrate intake. The general advice is to take about 15g of carbohydrate (CHO) for each 20min of moderately vigorous activity (50–70% VO_{2max}). This may be taken as complex CHO (e.g. bread, fruit) about 30min before the activity or as simple sugar (e.g. lemonade, cola) immediately before. This amount of CHO will generally protect people with diabetes from hypoglycemia but the required amount of CHO is quite variable and many people will become moderately hyperglycemic with the recommended amounts of CHO (**13**). Therefore, blood sugar levels should be checked at the end of the activity. If it is high, the amount of CHO could be reduced, say by 30%, on the next occasion. *For physical activity that is very strenuous or lasts more than an hour, adjustment of insulin dose becomes critical.*

3 *Insulin doses.* Most people with type I diabetes are taking an insulin regimen of (a) 3 doses of quick acting insulin with meals and a night time dose of intermediate acting insulin or (b) a morning and evening dose of quick acting insulin plus intermediate acting insulin.

- For exercise which is around an hour or longer it is usually appropriate to alter the insulin dose operating at that time (**10**). For 2h physical activity at say 60–70% VO_{2max} a reduction of 20–30% in the insulin dose acting at that time might be appropriate. Once again, blood glucose monitoring should be undertaken with modification of the insulin dose adjustment on future occasions according to the blood glucose response. As an example, if the physical activity was occurring in the late morning it would be appropriate to reduce the pre-breakfast quick acting insulin. If the activity was occurring in mid or late afternoon it would be appropriate to reduce the lunchtime quick acting insulin, for regimen (a) above, or the morning intermediate acting insulin, for regimen (b) above.

- *Note there are now two types of quick acting insulin.* Conventional quick action insulin (neutral or regular insulin) has an onset of acting at about 30min, a peak at 2–3h and lasts about 7h. A new genetically engineered insulin (Lispro, Humalog) has 2 amino acids in the B chain reversed, so it has a lesser tendency to form dimers or hexamers, with the result that it enters the bloodstream more rapidly and has a much quicker onset of action (about 10min) peak (about 1h) and an earlier decline in activity. This insulin can be injected just before eating (in comparison to neutral insulin which should be taken 30–40min before a meal), controls the rise in blood sugar more satisfactorily after feeding, and has a somewhat reduced tendency to cause hypoglycemia (**14**).

- Subjects who are taking ordinary neutral or regular insulin are less liable to exercise-induced hypoglycemia within 2h of taking a meal, but are more at risk 3–5h after a meal when the insulin is still working strongly but the effect of the meal has waned. People on Lispro insulin may be quite liable to hypoglycemia when exercise is undertaken within 2.5h of the injection as the activity of the insulin is vigorous in that timeframe. However, more than 3h after a meal they would be less at risk of hypoglycemia than people who are taking conventional quick acting insulin.

4 *Injection site.* Insulin absorption occurs more rapidly from an exercising limb and increases the likelihood of hypoglycemia (**15**) so an insulin injection should not be given into a limb that will be involved in exercise. In general the abdominal subcutaneous area provides the most consistent absorption and is not greatly influenced by exercise.

5 *Recognition and treatment of hypoglycemia.* People with diabetes may have trouble recognizing that they are hypoglycemic during strenuous activity as sweating, tremulousness, and other indicators of increased sympathetic activity may be related to the exercise itself or to hypoglycemia. Therefore, it is important that the athlete and their team-mates or trainer maintain a high index of suspicion and do a blood glucose level or give glucose at the earliest indication. The usual amount of sugar given for hypoglycemia (about 15gm, e.g. 7–10 jelly beans or 2–3 teaspoons of sugar) may be inadequate when glucose utilization is greatly increased by exercise and 2–3 times this amount is appropriate. If a coma should occur one cannot give sugar orally because of the possibility of inhalation. Intravenous (IV) glucose should be given as soon as possible. If an injection of glucagon is available and it is not possible to give IV glucose immediately, glucagon can be given subcutaneously or intramuscularly—but if prolonged exercise has depleted the hepatic store of glycogen the response to glucagon injection may not be adequate to restore or maintain the blood glucose level.

6 *Late hypoglycemia after exercise.* This is an extremely important issue (**16**). A vigorous bout of physical activity improves insulin sensitivity for a period of up to 15h. So, apart from the risk of hypoglycemia at the time of exercise, a person with diabetes who exercises vigorously can be more responsive to their usual insulin dose for 15h or so after exercise and be liable to troublesome hypoglycemia during that time. Therefore, it may be necessary to reduce the insulin doses operating many hours after the physical activity to avoid this problem. Many parents of diabetic children have returned home happy after a sporting event, having avoided hypo- or hyperglycemia during the day, but are chagrined when their child has a severe hypoglycemic reaction at 2am.

Very prolonged vigorous physical activity

People with type I diabetes undertaking such endurance events as marathons, triathlons, etc. may need a dramatic reduction of their insulin dose on the day they are competing—perhaps down to 15–25% or less of their usual dose (**17,10**). Fortunately, these people undertake prolonged training beforehand; with careful monitoring of their blood glucose response during training sessions it is usually possible to predict an appropriate dose of insulin for the event.

Oral hypoglycemic agents

As indicated above, people with type II diabetes generally have less blood glucose fluctuation with physical activity than people with type I diabetes. However, people with type II diabetes who are taking insulin or sulfonylurea tablets can become hypoglycemic (this should not occur with metformin therapy alone). Thus people on sulfonylurea therapy may need supplementary CHO, or a reduction of their dose of sulfonylurea on the day of exercise (**18**).

Diabetes mellitus (cont)

Responsibility of coaches, trainers, supervisors

It is most important that people who are training or supervising athletes with type I diabetes understand the need for the athlete to have access to food or sugary drinks—and they should be aware of the possibility of a hypoglycemic reaction, and the need to give sugar if the athlete shows any sign of mental confusion.

Sporting activities that may be dangerous (9)

There are a number of sports which may pose a substantial risk to the person themselves or others if mental confusion should occur due to hypoglycemia. Such activities might include racing cars, scuba diving, surfing in remote areas, mountain climbing, hang gliding, etc. Depending on the circumstances, it may be too dangerous for someone with type I diabetes to undertake such sporting activities. In other cases the risk may be acceptable if the diabetic person is accompanied by a team-mate who has a good understanding of his/her diabetic state and appropriate measures to deal with hypoglycemia.

Cardiovascular risk

Because of the threefold increase in cardiovascular (CV) risk in people with both types of diabetes, some experts recommend a CV stress test in any person with diabetes over the age of 35 if they are planning strenuous sporting activity. Because of expense and the relatively poor predictive index of exercise stress tests in people without chest pain, it may be reasonable not to undertake a stress test in people with diabetes if they are planning low level to moderate activity and can work into it gradually, provided one approaches the person as though they had known coronary artery disease, and they are carefully instructed to report immediately if they experience chest pain or undue dyspnea.

Foot care

One of the greatest dangers for people in middle age or older with diabetes is damage to or ulceration of the feet. This is of particular concern if the person has peripheral neuropathy or peripheral vascular disease (10)—but one must always remember that a diabetic subject without complications may get an infection due to a blistering of the feet. A diabetic patient with good blood glucose control is not at increased risk of infection; however, if an infection occurs the inflammatory process creates insulin resistance and results in hyperglycemia. High blood sugars, by disturbing neutrophil function and complement activity, reduce the immune response to infection and a severe or persistent infection may result. Therefore, in any person with diabetes, but especially older people, one must give careful attention to the feet and make sure that footwear is optimal for the activity to be taken. The help of a podiatrist may be invaluable.

References

(1) CR Kahn 1985 Pathophysiology of diabetes mellitus: An overview. In A Marble *et al* (ed) *Joslin's diabetes mellitus* 43–50. Lea & Febiger, Philadelphia

(2) C Bogardus *et al* 1984 Effects of physical training and diet therapy on carbohydrate metabolism in patients with glucose intolerance and non-insulin-dependent diabetes mellitus. *Diabetes* **33** 311–18.

(3) HB Simon 1984 Sports medicine. In E Rubenstein, D Federman (ed) *Current topics in medicine* 1–26. Scientific American Medicine, New York

(4) JL Ivy 1995 Exercise physiology and adaptations to training In N Ruderman, J Devlin (ed) *The health professional guide to diabetes and exercise* p7–26 American Diabetes Association, Virginia

(5) A Mourier *et al* 1997 Mobilization of visceral adipose tissue related to the improvement in insulin sensitivity in response to physical training in NIDDM. *Diabetes Care* **20** 385–91

(6) DG Carey *et al* 1996 Abdominal fat and insulin resistance in normal and overweight women. Direct measurements reveal a strong relationship in subjects at both low and high risk of NIDDM. *Diabetes* **45** 633–8

(7) JE Manson, A Spelsberg 1995 Reduction in risk of coronary heart disease and diabetes In N Ruderman, J Devlin (ed) *The health professional guide to diabetes and exercise* p7–26. American Diabetes Association, Virginia

(8) R Wing 1995 Exercise and weight control In N Ruderman, J Devlin (ed) *The health professional guide to diabetes and exercise* p7–26. American Diabetes Association, Virginia

(9) ST Cohen, AM Jacobson 1995 Psychological benefits of exercise In N Ruderman, J Devlin (ed) *The health professional guide to diabetes and exercise* p7–26. American Diabetes Association, Virginia

(10) K-L Choi, DJ Chisholm 1997 Exercise and insulin-dependent diabetes mellitus (IDDM): benefits and pitfalls. *Aust NZ J Med* **26** 827–33

(11) ME Levin 1995 The diabetic foot In N Ruderman, J Devlin (ed) *The health professional guide to diabetes and exercise* p7–26. American Diabetes Association, Virginia

(12) MY McNiven-Temple *et al* 1995 The reliability and repeatability of the blood glucose response to prolonged exercise in adolescent boys with IDDM. *Diabetes Care* **18** 326–32

(13) K Soo *et al* 1996 Glycemic responses to exercise in IDDM after simple and complex carbohydrate supplementation. *Diabetes Care* **19** 575–9

(14) JH Anderson Jr *et al* 1997 Reduction of postprandial hyperglycemia and frequency of hypoglycemia in IDDM patients on insulin-analog treatment. *Diabetes* **40** 265–70

(15) VA Koivisto, P Felig 1978 Effects of leg exercise on insulin absorption in diabetic patients. *N Engl J Med* **298** 79–83

(16) MJ MacDonald 1987 Post-exercise late-onset hypoglycaemia in insulin-dependent diabetic patients. *Diabetes Care* **10** 584–8

(17) AE Meinders *et al* 1988 Metabolic and hormonal changes in IDDM during a long-distance run. *Diabetes Care* **11** 1–7

(18) SH Schneider, NB Ruderman 1990 (Technical Review) Exercise and NIDDM. *Diabetes Care* **13** 785–9

Respiratory problems

Upper respiratory tract infections (URTI)

Adenoviruses and rhinoviruses primarily cause these infections.
Symptoms: a range of self-limiting symptoms can occur including
pyrexia, pharyngitis, cough, nasal congestion, and myalgias. **Treatment**: supportive therapy with optimal fluid management and rest.
Symptomatic therapy with nasal decongestants, cough suppressants,
and antipyretic agents may be used. Care must be taken to not
prescribe banned medications to athletes involved in competitive
events. **Impact on athletic performance**: providing that the athletes
do not suffer from pyrexia ($<38\,°C$) or myalgia, training can be
continued. However, caution must be exercised especially with respect
to fluid management and overexertion. Reconditioning may take a
few weeks. The depression in peak performance has been postulated
to be due to epithelial damage in the lungs due to viral infection.
Prevention of URTI: regular handwashing may prevent transmission
among athletes. There is little to no evidence to support prophylactic
treatment with megadoses of Vitamin C, or antihistamines.

Note: 'walking pneumonia' which is a lung infection caused by
Mycoplasma pneumonia with a 10–14 day incubation period and mild
symptoms (similar to influenza). It is the most common lung pathogen in the 5–35-year age group and is got from close contact.
Recovery is within 1–2 weeks and the antibiotic is erythromycin.[1]

Infectious mononucleosis

Is caused by the Epstein–Barr virus. **Presenting symptoms and signs**:
the illness can present acutely with a prodromal illness lasting for 3–5
days. This prodrome consists of myalgia, headaches, appetite loss,
malaise, and fatigue. The classic symptoms of the illness include a
sore throat with tonsillar enlargement. There is occasionally a
tonsillar exudate. A generalized lymphadenopathy can occur with
prominent anterior and posterior cervical nodes. *Abdominal signs* can
include splenomegaly and hepatomegaly. In addition a characteristic
morbilliform rash can occur. **Investigations**: diagnosis can be made
via serological tests (heterophil antibody absorption test). **Treatment**:
supportive and symptomatic therapy is indicated.

Complications:

- *Airway obstruction* due to massive tonsillar enlargement. Parenteral
  glucocorticoids can be used to treat this. However, nasotracheal
  intubation and emergency tracheostomy may be required.
- *Rupture of the spleen can occur*. This can occur spontaneously or
  due to an increase in intraabdominal pressure. Collisions during
  contact sports can also bring about rupture of the spleen. Splenic
  rupture requires surgical correction (splenectomy or splenorraphy).
- *Neurological complications include* cranial nerve palsies and encephalitis. A large proportion of people with neurological complications recover spontaneously
- *Hepatitis can occur*. Up to 90% of patients have elevated transaminases. However spontaneous recovery is usual.
- *Cardiac abnormalities* can occur including pericarditis and myocarditis.

1 R Berkow, A Fletcher (ed) 1987 *Merck manual* 15th edn. Merck & Co, Rahway NJ

Exercise-induced asthma

Is a condition commonly seen in the community. This condition is seen in 15% of the community and up to 90% of asthmatic patients. It also appears to occur more frequently in obese people. There is no allergen involved. **Pathophysiology**: the bronchospasm induced by exercise appears to be related to the inhalation of cool dry air. This airway cooling, which occurs during exercise due to the increased minute ventilation, is thought to cause a hyperosmolality in the epithelial cells. This in turn causes the release of histamine and leukotrienes, which cause the bronchospasm. There is also a bronchial vascular bed vasodilatation and sympathetic mediation via the vagus nerve, which contributes to the bronchospasm. Thus, this condition is classically seen when exercise is undertaken in cool dry climates. There is often a family history of asthma or atopy. Swimming, which involves the inhalation of moist warm air, rarely causes this condition. Exercise-induced asthma tends to be associated with intense exercise as opposed to continuous aerobic exercise.

Other stimuli that contribute to exercise induced asthma:
- Emotional stress
- Overtraining
- Pollutants
- Fatigue

Presenting symptoms: characteristic features of exercise-induced asthma are cough, dyspnea, wheezing, and chest tightness. Symptoms tend to occur 15min after exercise. A refractory period (up to 1 hour in duration) can follow during which bronchoconstriction cannot be induced. **Investigations**: measurement of the peak expiratory flow rate (PEFR) before and after 8min of running at the maximum speed the athlete is capable of. This can be measured outdoors or on a treadmill. Post-exercise levels of PEFR that is 10% or more lower than the pre-exercise levels is indicative of exercise-induced asthma. Hyperventilation challenge tests can also be used. This involves the inspiration of large amounts of dry air. The athlete's forced expiratory volume in one second (FEV1) is measured and the response to bronchodilator is recorded. If there is a negative result on this test, exercise induced asthma would be unlikely. **Treatment**: the symptoms described are generally responsive to inhaled β-agonists (salbutamol), which can be used shortly before exercise along with sodium cromoglycate prior to exercise. Sodium cromoglycate can also be used prophylactically if symptoms continue to persist. Other medications that can be used are listed in Table 4.9. Use of a facemask which covers both the mouth and the face may be considered when exercising in cold outdoor settings.

Impact of exercise-induced asthma on the athlete: competition in environments, which might provoke an attack of exercise, induced asthma will therefore involve planning. Running is a greater inducer of exercise-induced asthma compared to cycling, which in turn is worse than swimming. Deep water diving should be avoided as failure to surface quickly during an asthma attack may result in severe hypoxia. Infections can bring about or worsen asthma attacks. Thus, expedient treatment of infections is mandatory. For international competition, caution must be taken when prescribing medications and it must be remembered that most β agonists and decongestants are classified as banned substances. Medications that can be used are listed in Table 4.10. Exercise-induced asthma is not a condition that could prevent competitive sports.

Exercise-induced anaphylaxis

First described in 1979. The **clinical features** are skin warmth, flushing, and pruritis, urticaria, angioedema, laryngeal edema, bronchospasm, and hypotension. So far, no deaths associated with exercise-induced anaphylaxis have been recorded. *There is a strong correlation with atopy*. It classically occurs with exercise of moderate intensity. Females are affected more than males (2 : 1).There are family clusters. Jogging is most commonly associated anaphylaxis. A number of coprecipitating factors have been identified (exercise with heat, cold, humidity, following certain foods, alcohol, and medications). **Treatment of the acute episode** is as for anaphylaxis of other origins. Airway maintenance, circulatory support, and use adrenaline. Prevent by avoiding known coprecipitating factors or vigorous exercise if symptoms warrant. Prophylactic non-sedating antihistamines has been successful. Cromolyn has also been used prior to exercise.

Note: distinguish cholinergic urticaria (develop hives, small punctate lesions 2–4mm, from the heat of exercise and rarely go into shock, may need antihistamines) and exercise-induced urticaria (large skin lesions,1–2.5cm, which may progress to angioedema and anaphylaxis, may well need adrenaline).

Table 4.9 Other medications
used in exercise-induced asthma

- Theophylline
- Antihistamines
- Inhaled corticosteroids
- Calcium channel blockers
- Nedocromil

Table 4.10 International Olympic
Committee approved antiasthmatic
medications

- Oral theophylline
- Inhaled cromolyn
- Inhaled and oral albuterol
- Inhaled and oral terbutaline
- Inhaled and oral corticosteroids

Gastrointestinal problems

Complaints are not uncommon in endurance events. Those seen are: nausea, vomiting, diarrhoea, cramps, and gastrointestinal (GI) bleeding. It is necessary to understand the redistribution of blood flow in exercise. Esophageal contractions and lower esophageal sphincter pressure both decrease with exercise. Women and inexperienced athletes are more commonly affected.

Splanchnic blood flow in exercise

With exercise, blood is shunted from the splanchnic circulation to the working muscles. The extent of this depends on the intensity and duration of exertion (in strenuous exercise up to 80% reduction of flow to the GI system). The increase in the oxygen extraction by the GI organs does not compensate for this marked reduction in blood flow. *Dehydration* may further reduce splanchnic blood flow. Gut ischemia probably produces the GI symptoms associated with endurance exercise. *Factors that contribute to the high incidence of GT symptoms* in endurance athletes are use of NSAIDS, slow rate of gastric emptying with moderate/ severe exercise, diet (high in fiber), and pre-competition anxiety.

Nausea and vomiting with exercise is due to gut ischemia, gastric erosions (from NSAIDS), or poor gastric emptying from inappropriate pre-event meal (high proportions of fat or protein in a meal prior to exercise will reduce the rate of gastric emptying and so will high concentration carbohydrate drinks during exercise). Treatment is modify diet, avoid dehydration, use antacids or H_2 antagonists; an endoscopic examination may be necessary.

Abdominal cramps and diarrhoea are common. Treatment is good hydration, reduce pre-exercise fiber intake and deal with pre-competition nerves and endoscopy. Athletes may be affected by the GI diseases of the sedentary population (inflammatory bowel disease, infections, and bowel tumors, although regular exercise is associated with a lower incidence of bowel cancer).

Gastrointestinal bleeding

GI bleeding (often occult) is common with events such as an ironman triathlon (up to 85% such athletes have fecal blood loss). The site of blood loss is probably the upper GI tract (stomach) and the cause, gut ischemia and gastric erosions (from use of aspirin/NSAIDS). Possibly the mechanical effect of running on hard surfaces may contribute to gastric blood loss. Treatment is to withdraw NSAIDs and then conduct endoscopic evaluation. It is important to maintain/correct fluid status problems. *Consider the prophylactic use* of cimetidine or misoprostol in ultramarathoners.

Cardiac conditions

Cardiac symptoms vary according to the age of the athlete. **Symptoms and signs** of ischemic heart disease (chest pain and dyspnea) are not uncommon and need to be thoroughly investigated in the over-35 age group. Younger athletes may also present with cardiac symptoms (in under 35 years, palpitations, dizziness, syncope). May be benign and insignificant or the only warning sign of severe congenital cardiac defect. Sudden cardiac death (SCD) does occur during sport. **Investigate thoroughly**.

Palpitations

Are relatively frequent in athletes (resting ECGs commonly show frequent ectopic beats). However, these *ectopic beats should become less frequent* with exercise. Otherwise, investigate with an ECG, an exercise stress test or a 24h Holter monitor (if necessary to capture the rhythm). **Treatment** depends on the nature of the arrhythmia, the frequency of symptoms, and the underlying heart disease.

Dizziness and syncope

Dizziness after exercise is often seen (especially if the athlete suddenly stops when exercising upright; blood pools in the lower limbs with ↓CO causing dizziness or syncope especially in hot weather where maximal skin vasodilatation). Therefore, runners and cyclists should slowly jog or pedal after the event to avoid ↓VR.

Note: dizziness or syncope during heavy exercise is a serious symptom. Syncope (first exclude dehydration) during exercise should be thoroughly investigated with a full cardiac work-up— ECG, CXR, and echocardiography to exclude congenital cardiac defects, such as hypertrophic cardiomyopathy, HCM (the most common cause of sudden cardiac death during exercise of those under 30 years). Dizziness or syncope during exercise in the older age group maybe an arrhythmia (2nd IHD). Requires a thorough cardiac work-up.

The 'athlete's heart'

On an ECG, differentiate pathological changes from the typical ECG changes of the athlete's heart (the normal physiological adaptation to prolonged and intense physical training). These changes in cardiac dimensions depend on the type of training. Resistance athletes, weight lifters, show an increase in ventricular wall thickness from pressure overload (concentric enlargement). Endurance athletes have an increase in heart volume from volume overload (eccentric enlargement). Enlargement occurs by hypertrophy rather than hyperplasia with no (pathological) fibrosis.

ECG changes are:
- voltage criteria for LVH (and/or RVH)
- sinus (or junctional) bradycardia
- third or fourth heart sounds (gallop rhythm)
- soft ejection systolic murmur (from ↑SV; also seen in 40% young male athletes)
- frequent premature ventricular contractions at rest
- prolonged PR interval (1st and 2nd degree heart block are common in athletes at rest). This should shorten with exercise.
- wandering atrial pacemaker
- non-specific ST segment and T wave changes (seen with isometric/resistance exercises whereas endurance exercise produces voltage changes)

These *changes revert when exercise ceases* (initially the bradycardia followed by ECG changes). Extent of changes depend upon body type (heredity) and exercise intensity. The *echocardiogram* of highly trained athletes will show concentric hypertrophy with symmetrical thickening of both septa and posterior ventricular wall (but no interventricular outflow tract gradients). The echo is useful to differentiate from hypertrophic cardiomyopathy. *Other changes* are ↑SV (especially in endurance athletes, but unchanged ejection fracture, from ↑VO_{2max}),unaltered coronary resistance, and blood flow.

Note: detailed recommendations for athletic participation for athletes with cardiovascular disease(congenital/valvular/myopericardial/coronary heart disease, HBP, and arrhythmias) have been provided by the 26th Bethesda Conference.[1]

Sudden cardiac death

Causes

Sudden cardiac death (SCD) during (or within 1 hour of completion of) sport is rare. The estimated risk of death from exercise for apparently healthy adults is 1 per 187,500 person-hours and the death rate for male joggers is 1 per 396,000 man-hours of jogging (the incidence of cardiac arrest whilst jogging is 1 episode per year for every 18,000 healthy men).[2,3] Although it is 4–56 times the risk at rest, it is much lower for the regular exerciser.[4]

The cause is according to age. In the >35 years, it is CAD (in about 75% of cases; followed by conduction abnormalities, HCM and anomalous coronary arteries. For the <35 years it is HCM (up to 48%), LVH, anomalous coronary arteries (such as of the left coronary artery from the right sinus of Valsalva), aplastic coronary arteries, Marfan's syndrome, and conduction abnormalities (Wolff–Parkinson–White syndrome, prolonged Q-T syndrome, bradycardias). Mitral valve prolapse is no longer thought to be a cause of SCD. SCD is 14 times less common in female athletes.

Hypertrophic cardiomyopathy

A congenital condition in which there is asymmetric hypertrophy of the left ventricle and septum (>15mm). For some with HCM there is left ventricular outflow obstruction. However, the usual cause of death is usually ventricular arrhythmias. **Symptoms** include dyspnea, chest pain, palpitations, and exertional syncope. Check for a family history of sudden death with exertion (prior to 50 years). Physical examination may reveal a systolic murmur, louder with standing, squatting or a Valsalva maneuver, in those with outflow obstruction. The ECG is often non-specific, indistinguishable from that of the athlete's heart (however, a normal ECG is solid evidence against HCM).

1 JH Mitchell *et al* 1994 26th Bethesda Conference: Recommendations for determining eligibility for competition in athletes with cardiovascular abnormalities *Med Sci Sports Exerc* **26** S223-83 2 LW Gibbons *et al* 1989 *Am Heart J* **98** 572–9 3 PD Thompson *et al* 1982 *JAMA* **247** 2535-8 4 SP Van Camp 1992 *Clin Sports Med* **11** 273–89

Diagnosis. Only one-quarter of cases are diagnosed on physical examination, ECG, and CXR. Diagnosis is made with echocardiography (thickening of the septum >15 mm; the septum often >1.3 times the thickness of the free left ventricular wall). Where outflow obstruction, the echocardiogram will show systolic anterior motion of the mitral valve. **Treatment.** All moderate or vigorous exercise should be avoided in HCM. Beta-blockers and calcium antagonists may relieve chest pain and palpitations (?reduce the incidence of sudden death).

Critical risk factors are:

- Family history (SCD prior to 50 years)
- Sedentary lifestyle
- Diabetes mellitus
- HBP (systolic >160, diastolic >90)
- Lipid disorders
- Cigarette smoker

Exercise tolerance tests are useful for the symptomatic patient.

Marfan's syndrome

An autosomal dominant condition, is a possible cause of SCD <35 years (from aortic rupture/dissection caused by dilated aortic root, secondary to cystic medial necrosis). Check for Marfanoid features (long fingers, pectus excavatum/pectus cavinatum, high arched palate, ligamentous laxity, increased length of tubular bones, arm span often greater than height, kyphoscoliosis, lens dislocation/subluxation in 70%, striae distensae over abdomen) as well-suited to basketball, volleyball and high jumping (as tall). *Note* strong family history. Individualize advice. Echocardiogram is necessary to determine the presence of aortic root disease.

Coronary artery disease

Is the commonest cause of SCD >35 years. **Symptoms of exercise-related** dyspnea, chest pain, palpitations, or syncopal episodes need to be investigated with an exercise stress test and thallium 201 scanning or coronary angiography. Cardiac symptoms vary according to the age of the athlete. **Symptoms and signs of ischemic heart disease** (chest pain and dyspnea) are not uncommon and need to be thoroughly investigated in the >35 athlete.

Younger athletes may also present with cardiac symptoms (in <30 years: palpitations, dizziness, and syncope). May be benign and insignificant or the only warning sign of severe congenital cardiac defect. SCD does occur during sport. Investigate thoroughly thickening of both septa and posterior ventricular wall (but no interventricular outflow tract gradients). The echo is useful to differentiate from hypertrophic cardiomyopathy.

Exercise and high blood pressure

Exercise (aerobic, of moderate intensity at 60–90% of maximal HR[1] and 3 to 5 times/week for 20–60min duration) is useful in the management of HBP. Thought to work by reducing sympathetic tone (also consider the 'insulin hypothesis'). Low weight, high

---

1 Use predicted maximum heart rate, PMHR = 220 minus athlete's age.

repetition resistance weight lifting is also useful. Beware of the well-described hypertensive response to exercise (BP goes >200–225 systolic). The drugs commonly used to treat HBP need to be checked (diuretics may induce $\downarrow$K and exacerbate dehydration; beta-blockers may reduce exercise tolerance, $\uparrow$K$^+$ and worsen heat tolerance-selective beta-blockers are thought to be better; angiotensin-converting enzyme inhibitors, calcium channel blockers, prazosin and doxazosin have fewer side-effects with exercise).[1]

133

1 Joint National Committee on Detection, Evaluation and Treatment of High Blood Pressure: The 5th Report of the JNC. NHLBI NIH 30 Oct 1992. Bethesda, MD

Headache

Is common among all populations. The causes are as for the general population (migraine, cluster headaches, viral, sinusitis, and drug-related). There are headache types specific to athletes: benign exertional headache (seen in weight lifters), post-traumatic headache (boxing and the football codes), 'exertional migraine', cervicogenic headache (also seen in the non-sporting population).

Note: the history is vital.

Benign exertional headache

Follows relatively intense exertion (weight lifting and running). Cause may be related to a disturbance in cerebrovascular autoregulation. The onset of headache is acute and severe but it is brief (seconds or minutes) and followed by a dull ache for (hours). If recurrent, should be investigated as 10% so-called 'benign exertional headaches' have intracranial pathology (posterior fossa tumor, arteriovenous malformations, Arnold–Chiari malformations, aneurysms, and subdural hematomas). NSAIDs are useful, as is cervical massage, hydrotherapy, pre-activity use of paracetamol (acetaminophen) or ibuprofen; hypnosis and anxiolytics/antidepressants.

Post-traumatic headache

Minor head injuries are not uncommon in contact sports. Headache does follow concussion and may last for days/weeks. Post-traumatic headache has been described after trivial head traumas such as 'heading' the ball in soccer, called 'footballer's migraine'. If such headaches persist perform a thorough neurological examination with CT or MRI scan. Most have no abnormality on imaging and are diagnosed as having 'post-concussion syndrome' (where symptoms such as headache, poor concentration, dizziness, and fatigue persist for weeks following an episode of concussion). See chapter 5.

'Exertional migraine'

Is similar to a classical or common migraine but occurs at the end of exercise. Usually seen in patients with a history of non-exertional migraine. **Precipitated** by hot weather and dehydration. The headache (as for classical migraine) is preceded or accompanied by visual and sensory symptoms, nausea and vomiting, and is retroorbital. Treatment as for classical migraine (mainly pharmacological), identify and modify causes such as drugs (oral contraceptive pill, caffeine, vasodilators, alcohol), exercising in hot weather and inadequate hydration. Warm-ups are thought to adapt the sympathetic system.

Cervical headache

This is common in the sporting and non-sporting populations. Less intense than migraine. It is typically worse with neck movements and dull in nature, lasts for days without variation. Dizziness may be present. **Physical examination** includes neuro and cervical spine assessment. Cervical spine examination includes assessment of ROM, palpation for point tenderness over the spinous processes, facet joints and cervical muscules. Sometimes, symptoms can be provoked by palpation or neck movements. Posture may contribute from hyperextension of the cervical spine increasing the load on the facet joints. Correct with a neck flexor strengthening program with emphasis on chin retraction, mobilization of the intervertebral joints, and soft tissue treatment. If any suspicious features (such as nocturnal neck pain) x-ray and CT/MRI scan.

Fatigue

The **causes of fatigue** in an athlete are: overtraining, medications (e.g. beta blockers, sedatives); viral/post viral illness; CFS (chronic fatigue syndrome); nutritional factors; metabolic/endocrine causes (e.g. anemia/iron deficiency, diabetes, and hypothyroidism; pregnancy; and malignancy.

Take a thorough history (diet, training diary) which will often reveal the cause. From the training diary assess the progression of exercise duration/intensity and the frequency/duration of recovery periods. *Also check*: current medications; menstrual history; history of recent overseas travel; presence of systemic or localizing symptoms; social history (work and home situations); and whether any stressors. **Physical examination** of the 'tired athlete', should include a full cardiovascular, respiratory, and GI work-up. In particular, look for pallor, lymphadenopathy, hepatosplenomegaly, and enlarged thyroid. **Useful investigations include**: FBC, ESR, EUC, liver function tests, fasting plasma glucose; serum iron studies, Vitamin B_{12}, folate; thyroid function tests; pregnancy test; viral serology (EBV, CMV, toxoplasmosis, hepatitis A, B, and C).

Overtraining syndrome (staleness)[1]

Is typified by tiredness, irritability, poor motivation, sleep disturbances, depression, weight loss, frequent injuries and illness, muscle aches and heaviness, lowered immunity to infection and deteriorating performance ($\downarrow$max work output in terms of speed/endurance/power). Training fatigue leads to overreaching to overtraining syndrome, each stage characterized by overload.[2] The **diagnosis** is suggested by the history with the following markers: changes on psychological tests (use the Profile of Mood States, POMS: overtrained athletes record low scores for vigor and high scores for anxiety and depression), elevation of early morning HR (the hallmark with typical $\uparrow$5bpm, from $\downarrow$SV and $\downarrow$blood volume from fluid loss), $\uparrow$ventilation, $\uparrow$blood lactate, and deterioration in performance tests. There is no one pathognomonic blood test; there will be $\downarrow$serum testosterone/urinary cortisol ratio, $\downarrow$plasma glutamine levels, $\downarrow$urinary noradrenaline levels, $\uparrow$white cell count and $\downarrow$serum ferritin level. Immunological markers of overtraining may become available. **Treatment** is by reduction of training volume and intensity. First prevent by having training programs designed cyclically to incorporate alternative recovery periods and light training periods interspersed with the heavy sessions. This allows consolidation of gains and recovery of muscle tissue and requires close collaboration with coaches and relatives.

1 M B Mellion 1994 In MB Mellion (ed) *Sports medicine secrets* Ch35 p152. Hanlet & Belfus, Philadelphia 2 F Borselen *et al* 1992 The role of anaerobic exercise in overtraining. *NaH Strength Cond Assoc J* **14** 74

137

Chronic fatigue syndrome

CFS is a syndrome comprising a constellation of clinical manifestations (Table 4.11). The primary feature of this illness is fatigue. There are no pathognomonic features of this illness and diagnosis is essentially one arrived at by exclusion. **Etiology**: there is no firm evidence pointing towards a specific cause of the syndrome. There is some evidence pointing towards a viral etiology as well as an immune system defect. The viral hypothesis is suggested due to the observation that many CFS cases have been diagnosed after infection with EBV. In addition antibody titres to several viruses have been shown to be elevated in patients with CFS. Damage to the reticular activating system (RAS) of the upper brainstem has also been identified as a potential cause of the syndrome.[1] A molecular basis for CFS was postulated by the finding of increased aminohydroxy-*N*-methylpyrrolidine (chronic fatigue symptom urinary marker 1, or CFSUM1), tyrosine, β-alanine, aconitic acid, and succinic acid in urine samples.[2] Evidence of an endocrine abnormality has also been suggested due to the finding that CFS patients tend to have reduced levels of corticotropin releasing hormone and correspondingly high levels of ACTH.

Epidemiology: the syndrome occurs most often in women in the 25–45 year age group. Women are twice as likely to have CFS as men. **Diagnostic criteria:** the Center for Disease Control (USA) established diagnostic criteria,[3] which are an attempt to standardize the criteria for diagnosis. They comprise major, minor and physical finding criteria. To make a diagnosis both major criteria and greater than or equal to 6 minor and at least 2 physical criteria need to be documented. **Investigations**: there are no definitive investigations for this illness. Detailed and extensive work-ups are not desirable.

Management: there are several approaches that can be used in the treatment of CFS:
- Periodic assessment is important to detect an underlying disorder, which has so far escaped diagnosis.
- Symptomatic treatment with antipyretics, NSAIDs for headaches, antihistamines, and decongestants for rhinitis and sinusitis.
- Non-sedating antidepressants must be considered if a depressed mood or disturbed sleep pattern is reported.
- Avoidance of strenuous exercise or total avoidance of exercise (which might lead to deconditioning)
- Medical therapies, which have not been shown to be successful, include acyclovir, folic acid–cyanocobalomin injections, and high dose immunglobulin therapy
- Cognitive/behavior therapy has been used and been found to be successful when compared to relaxation methods. Outcomes were measured in terms of improvement in fatigue, mood, and functional impairment.

Nutritional factors

Inadequate nutrition is not an uncommon cause of fatigue in athletes. There may be: inadequate caloric intake/CHO intake/ iron intake or poor iron absorption. (See Chapter 16.)

1 CJ Dickinson 1997 *Eur J Clin Invest* **27** 257–67 2 NR McGregor 1996 *Biochem Mol Med* **57** 73–80 3 *Harrison's principles of medicine* 13th edn, p14—*Neurological disorders*, Table 388–2

Table 4.11 Working definition of chronic fatigue syndrome

Major criteria
- Persistent or relapsing fatigue or easy fatiguability that:
  - does not resolve with bedrest
  - is severe enough to reduce daily activity by >50%
- Exclusion of other chronic conditions (including psychiatric illnesses)

Minor criteria
- Symptoms
- Pyrexia
- Pharyngitis
- Lymph node pain in anterior or posterior cervical or axillary chains
- Unexplained generalized muscle weakness
- Muscle discomfort
- Prolonged generalized fatigue following previously tolerable exercise
- Generalized headaches
- Migratory non-inflammatory arthralgia
- Neuropsychiatric symptoms such as photophobia, irritability, confusion, depression, inability to concentrate
- Sleep disturbance
- Acute or subacute onset

Physical findings (documented for longer than 1 month)
- Pyrexia (mild 37.6–38.6°C)
- Non-exudative pharyngitis
- Palpable or tender posterior cervical or axillary lymph nodes

Anemia

In the athlete, this may be a false anemia (called 'sports anemia') which derives from expansion of the plasma volume with a resultant ↓hemoglobin concentration. Occurs from aerobic exercise and is a sign of fitness. True anemia occurs in athletes from iron deficiency (female athletes are prone from reduced dietary intake) and from GI bleeding. Correct with dietary supplement. (See Chapter 16.)

'Foot-strike' hemolysis occurs in heavy runners (stomping on hard road with thin soles), swimmers, and rowers. There is a ↓serum haptoglobin with normal blood film.

Pseudonephritis (stress hematuria)

Where red blood and white blood cells, along with hemoglobin, myoglobin, protein, and casts are found in the urine after exercise (especially events >10,000m). Usually microscopic. Clears after 24–48h rest (so is not significant).

Exercise and the immune system

There is some conflicting evidence regarding the effects of exercise on the immune system. Of what is known, major findings of practical importance, in terms of athletic endeavor include:

- Paradoxically, it seems that the immune system responds to increased physical activity and may be given some of the credit for exercise-related reduction in illness. In contrast, it has repeatedly been shown that intense exercise (>60% VO_{2max}) causes immunosuppression. In essence, the immune system is enhanced during moderate and severe exercise, and only intense long duration exercise is followed by immunodepression.[1]

- Acute exercise leads an increased total blood white cell count and an increase in neutrophil and natural killer (NK) cell activity and decreased salivary IgA.
- The effects of chronic exercise include suppressed concentration of lymphocytes, suppressed NK- and lymphokine-activated cytotoxicity, and much greater decrease in secretory IgA than in acute exercise. Whether or not the depression in the immune system activity occurs is dependent on the intensity and duration of exercise. It has been suggested that the 'overtraining effect' seen in élite athletes could be due to the window of opportunism for pathogens being longer and the degree of immunosuppression greater.
- It is suggested that severe immunodepression may occur if athletes do not allow the immune system to recover, but initiate a new bout of exercise while still immunodepressed. It has also been suggested that neutrophils serve as a last line of defense. The removal of this back-up system following extreme activity would be compatible with the propensity of 'overtrained' individuals to develop URTIs. However, it should be noted that in 'non-overtrained' individuals (i.e. those undertaking regular moderate physical activity) may have reduced URTI symptomatology.
- Work performance tends to diminish with most systemic infectious, and clinical case studies and animal data suggest that infection severity, relapse, and myocarditis may result when patients exercise vigorously. At least 2 sports-related deaths due to myocarditis have been reported during athletic activity.
- Data suggests that the incidence and mortality rates for certain types of cancer are lower among active subjects. The role of the immune system may be limited, however, depending on the sensitivity of the specific tumor to cytolysis, the stage of cancer, the type of exercise program, and many other complex factors.
- Mental stress, undernourishment, quick weight loss, and improper hygiene have each been associated with impaired immunity. Athletes who are undergoing heavy training regimens should realize that each of these factors has the potential to compound the effect that exercise stress is having on their immune systems.[2]
- As individuals age, they experience a decline in most cell-mediated and humoral immune responses. Two human studies suggest that immune function is superior in highly conditioned v sedentary elderly subjects.[3]

1 BK Pedersen *et al J Sports Med Physical Fitness* **36** 236-45 2 C McGrew *HIV/ AIDS in athletes ChVIII General medical problems* 3 DC Nieman 1997 (Mar) *Int J Sports Med* **18**(Suppl 1) S91–100

HIV/AIDS in athletes

Existing information suggests that the potential risk for such transmission is extremely low and that the principal risks athletes have for acquiring HIV and hepatitis B virus are related to off-the-field activities. Therefore, efforts to prevent transmission of blood-borne pathogens among athletes should emphasize prevention in off-the-field settings.[1]

In an HIV positive athlete the decision to advise continued athletic participation should be individualized and involve the athlete and the athlete's physician. Factors which should be taken under consideration include: the athlete's current state of health and the status of the HIV infection, the nature and intensity of the training. There is no evidence to suggest that exercise and training of moderate intensity is damaging to the health of HIV infected individuals, however it should be noted that helper T cell numbers and other markers of immune function are not improved either. In fact, high level training and competition may be deleterious.[1]

1 EE Mast *et al* *Annals Internal Med* 1995 (Feb 15) **122**(4) 283–5

Epilepsy

Studies indicate that epilepsy is infrequent during states of exercise. Exercise may actually be beneficial in the prevention of seizures. It is thought that genetic factors are involved in the etiology of low seizure thresholds in patients. In addition, hyperventilation, adrenaline release, and hypoglycemia may cause seizures. It is theorized that an increase in β-endorphins associated with exercise might inhibit seizures. Levels of anticonvulsant medication may be affected by exercise (by hepatic enzyme-inducing effects). This has not been conclusively shown in research to date. There is no evidence to suggest that athletes with epilepsy have a higher injury rate than non-epileptic athletes. Epilepsy can be well controlled by medication. However, breakthrough seizures can occur. These breakthrough seizures could potentially be due to metabolic abnormalities, head injuries, hyperthermia, sleep deprivation, and subtherapeutic anticonvulsant levels. Head CT should be performed to exclude head injuries or a focal brain lesion. Recommendations for athletes with seizures:

- Avoid contact sports if daily seizures occur
- Anticonvulsant therapy should be continued throughout adolescence to prevent recurrence after remission.
- Head injury should preclude the athlete from sports, which might result in further head injuries.
- Contact sports should be avoided if seizures are followed by a long post-convulsive state.
- Sports that are relatively contraindicated are car racing, boxing, motorcycling, and ski jumping. Horseback riding and high altitude mountain climbing should also be avoided in all athletic patients.
- An individualized approach to management is desirable based on the seizure pattern of the athlete.

Conclusion

Sports medicine is concerned with the treatment of medical problems in athletes as well as the diagnosis and treatment of injury. Regular physical activity has health-promoting effects, nevertheless athletes are do incur the same general illnesses of the larger population. The usual medical presentations of the sporting population have been described in this chapter. The author has seen disasters (severe complications and deaths of young athletes) who continued to exercise with minor respiratory illness (cardiomyopathy after URTI), collapse, and death whilst skiing during the jaundice phase of hepatitis. Early recognition and treatment will often enable a prompt and safe return to sport.

The team doctor (see Chapter 24) has a vital role in treatment of illness and injury (referring on when necessary); making decisions in regard to athletes eligibility to join the team and to return to play after injury. The doctor's responsibilities are first to the athlete (as patient), the team, family, and administrators. It is hoped that being a team doctor does not become a position of burden but of pleasure in being able to practice a broad spectrum of medicine (internal medicine, orthopedics, gynecology, pharmacology, and exercise physiology). Remember to always preserve the athlete's (patient's) confidentiality and practise to the best Hippocratic ideals.

Many teams find a primary care doctor and orthopedic surgeon ideal (most injuries are musculoskeletal). However, sports medicine physicians are best able to provide such comprehensive care.

Part II
Injuries

LAURIE GEFFEN, GINA GEFFEN, SAUL GEFFEN,
ANTON D HINTON-BAYRE

Introduction

Head injury is one of the most common forms of acquired neurological damage, particularly in young males. Head injuries are especially prevalent in contact sports that produce collisions, in sports where participants move or fall at high velocity, and in sports that involve the use of force imparting implements (1). The incidence is highest in combat sports, such as boxing, where the head is a legitimate target. However, head injury is also common in contact sports such as the various codes of football, especially gridiron, where the annual incidence may be as high as 10–20% of participants, and rugby, which has up to twice the risk of other (non-gridiron) football codes (2, 3). Other non-contact sports with a higher risk of head injury include motor racing, equestrian and gymnastic events, snow board and blade sports, and cycling. Sports where head injury is rare but potentially severe include golf, shooting, cricket, baseball, and field hockey.

The focus in this chapter is on brain injury. However, head injuries often involve significant damage to scalp, skull, meninges and blood vessels as well as the face, jaws, eyes, ears, and neck. While the initial assessment and management of head injury described in this chapter includes injuries to these other tissues and sites, the subsequent management of extracranial head injuries is dealt with in Chapters 6 and 7.

The most common form of head injury in sport is an episode of concussion (Latin: *concutere*, to shake violently), from which a full recovery is usual. However, any head injury can have immediate or delayed life-threatening consequences and serious long-term sequelae. As such, all head injuries require thorough systematic assessment by the sports physician (a) to recognize and manage the acute consequences, including the prevention of secondary brain damage, (b) to arrange the safe transfer of the injured athlete to an appropriate treatment facility when necessary, or (c) to ensure that the athlete is closely monitored for at least 24 hours and returns to participation only when fully recovered. Finally (d) prevention also needs to be addressed by the sports physician. This chapter has five main sections:

1 Mechanisms of brain injury, which provides a summary of the anatomical, physiological, and pathological issues that influence management and prevention.

2 Clinical features of brain injury, including symptoms and signs of concussion.

3 On-site assessment and management of head injuries.

4 Post acute assessment and management of concussion, which includes clinical and psychometric assessment of recovery and guidelines for the return to participation in sport.

5 Prevention measures including athlete preparation, protective devices and rule modifications.

Mechanisms of brain injury

Head injuries in sport usually result from direct impact of the head but can occur when the head is subjected to forces translated from elsewhere on the body. Brain injury may be *primary*, due to the direct application of physical forces damaging brain and associated vascular tissue, or *secondary*, arising from intracranial and extracranial complications of injuries to the head and other parts of the body (**4–6**).

Forces producing brain injury

- Forces acting on the brain produce three types of tissue stress: compressive, tensile, and shearing. *Compressor* forces tend to produce focal contusions and if relieved promptly produce the least long-term consequences. *Tensile* (stretching) forces act mainly on long fiber pathways and damage tends to be more diffuse (diffuse axonal injury). *Shearing* forces operate parallel to surfaces and can produce serious consequences by tearing brain and vascular tissue.
- Most forces are dynamic and result in propulsion and rotation of the brain within the cranium following impacts to either the head or body. Cerebrospinal fluid (CSF) dissipates focally applied forces and permits gliding of the hemispheres within the cranium.
- A forceful blow to the head usually produces maximal brain injury at the site of impact (*coup* injury) particularly if the head is stationary before impact. A moving head striking a non-moveable surface, as in falls or collisions, may also produce brain injury at the opposite pole of the cranium (*contrecoup* injury). This is because the brain lags behind in the moving cranium, thereby squeezing protective CSF away from the trailing pole (Fig 5.1).
- The magnitude of any force is the product of mass and acceleration (Newton's law). If the neck muscles are tensed at impact, the mass of the head approximates that of the whole body and acceleration (or deceleration) of the head is greatly reduced for any given force. Conversely, when the head is not braced, as in unanticipated blows or further blows in an already stunned state, a given force produces much greater acceleration of the head.

Pathophysiology of primary brain injury

- *Gliding of the brain* within the cranium is impeded at three main sites (1) dura mater—brain attachments (e.g. midline falx cerebri and tentorium cerebelli), (2) irregular and protuberant surfaces of the frontal and middle fossa of the base of the skull, (3) wherever CSF is dissipated by acceleration, especially at the poles of the frontal and temporal lobes.
- *Focal contusions* occur mainly at or at opposite sites of impact and comprise local petechial hemorrhages and necrotic damage, which are often accompanied by surrounding oedema and subarachnoid hemorrhage.
- *Propulsion and rotation* of the hemispheres on the relatively fixed brainstem may cause damage to ascending brainstem pathways, ranging from stretching with transient impairment of consciousness to tearing of subcortical fiber tracts with immediate unconsciousness and coma.
- *General cerebral oedema* due to a combination of local metabolic derangement, breakdown of the blood–brain barrier, and obstructions to venous outflow, leads to a rise in intracranial pressure (see below).

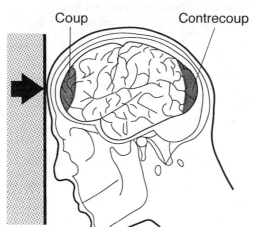

Fig. 5.1 Mechanisms of frontal trauma coup and contrecoup brain injury.

Mechanisms of brain injury (*cont*)

Pathophysiology of secondary brain injury

Head injuries may result in complications that are life threatening and can have serious long-term consequences. Because they are often remediable in their early stages, they require immediate attention.

Intracranial complications

Include skull fracture, intracranial hemorrhage, raised intracranial pressure, cerebral hypoxia, and infection.

1 Skull fractures may result in direct brain compression, intracranial bleeding, CSF leaks and infection. Brain injury may occur without a skull fracture; however, the presence of a skull fracture greatly increases the risk of intracranial bleeding and infection. The site of a fracture is also critical in anticipating complications (e.g. temporoparietal damage to meningeal vessels, frontal damage to sinuses). Fractures may be either of the vault or the base of the skull.

- *Vault fractures*, which may be linear or depressed, are usually associated with scalp hematomas or a localized area of swelling and tenderness.
- *Basal fractures* are harder to detect and usually involve intracranial bleeding. Periorbital hematomas, subconjunctival hemorrhage and CSF rhinorrhea are signs of an anterior fossa fracture; CSF otorrhoea, hemotympanum, and retromastoid bruising (Battle's sign) are signs of a petrous bone fracture.
- Close observation and radiological investigation are required for all suspected skull fractures. Opinions differ on the value of a routine computed tomography (CT) scan for all mild head injuries. Early CT scan and early discharge of patients with normal radiological and neurological findings has been advocated as being as safe and more cost effective than hospitalization for observation with CT scan performed only after clinical deterioration (7).
- *Intracranial hemorrhage* may result in local compression, raised intracranial pressure, and ischemia to the area of supply of the damaged vessel. All intracranial hematomas constitute a priority in the management of head injury because of their immediate threat to life and eventual recovery of function and because they may be surgically remediable. Hematomas may develop immediately or some time after the initial injury preceded by a lucid interval. **Delay in recognizing and treating intracranial bleeding is the most common cause of avoidable mortality and morbidity due to head injury.** Vigilance needs to be maintained for at least 24h. The four types of intracranial hemorrhage are:

  (i) *Extradural hematomas* result from shearing forces or skull fractures that tear blood vessels supplying the dura and skull. Hematomas may form rapidly (high pressure bleeding between dura and skull) and compress the brain leading to early loss of consciousness and localizing neurological signs or they may occur up to several hours following the initial injury.

  (ii) *Subdural hematomas* are the most common form of sports-related intracranial bleeding. Shearing and direct impact forces tear small veins resulting in low pressure bleeding between the brain and dura matter. Signs and symptoms may be subtle and develop insidiously over days or even weeks.

  (iii) *Subarachnoid hemorrhage* may result from any head injury, however mild. Severe headache and localizing signs usually develop rapidly.

(iv) *Intracerebral hemorrhage* occurs with major brain injury. Intraventricular hemorrhage may lead to subsequent blockage of CSF outflow. Brainstem hematomas are life threatening.

2 Raised intracranial pressure is a serious consequence of brain injury that may result from several causes including depressed fractures, hypoxia, hypercapnia, hyperperfusion, hypoperfusion, intracranial hemorrhage, and intracranial infection. Raised intracranial pressure leads to cerebral compression, which may be followed by herniation around the brainstem with venous obstruction and infarction. Signs include fluctuations in consciousness, fits and focal neurological deficits.

3 Two rare conditions are associated with life-threatening rises in intracranial pressure after even minor head injuries (4).

(i) *Malignant brain oedema syndrome* occurs in children and adolescents as diffuse brain swelling with extreme hyperemia. It may be due to loss of autoregulation but the mechanism is unknown. After even relatively minor head injury, there is a deterioration of consciousness resembling, in its rapidity, extradural bleeds in adults. Prompt intubation and measures to reduce intracranial pressure such as hyperventilation and osmotic diuretics are required. The mortality rate is high.

(ii) *Second impact syndrome* is a variant of malignant brain oedema syndrome that is seen in adults following even minor head trauma when still suffering symptoms of a previous head injury. Loss of autoregulation precipitated by an unknown mechanism leads to massive and diffuse hyperemia and oedema of the brain. Intracranial pressure rises within minutes and may lead to herniation and coma. Prompt measures to maintain respiration and reduce intracranial pressure as above are indicated. The mortality rate approaches 50% and morbidity is near to 100%.

4 Hypoxia due to loss of CNS control of airway patency and breathing may occur either following serious primary injury to the brainstem or may be secondary to raised intracranial pressure with brain herniation. Brain hypoxia may also result from extracranial complications (see below).

5 Infection (meningitis or brain abscess) may occur when the dura is penetrated. Direct contamination of the intracranial cavity may occur in compound depressed fractures of the vault, whereas contact with middle ear cavity and nasal sinuses may introduce infection in basal fractures.

6 Concussive convulsions seen within seconds of insult are to be distinguished from later epileptic seizures. Such concussive convulsions are rare, transient, and do not necessarily lead to the development of epilepsy (8).

7 Post-traumatic epilepsy may develop within days to months. It usually follows traumatic brain injury with prolonged periods of unconsciousness, and occurs in about 23% of hospital admissions of sports-related head injury (9).

Extracranial complications

Of head or associated injuries may interfere with brain metabolism and perfusion. Given the immediate dependency of brain tissue on its oxygen supply and the potential for remediation of many of the complications, recognition, and management of extracranial causes of secondary brain damage constitutes a clinical priority. Causes include *injuries interfering with ventilation,* such as chest, neck, or facial injuries that obstruct airways and affect chest movement, and *injuries interfering with brain circulation* by producing hemodynamic instability and hypovolemia.

Non-traumatic sports-related brain injury

There are two main causes of non-traumatic sports related brain injury (**10**).

Cerebral air embolism

- unique to underwater diving, second most common cause of death after drowning
- occurs in rapid ascents from >10m
- symptoms may occur within moments to hours of surfacing
- signs include: seizure, hemiplegia, diplopia, tunnel vision, vertigo, or dysarthria
- if diver surfaces unconscious, diagnosis is strong presumption
- seek to recompress subject as soon as possible

High-altitude cerebral oedema (see Chapter 26)

- accounts for up to 5% of deaths above 4000m
- symptoms develop within 72h and include ataxia, vertigo, confusion, and hallucinations
- immediate treatment is return to lower elevation and oxygenate
- monitor for signs of raised intracranial pressure and treat accordingly

Clinical features of brain injury

1 *The primary clinical features of brain injury are loss or alteration in consciousness, orientation, and responsiveness, followed by a period of post-traumatic amnesia.* Other clinical features will depend on the nature and severity of the injury and any supervening complications (4–6, 11)

2 Head injuries may be open or closed. *Open head injuries* may arise from skull fractures or as a result of a penetrating missile or implement, whereas *closed head injuries* usually result from blunt impacts or translation of dynamic forces to the head. There are no universally agreed clinical criteria for classifying the severity of closed head injury (12–14). *Gradings into mild, moderate, and severe categories* based on the duration of loss of consciousness, the period of post-traumatic amnesia and the initial Glasgow Coma Scale (GCS) score are shown in Table 5.1.

3 About 80% of head injuries are defined as mild as they result in post-traumatic amnesia of less than 24 hours duration (15). Approximately two-thirds of these mild head injuries occur as the result of a sporting injury (16).

Concussion

- The commonest consequence of a sports head injury is concussion.
- Concussion is a trauma-induced transient alteration in mental status that may or may not involve *loss of consciousness. Confusion* and *amnesia* are the hallmarks of concussion and may be immediate or delayed by several minutes. Other *neurological features* may include temporary disturbances of balance and vision (17).
- Depending on severity and recency of the trauma, athletes may display some or all of the *clinical features of concussion* listed in Table 5.2 (18).
- Signs and symptoms may occur immediately or take several minutes to evolve. Concussed athletes may be able to continue to play automatically with sensorimotor functions intact.

Table 5.1 A classification of severity of head injury (GCS)

Mild	Loss of consciousness	0–5min
	Post traumatic amnesia	<1h
	GCS score	13–14
Moderate	Loss of consciousness	5min–6h
	Post-traumatic amnesia	1–24h
	GCS score	9–12
Severe	Loss of consciousness	>6h
	Post traumatic amnesia	>24h
	GCS score	<9

Table 5.2 Acute clinical features of concussion

- Transient loss of consciousness (not obligatory)
- Confusion, including:
  - reduced vigilance
  - heightened distractibility
  - inability to think coherently
  - inability to sequence goal directed moments
  - disorientation for person, time or place
  - dazed facial expression.
- Amnesia, including
  - anterograde amnesia for events after the injury
  - retrograde amnesia for events before the injury
  - inability to acquire new memories.
- Other neurological features including
  - blurred vision or diplopia
  - slurred speech
  - dizziness
  - impaired balance or incoordination
  - nausea or vomiting
  - emotional lability
  - convulsions

On-site assessment and management of head injury

The sports physician may be required to triage and respond on site to **4 main categories** of head injury (see also Fig. 5.2):

1 Injuries requiring resuscitation of the unconscious athlete, stabilization, and transport to an appropriate clinical facility.

2 Injuries requiring withdrawal from contest and transport to an appropriate clinical facility.

3 Injuries requiring withdrawal from contest and monitoring on site and at home.

4 Injuries sufficiently minor to permit resumption but with monitoring.

The following description refers to injuries sustained in a team game and needs to be modified for the circumstances prevailing in individual sports.

Assessment and management of the unconscious athlete

This is an emergency that supersedes all other event considerations.

- Take charge of the situation and direct others in accordance with their training and the situation.
- Institute **resuscitation (DR ABC) procedure** (Table 5.3). Airway protection and maintenance takes precedence over possible spinal injury.
- If airway is clear, strong rhythmical breathing is present and pulse is normal, then 'log roll' into coma position, manually controlling head and neck, and check for other injuries using **primary survey protocol** (Tables 5.4 and 5.5).
- If the athlete has required resuscitation or has not recovered consciousness or has a GCS <14 within 3min, arrange **immediate transport to hospital** (Table 5.6).

Assessment and management of the head-injured conscious athlete

The following is based on recent recommendations for best practice on site (**17, 18, 20, 21**).

- If an athlete has had no loss of consciousness and is free from all symptoms and signs of concussion. They may be deemed to be fit to continue but should be rechecked in 10–15m to determine whether any symptoms have developed, including a gap in memory or somatic complaints and should be monitored closely for the rest of the event.
- If an athlete has lost consciousness, however briefly, or has any symptoms or signs of concussion, remove to sideline and conduct a *neurological screen* (Table 5.7) and *mental status examination* (**Table 5.8**) and (**20**). If neurological and mental status examinations are clear and there are no apparent signs or symptoms, conduct *physical tests* if return to participation is contemplated. Physical provocation tests should include two 20m shuttle runs out of play, 10 sit-ups, 10 push-ups, and 10 squats. Then check for complaints and assess capability to perform sport-specific tasks.

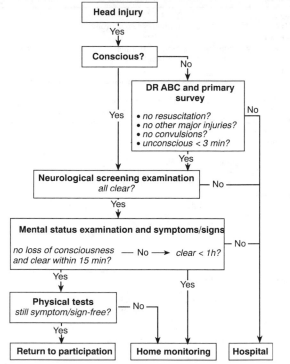

Fig. 5.2 Flowchart of on-site management of head injury

On-site assessment and management of head injury (*cont*)

Table 5.3 DR ABC procedure for resuscitation of unconscious athlete

Danger
- Remove athlete and self from dangerous environment.

Response
- Loudly say 'Hello, can I help you?' If athlete responds verbally then airway must be patent and some cognition is present.

Airway
- To clear: insert gloved finger into oral cavity and remove mouthguard, loose teeth, vomit etc.
- To open: place athlete on back then move mandible anteriorly (jaw thrust).
- If airway obstructed (full or partial) then slight cervical extension may help.
- If available oropharangeal airway (Guedel), supplemental O_2 and oral suctioning may be necessary.

Breathing
- Check color
- Listen to breathing rate and character.
- Check chest for movement and air entry.
- If not breathing start expired air resuscitation.

Circulation
- Check carotid pulse (if palpable systolic BP is >60mmHg)
- If absent commence cardiopulmonary resuscitation.
- Check for torrential arterial bleeding and treat.

Table 5.4 Primary survey

When resuscitated and in coma position:
- Inspect and palpate scalp (for wounds or skull fractures)
- Inspect and palpate face and anterior neck
- Check cervical spine alignment (run fingers along supraspinatus processes)
- Glasgow Coma Scale (*see Table 5.5*)
- Pupillary size, symmetry and reaction to light
- Check nose and ears for bleeding or CSF leak
- Inspect and palpate abdomen, pelvis, and limbs

Table 5.5 Glasgow Coma Scale (19)

Eye opening	
Spontaneous	4
To speech	3
To pain	2
None	1
Best verbal response	
Oriented	5
Confused	4
Inappropriate words	3
Incomprehensible sounds	2
Nil	1
Best motor response	
Obeys commands	6
Localizes to pain	5
Withdraws from pain	4
Abnormal flexion	3
Extension	2
Nil	1
Total score	3–15

Table 5.6 Transport of head injured athlete to hospital

- Complete resuscitation and primary survey
- Protect airway and cervical spine with sandbags or neck brace
- Treat and stabilize other injuries
- Arrange others to carry the injured athlete
- Travel with patient if paramedics unavailable

Table 5.7 Neurological screening examination

Eyes	visual acuity and fields, pupil size and reflexes, nystagmus
Ears	hemotympanum
Nose	rhinorrhea
Power	all limbs
Co-ordination	finger–nose touching, heel–toe walking, balance on one leg with eyes closed

Table 5.8 Mental status examination for concussion

Immediate memory
  5 words read to athlete and recalled on 3 successive trials, scored out of 15.

Processing speed
  Sentences read aloud for 2min, number correctly identified as true or false. Scores less than 38 indicate impairment.

Orientation:
  Query orientation for time, place, situation, scored out of 5.

Retrograde amnesia:
  Query event recall prior to trauma (may vary with time post trauma), scored out of 5.

Delayed recall
  Free recall of 5 items presented at immediate recall, scored out of 5.

Gradings of concussion and return to sport

- Gradings of concussion shown in Table 5.9 (not to be confused with gradings of severity of closed head injury, Table 5.1) are used to facilitate clinical decisions about mild head injuries, which constitute an overwhelming majority of sports head injuries.
- After a **grade 1** concussion athletes may return to play, providing mental status is normal and they are symptom- and sign-free, after physical exertion testing.
- If symptoms persist longer than 15min (**grade 2**), or if there was a brief loss of consciousness (**grade 3**), or if a second **grade 1** concussion has been sustained, return to participation should be prohibited that day.

Post concussion monitoring if not hospitalized

- Athletes with **grade 2 or 3** concussions should have their mental status rechecked every 15min, until they respond to all items appropriately on 3 consecutive occasions, indicating a continually lucid period of 30min.
- Record duration of post-traumatic amnesia, which is defined as the period of time following trauma when the athlete is disoriented, confused, and unable to lay down new memories reliably.
- If there is no further deterioration, and signs and symptoms are resolving, concussed athletes may be allowed to return home in the company of a responsible adult. If supervision is not available referral to hospital is advisable.
- Provide **written instructions for monitoring** in the next 24h (Table 5.10).
- Any of the criteria listed in Table 5.11 are an indication for **referral to hospital**. Negative changes in mental status (other than minor expansion of retrograde amnesia in the first few hours) or any deterioration in physical condition necessitates immediate transport to hospital.

Ongoing management of mild head injury

This is a contentious area because there are no agreed objective measures of individual recovery from concussion. *New guidelines for return to competitive sport* (Table 5.12) that have been designed to assist the decision about duration of absence from sport are based on the severity of the presenting injury, recent history of other concussions, and extent of recovery (**17**).

Clinical assessment of recovery

- **Milder injuries** commonly cause headaches, fatigue, dizziness, loss of concentration and impaired higher mental function for up to several weeks before recovery.
- **More severe nonfatal injuries** lead to long term changes in cognitive and emotional function including loss of intellectual capacity, memory, motivation and personality as well as more specific cognitive and behavioral deficits related to the location and depth and of lesions. Physical sequelae may include localized neurological deficits and post-traumatic epilepsy.
- **CT or MRI scans** (even if obtained earlier) may be required if symptoms persist longer than 1 week or worsen.

Table 5.9 Grading concussion

Grade 1
- transient confusion
- no loss of consciousness
- concussive symptoms and/or mental status abnormalities fully resolve within 15 minutes.

Grade 2
- as for Grade 1 except symptoms and abnormalities persist for longer than 15 minutes

Grade 3
- any loss of consciousness whether it be brief (seconds, Grade 3a) or prolonged (minutes, Grade 3b)

Table 5.10 Sports Head Injury Card

Name

Time of concussion   Date

Watch closely for the next 24 hours

Take to hospital immediately if:
- they vomit
- severe headache develops or increases
- they become restless or irritable
- they become dizzy, drowsy, or cannot be aroused
- they have a fit (convulsion)
- anything else unusual occurs

For 24 hours after injury they should:
- rest quietly
- not drive a vehicle or operate machinery
- not consume alcohol or non-prescribed drugs

Medical advice should be sought before returning to sport

Table 5.11 Criteria for referral to hospital

- Loss of consciousness greater than 3 minutes
- Post traumatic convulsion
- Focal neurological signs
- Symptoms of marked cerebral irritation persisting longer than 1 hour
- Any deterioration of mental status, particularly the development of drowsiness following a lucid period
- More than one episode of concussion in any one playing session
- Non-availability of responsible adult to monitor for next 24 hours.

Table 5.12 Guidelines for return to competitive sport

Grade of concussion	No. of concussions (within a calendar year)	
	Initial concussion	Repeat concussions
1	Same day if asymptomatic within 15min	1wk or longer*
2	1wk asymptomatic	2 wk or longer*
3a	1wk asymptomatic	1 month or longer*
3b	2wk asymptomatic	1 month or longer*

* Period may be prolonged depending on frequency and severity of previous concussions.

Gradings of concussion and return to sport (*cont*)

Post-concussion symptoms

- Symptoms may be classified as **acute** (minutes to hours), **prolonged** (days to weeks), or **chronic** (months to years). *Acute symptoms* are presented in Table 5.2. *Prolonged symptoms* include persistent lowgrade headache, concentration, and memory deficits, sleep disturbance, reduced alcohol tolerance, irritability and lowered frustration tolerance, sensitivity to light and noise, tinnitus, easily fatigued, anxiety and/or depressed mood, specific cognitive dysfunction. *Chronic symptoms* include those listed for prolonged symptoms, but are usually accompanied by changes to behavior, secondary changes in mood/affect, and family and/or social problems (**18**).
- Acute and prolonged symptoms require monitoring to determine when an athlete may return to participation. In the absence of any generally accepted clinical measures that assess extent of recovery the protocol detailed in Table 5.13 is recommended.
- Chronic post-concussive sequelae may be minimized through counseling player, coach, and parents of the likely course of recovery and likely negative effects of early return to high-risk activities.
- The unrealistic expectations of athlete, family, peers, or work colleagues have been linked to the onset and persistence of post-concussive complaints. Graded return to work or school activity minimizes the effects of symptoms and maximizes opportunity for recovery.

Cumulative effects of concussion

Successive episodes of concussion may have cumulative effects.

- Post-concussive symptoms, such as poor co-ordination or balance, impaired concentration, judgment, and fatigue may predispose the player to further head or other injuries. An athlete with a history of concussion is up to four times more likely to receive a further concussion (or injuries) than an athlete with a clear history (3). **Appendix A** provides a structured interview covering previous sports head injuries.
- Psychometric tests indicate greater initial impairment and extended recovery of mental functions in individuals with previous episodes of concussion (**22**).
- A second, even lesser, insult may have a disproportionately large effect. Repeated concussion predisposes athletes to a catastrophic outcome (*second impact syndrome*) if the brain has not sufficiently recovered (**23**).

Chronic traumatic encephalopathy

Repeated concussion, which is most common in professional boxers, may lead to the permanent structural changes of *chronic traumatic encephalopathy* (estimates vary from 17% to 55%) (**24**).

- MRI and/or CT scans providing evidence of atrophy or structural abnormality are an indication for cessation of all high-risk sports or activities.
- Signs and symptoms range from mild neurologic dysfunction to dementia, and evolve slowly but may emerge more rapidly following a significant incident.

Table 5.13 Recommendations for progressive return to activity

- Training should not commence when symptomatic at rest
- Training should cease upon development or recurrence of symptoms (requires systematic questioning)
- First day asymptomatic, allow brisk walk for at least 20min. If still asymptomatic, allow light exercise (20min), then check for symptoms
- Day 2–day 7, continue to monitor graded increases in training
- No full exertion until asymptomatic for at least 1 week with progressive loading
- If symptoms persist or develop, a full medical examination is required

- The full *dementia pugilistica* syndrome occurs over several years in a minority of boxers and is more closely related to the number of bouts rather than knockouts.

Psychometric indices of impairment and recovery of function

- Delayed onset of retrograde amnesia may occur within 10–15 min, and the amnesia may initially extend to a period of several hours before reducing (25).

- Various *post-traumatic* amnesia scales are available to measure the severity of head injury but they were designed for hospital rather than on-site testing (**26–29**), and for amnesia lasting longer than 24h. Since the duration of post-traumatic amnesia is rarely more than a few hours in most sports head injuries, a more suitable instrument for measuring severity of sports concussion is repeated administrations of the *mental status examination* (**Table 5.8 and Appendix A**) (**20, 25**).

- *Psychometric measures* of attention, psychomotor speed, judgment and decision making, and memory have been extensively studied as a means of providing objective measures of subsequent recovery of function after the period of post-traumatic amnesia resolves. Currently the most widely used are the *Digit Symbol Test* (**30**) and the *Paced Auditory Serial Addition Task* (**31**). However, the Digit Symbol Test has proved relatively insensitive compared to a more recent test, which involves judging whether sentences are true or false (**32**). It is recommended that the following three psychometric tests are used to monitor recovery of mentation from concussion: (i) Digit Symbol Subtest of the WAIS-R (**30**), (ii) Symbol Digit Modalities Test (**33**), and (i) the Speed of Comprehension subtest of the Speed and Capacity of Language Processing Test (**32**) at weekly intervals until performance returns to normal levels.

- Performance levels of élite athletes on most tests of speed of information processing are often better than comparable population norms. Since reference to regular norms could thus result in premature return to participation, it is desirable for professional athletes in high-risk sports to have at least two baseline preseason measures on alternate forms of the three tests (**34**).

- Detailed psychometric testings (**35–37**), brain electrophysiological measures (**38**), and computerized dynamic posturography (**39**) have demonstrated recovery of cerebral function from concussion usually resolves within 1 week to 3 months. However, reliable correlations between measures of severity of concussion and rate of recovery have yet to be established. Until then, the exclusion guidelines listed in Table 5.13 should be considered in conjunction with the results of individual-based testing.

Prevention of sporting head injuries

Given the potentially irreversible effects of head injury, even after apparently minor trauma, the sports physician has particular obligations to institute and advocate preventative measures aimed reducing the severity of head trauma, minimizing secondary brain damage arising from the initial incident and lowering the incidence of recurrent head injures (**40**).

Devices reducing the severity of initial injury

The use of protective devices, such as mouthguards and helmets, can reduce the degree of brain injury sustained for a given force and also afford protection against associated injuries of the skull, face, scalp, and jaws (see Chapter 24).

Mouthguards

- Mouthguards protect teeth, facial bones, and mandibles. Further, they open the temporomandibular joint (double type more so than single) and thereby decrease the force transmitted to the base of the skull by a mandibular blow.
- Fitted mouthguards moulded by taking a cast are superior to the heat and mould variety.
- Fitted single upper are recommended for contact sport, whereas fitted double (upper and lower) are necessary for combat sports.
- Non-fitted mouthguards are probably better than nothing

Helmets

There are two basic types, soft and rigid (often with soft inner). *Soft helmets* have been shown to reduce scalp and eyebrow injuries, but their efficacy in preventing brain injury is unproven. There are many types of *rigid helmets* and they can provide substantial protection to the head and face. As a general principle, the use of rigid helmets is recommended (and in some sports mandatory) unless there are compelling reasons for their avoidance, such as injuries to other athletes.

Although helmets provide protection against direct blows, they have at least three disadvantages:

1 Helmets increase size of the head, thereby permitting a blow which would otherwise have missed to connect. The increase in diameter of the head can also increase the rotational component of a blow.

2 Helmets can obstruct vision (especially if not correctly fitted) thereby hindering avoidance maneuvers.

3 Helmets may give a false sense of security, encouraging the athlete to perform more recklessly.

Selection and conditioning of individual athletes

- Selection and conditioning of athletes for particular sports and for roles within them is best directed at selecting appropriate physiques for particular sports and roles within them and at improving general physical fitness.
- It is not possible to condition the brain to resist external force; on the contrary, damage from repeated trauma, however minor, tends to be cumulative.
- In certain sports and roles within them that have a higher risk of head injury, neck-strengthening exercises may have a protective effect by reducing acceleration of the head following blows to the head or body and by protecting against cervical spine injury.

Rules regulating play and individual participation

It is one of the sports physician's roles to advocate for rule changes that reduce the chance of head injury. Such rules can be designed to reduce initial injury and prevent recurrence, by regulating both the contest and individual athlete participation.

- Hard objects in the arena of play should be padded wherever possible.
- Rules requiring the use of protective devices are desirable.
- Rules that require the presence of trained personnel with first aid qualifications are highly desirable in high-risk sports.
- Rules that permit immediate assistance to injured athletes are essential.
- Rules that prevent head-injured athletes from resuming immediately without appropriate screening are essential.
- Rules that provide for mandatory exclusion periods following documented head injuries are desirable.
- Rules making the head an illegitimate target in contact sports are highly desirable. Combat sports that encourage blows to the head such as boxing and martial arts, provide a moral dilemma. Do sports physicians who attend such sports in order to assess and manage head trauma, nevertheless lend sanction to them?

Education of athletes and officials

The sports physician not only has a clinical and an advocacy role as described above but also has a responsibility to educate those involved with the sport about its risks, the recognition of head injury and its consequences, and the procedures for its assessment and management.

References

(1) LB Lehman, SJ Ravich 1990 Closed head injury in athletes. *Clin Sports Med* **9** 247–1.

(2) H Seward *et al* 1993 Football injuries in Australia at the élite level. *Med J Austral*, **159** 298–301

(3) SG Gerberich *et al* 1983 Concussion incidences and severity in secondary school and varsity football players. *Am J Public Health* **73** 1370–5

(4) RC Cantu, 1992 Cerebral concussion in sport: Management and prevention. *Sports Med* **14** 64–74

(5) LA Bruno *et al* 1987 Management guidelines for head injuries in athletics. *Clin Sports Med* **6** 17–29

(6) G McLatchie, B Jennett 1994 Head injury in sport. *BJM* 308 1620–4

(7) T Ingebrigtsen, B Romner 1996 Routine early CT-scan is cost saving after minor head injury. *Acta Neurol Scand* **93** 207–10

(8) PR McCrory *et al* 1997 Retrospective study of concussive convulsions in élite Australian rules and rugby league footballers: phenomenology, etiology, and outcome. *BMJ* **314** 171–4

(9) AJ Ryan 1991 Protecting the sportsman's brain (concussion in sport). *B J Sports Med* **25** 81–6

(10) JM Moriarty, SM Simons 1994 Sports neurology. In RJ Johnson, J Lombardo (ed) *Current review of sports medicine*. Current Medicine, Philadelphia

(11) JC Maroon *et al* 1992 Assessing closed head injuries. *Physician Sports Med* **20** 37–44

(12) ED Bigler 1990 Neuropathology of traumatic brain injury. In ED Bigler (ed) *Traumatic brain injury* Pro-ed, Austin, Tx

(13) B Jennet, G Teasdale 1981 *Management of head injury*. FA Davis, Philadephia

(14) RW Rimel *et al* 1982 Moderate head injury: completing the clincial spectrum of brain trauma. *Neurosurgery* **11** 344–51

(15) HS Levin *et al* 1989. *Mild head injury*. Oxford University Press, New York

(16) P Wrightson, D Gronwall 1980 Time off work and symptoms after minor head injury. *Injury* **12** 445–54

(17) Quality Standards Subcommittee, American Academy of Neurology 1997 Practice parameter: The management of concussion in sport. *Neurology* **48** 581–5

(18) JP Kelly, JH Rosenberg 1997 Diagnosis and management of concussion in sports. *Neurology* **48** 575–80

(19) G Teasdale, B Jennet 1974 Assessment of coma and impaired consciousness, a practical scale. *Lancet* **ii** 81–4

(20) M McCrea *et al* 1997 Standardized assessment of concussion in football players. *Neurology* **48** 586–8

(21) R Roos 1996 Guidelines for managing concussion in sport: A persistent headache. *Physician Sports Med,* **24** 67–74

(22) D Gronwall, P Wrightson 1975 Cumulative effects of concussion. *Lancet* **2** 995–7

(23) RC Cantu, R Voy 1995 Second impact syndrome: A risk in any contact sport. *Physician Sports Med* **23** 27–34

(24) EA Shores *et al* (1986) Preliminary validation of a clinical scale for measuring the duration of post-traumatic amnesia. *Med J Austral* **144** 569–72

(25) D Maddocks *et al* 1995 The assessment of orientation in following concussion athletes. *Clin J Sports Med* **5** 32–5

(26) HS Levin *et al* 1979 The Galveston Orientation and Amnesia Test: a practical scale to assess cognition after head injury. *J Nerv Ment Dis* **167** 675–84.

(27) MF Mendez 1995 The neuropsychiatric aspects of boxing. *Int J Psych Med* **25** 249–62

(28) G Forrester, G Geffen 1995 *Julia Farr Centre—Post Traumatic Amnesia Scales Manual*. Glenelg Press, Adelaide

(29) G Forrester *et al* 1994 Measuring post-traumatic amnesia (PTA): An historical review. *Brain Injury* **8** 175–84

(30) D Wechsler, 1981 *Wechsler Adult Intelligence Scale—Revised*. Psychological Corporation, New York

(31) D Gronwall 1977 Paced auditory serial-addition task: A measure of recovery from concussion. *Percept. Motor Skills* **44** 367–73

(32) A Baddeley *et al* 1992 *The Speed and Capacity of Language Processing Test*. Thames Valley Test Company, Bury St Edmunds, UK

(33) A Smith 1982 *The Symbol Digit Modalities Test*. Western Psychological Services, Los Angeles

(34) AD Hinton-Bayre *et al* 1997 Mild head injury and speed of information processing: A prospective study of professional rugby league players. *J Clin Exp Neuropsychol* **19** 275–89

(35) AD Hinton-Bayre *et al* Impairment and recovery of speed of information processing after mild head injury: A prospective study of rugby league players. *Int Perspect Traum Brain Injury* 1997 J Ponsford, P Snow, V Anderson (ed) Australia Academic Press: Melbourne p291–8

(36) D Maddocks M Saling 1996 Neuropsychological deficits following concussion. *Brain Injury* **10** 99–103

(37) SN Macciocchi *et al* 1996 Neuropsychological functioning and recovery after mild head injury in collegiate athletes. *Neurosurgery* **39** 510–14

(38) EA Montgomery *et al* 1991 The psychobiology of minor head injury. *Psychol Med* **21** 375–84

(39) KM Guskiewicz *et al* 1996 Effects of mild head injury on postural stability in athletes. *J Athletic Training* **31** 300

(40) AP Garnham, 1992 Injuries to the head, eye and ear. In J Bloomfield *et al* (ed) *Textbook of science and medicine in sport* Blackwell Scientific, Melbourne

Appendix A
Previous sports head injuries—structured interview

Explain the nature of concussion.

A concussion can result from a direct blow to the head or even from the heavy contact of bodies, without actual head contact. You may have been concussed if you were knocked unconscious or if you were unable to remember part of a game clearly (that is, you had a gap in your memory). You may have just been confused or disoriented for a period of time. After a concussion you may have experienced headaches, blurred vision, nausea, dizziness, tiredness, irritability, loss of coordination, or difficulty concentrating or remembering things

Over your sporting career have you ever been concussed during an event?

If **Yes** go to (1)

If **No** go to (14)

(1) How many times have you been concussed?

(2) How long ago was your most recent concussion (weeks, months, years)?

(3) Were you knocked unconscious? If **Yes** how long?

(4) Was there a period of time where you were confused or disoriented or you could not remember the incident or you had a gap in your memory? If **Yes** how long?

(5) How many times have you been actually been knocked unconscious?

Ask (6)–(10) only if a player has had more than one concussion

(6) When was the last time you were knocked unconscious?

(7) What was the longest period of time you have been knocked unconscious?

(8) How many times have you had a memory gap after a concussion?

(9) What was the longest gap in your memory after a concussion?

(10) In which years did each of your concussions occur?

Restart here if only one concussion.

(11) Have you missed any games due to concussion? If YES how many?

(12) Have you ever been off work or other activities because of a concussion? If YES how long?

(13) Do you believe you have changed in any of the following ways as a result of your head injuries?

Rate each: 0 'no' to 4 'greatly'

Mental—attention, memory, decision making, follow conversation, detailed instructions, fatigue easily.

Physical—fatigue more easily, increased sleep.

Emotional—depressed, anxious, irritated more easily.

Social—enjoy leisure activities, relationships, friends, family commitments.

Work—maintaining workload, increasing productivity.

Playing ability—fatigue, decision speed, reaction time, skills under pressure.

Begin here if no previous sports-related concussion.

(14) Over your career how many non-head injuries have you had that required you to miss a game

(15) How many games have you missed due to non-head injuries?

(16) Have you ever received a head injury outside of competitive contact sport?

If the athlete says **Yes**, . . . *record length of unconsciousness, post-traumatic amnesia, and other clinical symptoms*

6 Eye and face

LAWRENCE TRIEU

180

1 NR Galloway 1990 In MA Hutson (ed) *Sports injuries: recognition and management* p25–9. OUP 2 E Hollenbach, I Ho 1997 In E Sherry, D Bokor (ed) *Sports medicine—problems and practical management* p91–103 GMM, London
3 L Lim 1997 In E Sherry, D Bokor (ed) *Sports medicine—problems and practical management* p83–90 GMM, London

Section I The eye

Introduction

Although the eye accounts for only 0.002% of the body's surface area[1] and has many protective mechanisms including rapid reflex lid closure, production of tears, and protection by bony orbital ridges, eye injuries due to sport are nevertheless common, accounting for 1–2% of all sports injuries. High-risk sports include basketball, squash, and contact sports such as football and boxing. A thorough examination is required for all eye injuries, even those that appear to be minor. All serious eye injuries and ideally all eye injuries should be examined by an ophthalmologist, but this is not always possible or practical. The clinician dealing with eye injuries must therefore have a thorough knowledge of the anatomy (Fig. 6.1) and physiology of the eye, and be able to treat minor eye injuries whilst being able to recognize and refer serious injuries to an ophthalmologist.

1 NP Jones 1989 *Sports Medicine* **7** 163–81

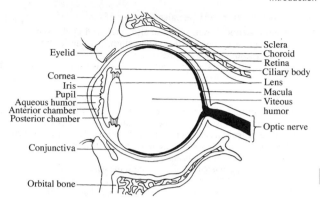

Fig. 6.1 Anatomy of the eye

Assessing an eye injury

Necessary equipment (see also Chapter 25)
- Ophthalmoscope, torch, visual acuity card, and eyelid speculum.
- Sterile single-use vials of fluorescein stain, mydriatic drops, anesthetic drops, and saline for irrigation.
- Sterile eye pads, eye shield (plastic/metal), cotton-tipped swabs, and tape.

History

In all eye injuries a thorough history detailing the mechanism of injury is vital. Of most importance is visual status—whether there has been any decrease in visual acuity after the injury. It is also important to ask what the patient's visual acuity prior to the injury was like. A detailed history should include:

Symptoms experienced. Ask the patient whether there is pain, blurred vision, double vision, or a decrease in visual acuity. Photophobia is suggestive of traumatic iritis, whereas floaters and flashing lights suggest a retinal detachment, tear, or vitreous hemorrhage. Diplopia is associated with blowout fractures. Loss of consciousness or altered mental status suggests significant trauma and additional injuries. Ask whether there has been any discharge, tearing, itching, burning, redness, headache, or altered facial sensation.

Mechanism of injury—velocity of injury causing particles, nature of particles involved, blunt injury v projectiles, whether protective equipment was worn at time of injury.

Ophthalmic history—previous eye injuries and eye problems, and whether spectacles or contact lenses are worn normally.

General medical and surgical history

Eye examination

In order to perform a satisfactory eye examination a clean location with good illumination is required. A thorough eye examination should always be performed with the unaffected eye used for comparison. The following routine is suggested:

- *Visual acuity* should be tested first as other examinations may require the instillation of mydriatics. The exception to this rule is chemical injury where irrigation of the eye takes precedence over examination. Visual acuity is tested using a Snellen chart or card. If unavailable a newspaper should be used. Each eye should be tested individually, while the other is covered by a small card or the palm of the hand, using the best corrected vision (if glasses are normally used by the patient these should be worn during the test). A patient unable to read the largest letter should be asked to count the number of fingers the examiner holds up. If this cannot be done then the perception of hand movement should be tested. Failing this perception of light using a torch should be tested.
- *Inspect the eyelids* for lacerations, hemotoma, and bruising.
- *Evert the eyelids* (instruct the patient to look down with their chin elevated) and inspect the conjunctival sac for signs of trauma and for foreign bodies. (See Fig. 6.2.)

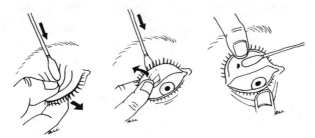

Fig. 6.2 Eyelid eversion to remove a foreign body

185

- *Examine the cornea and sclera* for surface irregularities, perforations, subconjunctival hemorrhages, iris prolapses, and foreign bodies. A magnifying lens or ophthalmoscope should be used. Fluorescein dye may aid in outlining corneal abrasions, which appear bright green under blue cobalt light.
- *Examine the anterior chamber.* Any haziness, the presence of blood and the depth should be noted. Examine the optic disk and retina. Look for the red reflex (reduced with retinal detachment, hemorrhage, or cataract). A thorough ocular examination should also include examination with a slit-lamp.
- *Inspect pupils.* Note size and shape. Test light reflexes—direct and consensual responses, and perform the swinging torch test.
- *Compare the iris colors* of each eye and look for iridodonesis (trembling of the iris with quick visual movements due to lack of support, e.g. in lens subluxation).
- *Examine visual fields* carefully and note any defects.
- *Examine the face* looking for signs of orbital fractures, nerve palsies, and altered face sensation.
- *General examination.* Ensure that no other more urgent injuries have been sustained.

Types of injuries (see Fig. 6.3)

Orbital hemorrhage (black eye)

May occur after blunt trauma to the orbital region. **Clinical features**: proptosis of affected eye, hemorrhage into the eyelids and beneath the conjunctiva, and restriction of eye movements. In cases of severe hemorrhage, there may be visual loss due to interruption of vascular supply to the optic nerve and retina, whereupon the patient should be **transported urgently with head elevated and ice pack applied, to a hospital with an ophthalmology department**. **Treatment**: if the eye is difficult to examine or the lid is swollen shut, do not force it open. Instead, an ophthalmologist should be consulted. In most cases, the swelling is usually self-limiting and the interstitial blood resorbed within a few weeks. Ice packs should be applied during the first 24h.

Lid lacerations

May be the result of sharp objects, blunt trauma, or an object catching the lid and causing a tear. **Treatment**: control bleeding with direct pressure and assess extent of injury. A thorough ocular examination must be performed to exclude ocular injury and any foreign body in the eye must be identified and recorded. The eye should be padded and the patient referred for surgical repair of the laceration to minimize cosmetic deformity. **Complications**: lacerations near the medial canthus may also involve the lacrimal canaliculus and if not repaired, the patient may have permanent tearing.

Conjunctival foreign bodies

Are very painful and are usually the result of dirt or mud thrust into the eye when there is contact with the ground after a tackle in a contact sport. They are most commonly located under the upper eyelid. **Treatment**: removal of the foreign body by irrigation with sterile saline and light brushing with a cotton bud. The upper and lower eyelids are everted by asking the patient to look downward whilst the examiner pulls the lid away from the eyeball (Fig. 6.2). Ophthalmologic consultation should be sought if the foreign body is not removed easily.

Corneal foreign bodies

These arise from the same mechanism as conjunctival foreign bodies. In most cases the foreign body is readily removed by irrigation with saline and use of a cotton bud. If the foreign body is embedded the eye should be anaesthetized and stained with fluorescein dye to assist with examination and treatment. **Treatment**: should be performed by an ophthalmologist if available (if the foreign body overlies the pupil it must be referred to an ophthalmologist for removal). The patient's eyes should be stabilized by asking him/her to fix on an object in the distance. The foreign object is removed by carefully scraping with a sterile 24-gauge needle held at a tangent to the cornea under magnification and bright illumination. Chloromphenicol ointment should be applied and the eye padded.

Corneal abrasions

One of the most common ocular injuries in contact sports and also seen in leisure activities. Frank injury (blown dust particles and

Hyphemia

Subconjunctival hemorrhage

Penetrating injury

Marginal laceration

Fig. 6.3 Types of eye injury

fingernails), wearing of contact lenses for extended periods of time, chemicals, and ultraviolet light may cause denuding of the corneal epithelium. **Symptoms**: may include severe pain, blurred vision, photophobia, lacrimation and blepharospasm. **Signs**: decreased visual acuity if the central cornea is extensively denuded. Careful examination with a slit-lamp and fluorescein dye to aid in revealing the extent of the injured area is indicated. The eyelids should also be everted to ensure foreign bodies are not present. **Treatment**: antibiotic drops such as chloromphenicol and daily review for the presence of infection until the fluorescein stain is no longer visible. Corneal abrasions normally heal within 48h. Contact lenses must not be worn until healing is complete. If the abrasion persists for more than 48h or increases in size, consultation with an ophthalmologist is advisable. **Complications**: ulcer formation and infection.

Conjunctival lacerations

Result in severe tearing pain, photophobia, blepharospasm. Do not forcibly open the eyelids, squeeze the eye closed, or put pressure on the eye as this may cause further damage by increasing the intraocular pressure. If the eye can be opened easily, an irregular pupil may be seen, along with a shallow anterior chamber and an iris adherent to the wound outside. Lightly pad and transfer to a hospital with an ophthalmology department.

Subconjunctival hemorrhage (SCH)

May result from trauma, severe hypertension, blood dyscrasias, or can occur spontaneously.[1] It also occurs in sports such as weight lifting and scuba diving where there is a change in intravascular pressure, and in mountain climbing where there is strenuous exertion under conditions of reduced oxygen saturation. **Symptoms**: in cases of extensive hemorrhage, photophobia and decreased visual acuity may be present, otherwise this condition is usually asymptomatic. **Signs**: a SCH appears as a bright red area in the white conjuctiva. **Treatment**: BP should be measured and hypertension if present, investigated further. In cases of trauma, a thorough eye examination should be performed. In most cases no further action other than reassurance of the athlete is required as SCH is a benign condition which resolves without treatment within 2 weeks of onset.

Chemical burns

An ocular emergency. May be the result of lime used in line markings on playing fields or chlorine and other swimming pool chemicals. **Treatment**: first aid involves holding the eyes open and irrigating with water for 20min. The eyelids must be everted to ensure that the chemical is completely removed. Neutralizing agents should be used if available. The initial injury may appear deceptively mild but later examination may reveal generalized superficial corneal scarring and injury which may require hospital treatment. **Complications**: iritis, uveitis, secondary glaucoma, and phthisis bulbi.

1 LP Fong 1994 *MJA* **160** 743–50

Hyphema

Is a collection of free blood in the anterior chamber of the eye, arising from bleeding of the small vessels of the iris as a result of blunt trauma to the eye (e.g. being struck by a ball). It is by far the most common sports-related intraocular injury requiring hospital admission. **Symptoms**: *Immediate*: pain, blurring of vision. *Within minutes*: photophobia, redness. The patient may also feel drowsy due to concussion or due to the hyphema itself. **Signs**—at the time of injury a hazy anterior chamber is seen, which with rest settles to form a fluid level. The iris appears muddy in comparison to the unaffected eye, and the pupils are irregular and slow to react to light. A corneal abrasion may also be present. **Treatment**—although most hyphemas self-resolve by absorption within a few days, in about one-eighth of cases rebleeding occurs. Hence, immediate referral to an ophthalmologist is necessary. Treatment involves padding of both eyes, and absolute bedrest (usually with sedation) for 5–6 days. The patient should be instructed to avoid aspirin. **Complications**: ocular hypertension, secondary glaucoma, bloodstaining of the cornea, and permanent visual impairment. In some patients, antiglaucoma medical therapy and surgery may be required.

Posterior Chamber Injuries

Macular injuries

Concussion of the globe with a contrecoup force may cause macular oedema resulting in the formation of a macular cyst. Severe impairment of central vision results, which may become permanent if the cyst ruptures and causes a macular hole. There is no treatment.

Choroidal injuries

Are usually the result of a blow to the eye by a blunt object such as a squash ball. Visual acuity is markedly reduced in the affected eye if splitting of the macular area occurs. On examination circumscribed white areas concentric to the optic disk can be observed. Choroidal hemorrhages without rupture can also occur, resulting in necrosis of the choroid and retina in the area involved. In both conditions there is no specific treatment, but ophthalmologic consultation should be sought and prolonged rest is necessary for healing.

Injuries to the lens

Occur after blunt trauma. Cataract formation due to opacification of the crystalline substance of the lens may follow immediately, or after a few days, weeks, or months. Severe blows can cause the lens to rupture and allow aqueous humour from the anterior chamber to enter the lens and lead to formation of a cataract (usually in the shape of a rosette in the subcapsular area). Treatment of cataracts involves removal of the lens. Contact lenses are used to restore refractive power.

Lens dislocation

After blunt trauma or a collision in a contact sport the lens zonule may rupture and allow the unanchored lens to displace itself into the vitreous or migrate anteriorly into the anterior chamber. **Symptoms**:

partial dislocations are usually asymptomatic. Complete dislocations result in blurred vision which may also be accompanied by monocular diplopia and pain. **Signs**: the classic sign is quivering of the iris when the patient moves the affected eye (iridodonesis). Other signs include decreased visual acuity and a decentred lens. **Treatment**: immediate ophthalmologic consultation is advisable. Surgical removal of the lens may be required. **Complications**: iritis and glaucoma.

Retinal injuries

Are sustained by blunt trauma to the eye and may occur independently of anterior segment injuries. All retinal injuries require referral to an ophthalmologist.

Retinal hemorrhage and oedema

The macular area is usually involved, resulting in blurred central vision. On examination a whitish elevated retina is seen and there is a decreased pupillary reflex.

Retinal detachments

Commonly follow a blow to the eye. The temporal quadrant is most commonly affected. **Symptoms**: flashes of light, floaters, or curtains coming down over the field of view are commonly reported. In some cases there is a delay of weeks after the injury before the onset of symptoms. **Signs**: an early detached retina appears elevated and progresses to a grey color. The overlying retinal vessels appear almost black. The red reflex becomes grey and there is a decreased pupillary reflex. **Treatment**: **an ocular emergency** requiring immediate treatment by an ophthalmologist. Successful recovery requires early treatment because if the detachment is allowed to progress to involve the macular area, there will be a degree of permanent loss of central vision even if the retina is successfully reattached later. The majority of detachments are now surgically treated with a laser.

Optic nerve injuries

May result from severe direct injuries to the eye but more commonly follow blunt injury to the head producing permanent blindness. The visual loss is usually the result of shearing of the nutrient vessels to the nerve rather than a fracture of the optic canal. On examination there is an abnormal pupillary response to light and a pale, swollen disk can be seen though the ophthalmoscope.

Orbital injuries

Blowout orbital fractures are sustained after blunt trauma to the eye, usually the result of being hit by a squash ball or being punched or kicked. The eye is forced back into the orbit and this causes a sudden increase in intraorbital pressure and a blowout fracture of the weakest part of the orbit, the thin orbital floor. Herniation of intraorbital contents may then occur through the defect in bone. The orbital margins, however, usually remain intact as the thicker bone there offers higher resistance. **Clinical features** include:

- *Weakness in ocular movement*—elevation is particularly affected because of entrapment of the inferior rectus and inferior oblique muscles. For the same reason diplopia, which is commonly present, is more marked on vertical gaze.

- *Enophthalmos*—usually with a downward displacement due to orbital herniation into the maxillary sinus.
- *Paresthesia or anesthesia*—around the cheek below the eye due to injury of the intraorbital nerve.
- Other signs may include ecchymosis, oedema, and subcutaneous emphysema.

  Treatment[1] is as follows:
- On diagnosis antibiotics should be started to prevent orbital cellulitis.
- Examination of the eye by an ophthalmologist and investigation of the fracture with x-ray and CT scan is mandatory.
- In some cases, the trapped inferior ocular muscles can be freed by elevating the eye with forceps after topical anesthesia, otherwise surgical exploration and repair will be necessary.

Medial wall orbital fractures

Occur in a similar manner to orbital blowout fractures but are less common. **Clinical features** may include:

- *Subcutaneous emphysema* around the nose and eyelids which can be accentuated if the patient blows his/her nose. However, this should be diskouraged as infected sinus contents could be blown intraorbitally.
- *Epiphora* if there is involvement of the nasolacrimal duct and it is occluded. Secondary dacryocystitis may follow later.
- *Weakness of lateral eye movements and diplopia* during lateral gaze if the medial rectus muscle is entrapped.

  Treatment: x-rays may demonstrate clouding of the maxillary sinus, herniated contents in the maxillary sinus, air in the orbit and rarely, the fracture itself. CT scans offer higher resolution and should be performed when there is doubt. Treatment is usually conservative unless there is entrapment of the medial rectus muscle in which case surgical repair is indicated. Antibiotics should be prescribed to prevent orbital cellulitis, the eye padded and the patient instructed not to blow his/her nose. The fracture will unite in most cases, otherwise surgery is required.

Penetrating injuries

Must always be suspected and excluded in all ocular injuries. The following conditions and signs suggest that a penetrating may have occurred: hyphema, subconjunctival hemorrhage, asymmetrical depth of the anterior chamber, and difference in intraocular pressure. If a penetrating injury is suspected urgent ophthalmologic referral is indicated as the longer the delay the greater the risk of the lens being damaged or the ocular contents being extruded or infected. Further damage can also be caused by attempting to remove the object or forcefully open the eye for examination. The patient should be transported to hospital supine and the injured eye supported by light padding. The unaffected eye should also be padded to prevent damage from conjugate movement. A CT or skull x-ray should be performed to exclude an intraocular foreign object.

1 LA Forrest *et al* 1989 *Am J Sports Med* **17** 217–20

Prevention of eye injuries

Many eye injuries are preventable. All too often, eye injuries occur because advice is ignored or because of careless regard for the rules of a particular sport. The role of the sports medicine physician in prevention therefore not only involves giving advice about forms of eye protection but to ensure that that this advice is followed. Strict enforcement of rules by umpires, referees, and governing bodies will also prevent many eye injuries and make the sport safer.

Spectacles and goggles

Adequate visual acuity is necessary not only for effective performance but also for the prevention of injuries to the eye. Spectacles or goggles, in addition to correcting vision, should also afford adequate eye protection for the sport concerned. Many spectacles and goggles are available which have been specifically designed for use in sports, and should be encouraged to be worn wherever there is a risk of eye injury. Prescription lenses should ideally be made of polycarbonate lenses with a thickness of at least 3mm at the center as these withstand not only the impact of a squash ball but also a gunshot. If the prescription is too high for polycarbonate CR39[TM] plastic[1] is the best alternative.[2] Glass lenses even of the 'toughened' or 'safety' types should never be used. A sturdy polycarbonate frame with a steep posterior lip should be used, so that the lens does not dislodge posteriorly. Use of metal frames is not advisable as they can cut the face and also cause eye injuries. Those not requiring a prescription should wear a wraparound eyeguard with good lateral protection.

Contact lenses

Have become popular among athletes as they overcome the disadvantages of spectacles that may have heavy frames, become knocked off, or fog-up. However, there are some disadvantages though: hard contact lenses may break and injure the eye, and should not be used in any contact sport (soft lenses appear to be safe), while all lenses may become displaced from the eye and lost on the playing field. In addition, contact lenses offer no protection whatsoever from eye injury so it is still important to wear eye protection during all high-risk sporting activities.

Refractive surgery

To rehabilitate visually refractive errors of the eye continues to evolve at a significant pace and will play an increasingly important role on the sporting field as its advantages are more widely realized. One of the first corrective refractive procedures was radial keratotomy, used to correct ametropia, which involved carefully planned incisions in the cornea. More recently, techniques such as photo-astigmatic refractive keratectomy, photo-therapeutic keratectomy (PTK), and photo-refractive keratomy (PRK) using a laser to ablate and recontour the corneal surface have been developed. They will be increasingly employed to correct myopia, hyperopia, astigmatism, and age-related presbyopia as the safety and effectiveness of these techniques improve.

1 CR39 is a registered trademark of PPG Industrial   2 TJ Pashby, RC Pashby 1994 In FH Fu, DA Stone (ed) *Sports injuries: mechanisms, prevention, and treatment* p833–51. Williams & Wilkins, Baltimore

Face protection (see also Chapter 24)

In certain sports (e.g. cricket, American football, ice hockey) it is important not only to protect the eye but facial structures as well with protective helmets and faceguards. It is imperative that these offer adequate eye protections as well.

Athletes with high risk of eye injuries

Athletes with certain eye conditions are at a very high risk of eye injury and should be evaluated by an ophthalmologist prior to participating in a high-risk sport. These problems are:

- one good eye
- severe amblyopia (lazy eye)
- history of retinal detachments or tears
- diabetic retinopathy
- Marfan's syndrome
- homocystinuria
- severe myopia (>6 dioptres) as an elongated globe is a strong risk factor for retinal detachment
- recent eye surgery

Protective eyewear should be encouraged to be worn whenever playing a sport that could lead to eye injury, and if possible persons with these conditions should be discouraged from participating in high-risk sports altogether.

Section II: The face

Introduction

Maxillofacial injuries in sport are usually the result of direct trauma and include fractures of the facial skeleton, intra- and extraoral lacerations, and dental trauma. Although face masks, helmets and mouthguards have reduced the number of facial injuries in sports such as American football, cricket, and ice hockey[1], the incidence of facial injuries is still significant.

1 RF LaPrade *et al* 1995 *Am J Sports Med* **23** 773–5

Fractures of the mandible

Are the most common maxillofacial injury from sport and are usually the result of a direct blow. Mandibular fracture patterns include condyle, angle, body, symphysis, ramus (rare), and coronoid process (rare).

Condylar fractures

The condyle is the most common site of mandibular fracture. Most fractures are subcondylar fracturing through the weak area at the neck of the condyle. The fracture may be undisplaced, displaced (anterior-medially due to pull of the lateral pterygoid muscle, condyle remains within the glenoid fossa), or dislocated. **Symptoms**: pain and tenderness from the temporomandibular joint (TMJ), exacerbated if the patient opens his/her mouth or clenches his/her teeth. **Signs**: swelling in front of the ear, alteration of the natural bite (occluded) position with gagging of the posterior molars, deviation in mandibular movements on opening towards the side of the fracture. **Investigations**: the diagnosis is frequently missed. The orthopantomogram (OPG) and posterior-anterior (PA) mandible x-ray must be carefully studied by outlining the contour of the condyles bilaterally. **Treatment**: maintenance of the airway is the first priority in fractures of the mandible. If the patient is conscious they should be advised to support the lower jaw with their hands in a forward sitting position. If the fracture is comminuted or displaced then a bandage or cervical collar may be applied taking care not to compromise the airway by causing backward displacement of the mandible. Unconscious patients should be placed in a lateral ('coma') position so that blood and saliva can drain from the mouth. The mouth should be cleared of any dislodged teeth, dentures, blood, and other foreign bodies then the head tilted and jaw supported.

In children, management of condylar fractures is non-surgical because remodeling occurs with complete regeneration of the normal condylar anatomy. Jaw exercises to achieve normal occlusion is usually all that is required. If normal occlusion is not consistently attainable then intermaxillary fixation for 2 weeks followed by a period of guiding elastics may be required.

In adults, management of subcondylar fracture is controversial. There are opposing views on whether displaced condylar fractures should be treated by open or closed reduction. Lim[1] suggests that open reduction should be reserved for gross fracture dislocations and when correct occlusion cannot be attained by closed reduction. In the majority of cases of condylar fracture in adults there is minimal alteration to the occlusion position. The patient is able to achieve a correct occlusion with a minimum of effort and simple jaw exercises may be all that is required to achieve a consistent occlusion. Good results have been achieved by both conservative management and open reduction but it seems preferable to avoid surgery if it is possible to do so without compromise to the outcome. If the occlusion is not readily achieved then this is an indication for closed reduction. Arched bars are placed and the patient is placed into intermaxillary fixation for a period of 2 weeks after which it is released and guiding elastics used for a further 2–4 weeks.

1 L Lim In E Sherry, D Bokor (ed) *Sports medicine problems and practical management* p83–90. GMM London

Fractures of the angle

The angle is the second most common site of mandibular fracture, usually occurring through the unerupted lower third molar. A concomitant body fracture or subcondylar fracture contralaterally may be present. Bilateral angle fractures are not common. **Symptoms**: the patient will state that their bite feels different from normal (change in occlusion). There may also be altered sensation of the lower lip and chin due to injury to the inferior alveolar nerve. **Signs**: the teeth do not interdigitate well into the occlusion.

Fractures of the body

Fracture of the body of the mandible may be midline (symphyseal), lateral to the midline (parasymphyseal), or midbody (molar and premolar area). Symphyseal fractures usually present with little displacement. They are difficult to demonstrate on x-ray.

Parasymphyseal fractures usually present with considerable displacement and can be very mobile. **Clinical features**: there is pain and diskomfort as well as swelling and ecchymosis. There may be loose teeth present on either side of the fracture. **Treatment**: with undisplaced surgery is not usually required. Treatment is with antibiotics, a soft diet and regular review. The treatment for displaced fracture is open reduction and fixation. While the patient is awaiting definitive surgery, stabilization of the fracture with a simple wire passed interdentally and on either side of the fracture can improve patient comfort. Postoperative care includes antibiotics, a soft diet, strict oral hygiene and avoidance of contact sports for at least 6 weeks.

Midbody fractures are usually unilateral and present with very little displacement since the muscles on either side of the fracture site have a counteracting action on each other.

Fractures of the maxilla

Are usually caused by direct trauma to the middle third of the facial skeleton and are much less common than fractures of the mandible. They are classified according to the system devised by René Le Fort in 1900 from cadaver experiments, as Le Fort I, II, and III, depending on the involvement of the maxillary, nasal, and zygomatic bones. **Clinical features**: the signs and symptoms of Le Fort I and II fractures appear very similar and can only be differentiated with careful examination by palpation and x-ray of the zygomatic bone which is not fractured in a Le Fort II fracture. They include bilateral circumorbital and subconjunctival ecchymosis ('racoon eyes'), facial oedema, mobility of the third of the face, paresthesia in the distribution of the infraorbital nerve, CSF rhinorrhea indicating fracture of the cribiform plate, diplopia, and enopthalmos. In all Le Fort fractures lengthening of the face also occurs because the middle third of the facial skeleton is displaced downward and backward causing an anterior open bite occlusion due to retropositioning of the anterior incisors behind the lower incisor teeth. **Treatment**: maxillary fractures can cause life-threatening embarrassment to the airways. Initial treatment therefore should be to ensure maintenance of the airways. Unconscious patients should be placed in the coma position whereas conscious patients nursed in the forward sitting position, as is the case with mandibular fractures. In some cases endotracheal intubation may be necessary. The patient should then be urgently transferred to a hospital for definitive surgical treatment which may involve closed reduction or open reduction and fixation with screws, wires, or plates.

Zygomaticomaxillary complex fractures

Are the second most common fracture of the facial skeleton due to sporting accidents, occurring from direct trauma to the cheek in sports such as hockey, baseball, and boxing. **Clinical features**: periorbital swelling and bruising, flatness of the cheek, limited mandibular opening, and tenderness to palpation at the maxillary buttress. If there is a concomitant orbital fracture then there may be paresthesia in the distribution of the infra-orbital nerve, diplopia, enopthalmos, and limitation of ocular movement. **Investigations**: coronal CT scan, x-ray (occipitomental and submentovertex). **Treatment**: *the first priority* is to assess the globe and protect it from any further injury, as ocular injuries occur in 5% of fractures of the zygoma. The patient should be transported to a hospital for definitive treatment which in most cases will involve open reduction and internal fixation. For minimally displaced fractures, a simple elevation of the zygoma via a Gilles' temporal approach may be all that is required.

Nasal fractures

Fractures of the nasal bone and cartilage are usually caused by a direct blow and can be either high or more commonly low velocity type fractures. **Clinical features**: pain, epistaxis, nasal swelling, crepitus over the nasal bridge, nasal deviation and deformity, and nasal airway obstruction. **Investigations**: radiographs of the nasal bone views may be of help. **Treatment**: secure the airways and control bleeding with external pressure and intranasal packing. Undisplaced fractures do not require any further treatment whereas displaced fractures should be reduced if there is obstruction of the nasal passages, or for cosmetic reasons.

Temporomandibular joint injuries

Blows to the TMJ area can produce a variety of injuries including hemarthrosis, capsulitis, meniscal displacement, and intracapsular fracture of the head of the condyle. TMJ dislocation results if the mandible is hit while the mouth is open. Some injuries may be occult with complications arising months after the traumatic event. **Clinical features**: limitation of mouth opening with pain or deviation, malocclusion, clicking, pain and difficulty closing the mouth. **Treatment**: rest with limitation of mouth opening for 1 week, a soft diet, and NSAIDs or surgery (arthroplasty). A dislocation can be reduced by grasping each side of the jaw with thumbs inside the mouth as far back as possible (away from teeth) and pushing down and posteriorly. After surgery, the patient should be advised to avoid contact sports for at least 2 months and use a mouthguard until participation in such sports is resumed.

Dental injuries

Teeth may be impacted, displaced, avulsed or broken through collisions with other participants during contact sports or from direct
trauma with equipment such as bats, sticks, and balls. In all cases of
facial trauma a thorough examination of the oral cavity should be
performed and if a tooth or tooth fragment can not be located then x-
rays of the chest and abdomen should be performed.

7 Spine

JOHN D YEO

Biomechanics

Anatomy of the spinal cord

Within the human spinal canal the spinal cord extends from the base of the brain to the conus medallaris usually at the level of the L1/L2 vertebrae when the nerve roots become the cauda equina. The spinal cord is a soft, pliable mass of nerve fibers and cells supported by glial tissue and enmeshed in small blood vessels. The cord contains myelinated 'long' tracts and interconnecting fibers described as the 'white matter' surrounding the central 'grey matter' comprising mostly unmyelinated nerve fibers with supporting glial tissue and a very intense small blood vessel network. Blood flow to the spinal cord is mainly provided to the anterior two-thirds of the cord by the anterior spinal artery which arises from two branches of each vertebral artery over the medulla and runs superficially in the anterior sulcus to synapse eventually around the lower end of the spinal cord with the descending branches of the posterior spinal arteries which arise from the posterior inferior cerebellar arteries. Posterior spinal arteries provide blood flow to the posterior third of the spinal cord.

These small spinal arteries require additional assistance from the major supplementary arterial supply usually at two levels of the spinal cord (T1 and T11), from the corresponding intercostal arteries.

Nerve fibers in the posterior columns of white matter are essentially traveling cephalward and are uncrossed until higher in the CNS carrying sensory modalities for proprioception, vibration, some touch, and appreciation of moderate degrees of temperature variation. Tracts in the anterior column of white matter are mainly traveling caudalward to synapse either directly with anterior horn cells or with other interneuronal pathways. In the lateral column there is a mix of fibers going 'upwards and downwards'. The lateral column contains the lateral corticospinal pathway (pyramidal pathway) for control of motor power and anteriorly is the main tract for pain (spinothalamic) which are mostly crossed fibers. In the cervical spinal cord the nerves in this tract have a laminated arrangement with the most distant fibers traveling towards the distal end of the body (sacral) and the cervical traveling more central within the tract. Anteriorly to the pain pathway is the main pathway for temperature and further anteriorly again is the pathway for touch. Touch appears to be transmitted in the anterior and posterior columns. The corticospinal pathway also has a layered orientation with those motor fibers destined to synapse with anterior horn cells in the lower spinal cord (lumbosacral) traveling in the more superficial layers of the tract in the cervical region. There remains a complex arborization of synapsing fibers within the spinal cord and many interneuronal pathways are necessary to achieve balanced efferent and afferent activities within the human spinal cord. The spinal cord tends to occupy only 50% of the ligamentum denticulatum and in the intervertebral foramina.

The dura mater is also attached firmly to the base of the skull and at the second fused segment of the sacrum in the adult (filum terminale).

There is therefore a lateral attachment of the spinal cord to both sides of the spinal canal. The spinal cord within the dura is a mobile organ which tends to be held more tightly in the flexed position of the spine and in a more relaxed position when the spine is extended.

The spinal canal is formed by 26 vertebrae, 24 usually being separate from each other but attached with intervening disks, ligaments, and muscles. The coccyx is attached to the lower end of the sacrum and usually comprises 4 small fused vertebrae of a vestigial 'tail'. The sacrum usually consists of 5 vertebrae also fused together. The stable spinal column is maintained with a cervical lordotic curve, a thoracic kyphotic curve, and a lumbar lordotic curve. There are fixed kyphotic curves in the fused sacrum and coccyx.

The spinal vertebral column (Fig. 7.1) can be subdivided into the Denis 3-column classification, with an *anterior column*, which includes the anterior longitudinal spinal ligament (ALL), the anterior annulus of the disk, and the anterior third of the vertebral body; the middle column under this classification includes the posterior spinal longitudinal ligament (PLL), the posterior annulus of the disk and the posterior two-thirds of the vertebral body; the *posterior column* involves the posterior bony arch with the spines, laminae, and pedicles, and attached ligaments including supraspinous, interpinous, ligamentum flavum, and capsules of the posterior facet joints.

The muscles immediately surrounding the spinal column and attached to the vertebrae are of great importance in maintaining stability. In addition to those muscles which are closely applied to the vertebrae, there is the additional 'wider circle' of muscles which includes the larger spinal muscles (e.g. trapezius, latissimus dorsi, and the abdominal muscles).

Each disk has a firm annulus fibrosus surrounding the nucleus pulposus, which is a softer, pliable material, and each disk is firmly attached to the adjacent surfaces of the vertebrae above and below. The posterior spinal longitudinal ligament is loosely attached to the disks. The annulus fibrosus has a nerve supply from the sinu vertebral nerve of Luschka.

Injury

Damage to the spinal cord can either occur from direct injury to the spinal cord tissue, including nerves, cells and supporting tissue (glia) within the spinal membranes or through injury to the blood vessels essential for cord function. Damage can occur to the anterior spinal artery, posterior spinal arteries, and the circumferential arteries which give off radiate branches running into the deeper central regions of the spinal cord. There is also a complex network of very small vessels, particularly within the grey matter which can be injured. There is now evidence to suggest further progressive damage will occur to nerves in the spinal cord within hours of the initial injury due to changes which occur in microvascular tissue within both grey and white matter. The exact nature of these progressive pathological changes has yet to be fully identified. A lack of efficient blood flow to the partly damaged nerve tissue can lead to additional ischemia and further damage to nerves which may have otherwise survived the initial direct injury.

Damage to the spinal cord is described as 'complete' if laceration or severe bruising has occurred at the level of the lesion. In adults, this injury is frequently associated with disturbance of the bony canal following fracture or fracture dislocation. In children there is often no obvious radiological evidence of significant damage to the vertebral column. Less serious injuries are described as 'incomplete' spinal cord

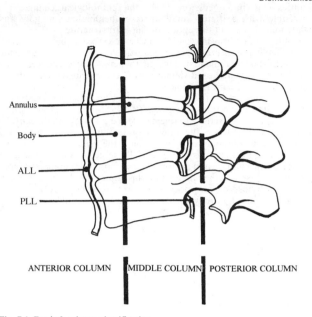

Annulus

Body

ALL

PLL

ANTERIOR COLUMN MIDDLE COLUMN POSTERIOR COLUMN

Fig. 7.1 Denis 3-column classification

injuries (e.g. in concussion where the pathological changes are reversible with scattered small areas of hemorrhage in grey and white matter without disruption of the cord structure).

Contusion, or bruising, which can be described as being (I) 'mild' where hemorrhages are larger in number and size than in concussion and with some permanent damage to nerve fibers and cells; (II) 'moderate' with increased damage and severe bruising resulting in complete loss of cord function.

The various areas of the spinal cord can be damaged resulting in specific clinical syndromes (e.g. the *Brown-Séquard syndrome* where damage is confined mostly to one half of the spinal cord); the *anterior column syndrome* where the anterolateral columns are often affected by damage to the anterior spinal artery; the *central cord syndrome* where the grey matter is the essentially affected area resulting in central cystic changes and profound loss of anterior columns without significant loss in other areas and this injury produces severe disability with loss of proprioception, even though there is usually significant voluntary movement below the level of the lesion.

Damage to the spinal vertebral column

Bones

Fractures in the vertebral bodies are described as *wedge fractures*, from flexion and compression injuries; *extension fractures* are associated with 'shearing' translational injuries; *compression fractures* is a burst injury to the vertebral body with retropulsion; a *slice injury* which can occur as a flexion and rotation causing damage to the vertebral body and interspinous and supraspinous ligament between the vertebrae.

Spondylolysis (Fig. 7.2) occurs with a defect in the pars interarticularis of the vertebral body. If the defect is bilateral possible shift may occur in the anterior and middle column segments of the spine following separation from the posterior spinal column segment. This is described as spondylolisthesis (Fig. 7.3) and identified as *grade 1* (i.e. 25% of the shift forward of one vertebra in relationship to another), up to greater than 50% of the vertebral displacement (*grade 4*). Ligaments and joint capsules are usually damaged including the interspinous ligaments, facet joint capsules, posterior longitudinal and anterior longitudinal ligament to allow subluxation of facet joints with the anterior vertebral subluxation. These injuries can be found in fast bowlers, baseball pitchers, gymnasts and weight lifters.

Damage can occur to the intervertebral disks (Fig. 7.4) resulting in mild bulging of the annulus, increasing to bulging with tearing of the fibrous annular tissue if more severe. Rupturing of the disk results when the nucleus pulposus herniates through a break in the annular wall frequently impinging on nearby spinal cord, cauda equina, or emerging nerve roots.

Damage to specific vertebrae

The C1 and C2 vertebrae (atlas and axis) damage. Fracture of the C1 ring secondary to axial compression can result in a Jefferson-type fracture. Rupture of the transverse ligament of the atlas produces instability. Consider potential instability if the atlantoaxial space is greater than 3mm in flexion in the adult and 4mm in a child. *Fractures of the odontoid* frequently produce pain which radiates posteriorly into the occipital area. The odontoid fractures are divided into *type 1* where there is a small segment of the odontoid fractured; *type 2* where the base of the odontoid is fractured; and *type 3* where the fracture extends from the base of the odontoid into the body of the C2 vertebra.

A 'hangman's fracture' (traumatic spondylolisthesis) occurs through the pedicles of C2 following hyperextension of the head and neck.

Damage to muscles, ligaments and tendons

Mild damage to muscles involves overstretch or direct bruising with more severe injury when muscle fibers are torn or disrupted at the insertion of the tendon. The ruptured fibers in the muscle belly will retract and ultimately heal with less elastic scar tissue.

The post-traumatic inflammatory process can localize at the insertion of muscles, tendons and ligaments near bone and is described as *enthesopathic inflammatory process* which can lead to calcification.

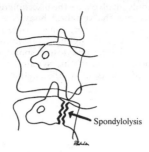

Fig. 7.2 Spondylolysis

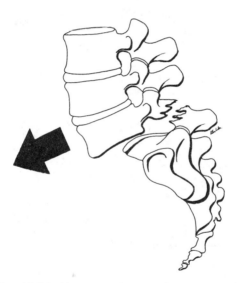

Fig. 7.3 Spondylolisthesis: Pars stress fracture with slip

Damage to the spinal vertebral column (*cont*)

The sites commonly involved are the insertion of the outer layer of the annulus fibrosus into the vertebral body, sometimes causing bony bridges between adjacent vertebrae (syndesmophytes). Injury to musculoskeletal tissue may highlight previously undiagnosed spondylarthropathies, including ankylosing spondylitis, spondylitis associated with psoriasis, enteropathic syndromes, Reiter's disease and arthritis associated with positive 'rheumatoid factor'.

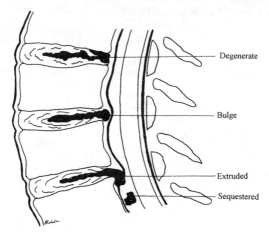

Fig. 7.4 Damage to intervertebral disks

Assessing the problem

Analysis of the patient with a spinal injury

When the patient is unconscious

If there is an associated head injury and the patient is unconscious, also consider spinal injury particularly involving cervical spine. Observe whether breathing is diaphragmatic. When intercostal muscles are weakened or paralysed from cervical spinal cord injury there will be a 'paradoxical'-type respiration with indrawing of the weakened intercostal muscles and prominent movement of the diaphragm. (Phrenic nerve supply is usually from C3, C4, C5 levels.)

Mid and lower cervical spine[1] (Fig. 7.5)

- *Compression fractures* Include wedging of anterior vertebral margin, secondary to flexion injury. Treatment: Sterno Occipital Mandibular Immobilisation (SOMI) brace immobilization. If associated with posterior instability—require fusion (greater than 50% of anterior vertebral height and associated posterior ligament injury).

- *Unilateral facet fracture/dislocation* Flexion rotation injury. Less than 33% subluxation on lateral x-ray. Neurological deficit usually root lesion or Brown–Sequard syndrome.

- *Bilateral facet fracture/dislocation* Flexion distraction injury with greater than 50% subluxation on lateral x-ray. Spinal cord injury is commonly associated with this injury. Treatment requires reduction, posterior stabilization, and fusion. Preoperative evaluation with CT scan is required. MRI is required to exclude disk protrusion behind superior vertebral body in all cases of bifacetal injury to prevent compression of spinal cord by disk material following reduction of dislocation as profound neurological deficit may result.

- *Burst fracture* Axial compression injury with fracture displaced into spinal canal. High incidence of spinal cord injury. Non-operative treatment may produce kyphosis and late neurological deficit generally requires anterior vertebrectomy and fusion.

- *Clay shoveller's fracture* Avulsion injury of spinous process (C7, C6, or T1). Stable, requires soft collar immobilization for comfort. Flexion extension radiographs required to exclude instability.

- *Neurological deficit without fracture* Occurs in patients with congenital narrowing of spinal canal and central disk protrusion, hyperextension injury or following spontaneous reduction of dislocation. MRI mandatory for evaluation.

- *Children's spine injuries* Are rare and when they do occur are at the C1–C2 level. It is often a soft tissue injury with subluxation. Vertebral growth plates may be damaged with later spinal deformity. Spinal cord injury can occur with a normal x-ray (SCIWORA).

- *Thoracolumbar spine* Is least susceptible to injury. The rib cage coupled with relative sagittal orientation of the facet joint protects the thoracic spine against injury. However, the thoracolumbar junction is the fulcrum between the mobile lumbar spine and relatively immobile thoracic spine and is very susceptible to injury.

The spinal cord usually ends at the L1/2 interspace. Structural

1 I Farey, C Huynh 1997 In E Sherry, D Bokor *Manual of sports medicine* GMM, London

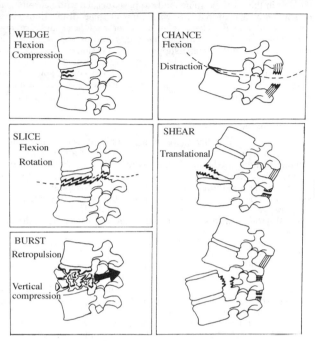

Fig. 7.5 Type of spinal fractures

damage in the thoracic spine tends to be associated with neurological deficit. Only 3% of patients with lumbar spine dislocations have neurological deficit. These tend to be at root level and are less debilitating. However, clinical instability of lumbar fractures is common. The lumbar spine supports high physiological loads. Late deformity, pain, and occasionally neurological deficit may develop following lumbar fractures. The 3-column concept of the spine allows stability to be assessed. Instability is present when 2 or 3 columns are disrupted. **Treatment** (*general* and *specific* is outlined in Tables 7.1 and 7.2.

When the patient is conscious

Ask the patient whether there is any pain and where this pain is located. Whether the patient can move upper or lower limbs, and whether there is any loss of feeling. When pain is present from injury to the spinal column or adjacent muscles ligaments or capsules, inevitably there is inhibition when movements precipitate or aggravate pain. The resulting restricted movement is therefore not necessarily the result of involvement of the spinal cord.

In all patients with suspected spinal injury consider the following important clinical signs:

- *Spinal Shock* All patients with significant spinal cord injury will have a period of spinal shock which may last as long as 2 days and occasionally for several weeks. This phenomenon produces loss of neuronal and reflex activity at and below the lesion, and is a pathophysiological phenomenon producing difficulties for the clinician who is attempting to identify the degree of underlying pathology within the apparently injured spinal cord. Complete spinal cord injury cannot be diagnosed until spinal shock has passed. Spinal shock has resolved when the bulbocavernosus reflex returns (anal sphincter contracts after squeezing the glans penis or by tugging on the urinary catheter).
- *Deformity* Fracture and fracture dislocations often do not produce obvious deformity. Fractures of the vertebrae can follow flexion, rotation, and compression injuries. Soft tissue damage, such as bruising or laceration to the face and skull, help to identify specific forces that produced the spinal injury. In children, frequently there is little evidence of external injury or bony displacement, although profound loss of motor power and sensory function has occurred from the spinal injury.

The site of the spinal cord lesion will eventually be identified as an 'upper motor neurone' lesion producing spastic tetraplegia or paraplegia or a 'lower motor neurone' lesion involving the central nerve cells, emerging nerve roots, or cauda equina with persisting flaccid paraplegia. Some patients remain with a 'flaccid' upper motor neurone-type lesion, where there is significant damage to length of spinal cord, such as in a gunshot wound or where there is obstruction to a main artery supplying the spinal cord (e.g. ruptured aortic aneurysm).

Table 7.1 General treatment of thoracolumbar spine injuries

- In general for *stable fractures* (well aligned, less than 30 kyphosis, and no neurological deficit) is rest, followed by bracing.
- *Unstable injuries*, or those with neurological deficit, usually require surgery to stabilize the fracture/dislocation to preserve or improve neurological function and to prevent late pain, instability, and neurological deficit.

Table 7.2 Specific treatment of thoracolumbar spine injuries

Injury	Mechanism/ Type	Treatment	Comment
Compression (wedge)	Flexion	Bedrest/orthosis (<50% loss of vertebral height)	Neurological deficit uncommon. Stabilization and fusion if associated posterior instability
Chance fracture	Flexion, distraction bony, and ligamentous involvement	Bedrest, hyperextension, orthosis, or stabilization and fusion	Neurological deficit uncommon. Duodenal or pancreatic injury common
Shear fracture and slice dislocations	Flexion/ rotation	Spinal stabilization and fusion	Neurological deficit common
Burst	Axial compression	Controversial Deficit Surgical decompression and fusion	
			No neurological deficit
		Bedrest/orthosis (unless kyphosis >300 and canal intrusion >50%	

Clinical analysis of sensory and motor disturbance (Figs. 7.6–7.8)

If spinal cord damage is considered likely then the clinical examination must include an assessment of the *dermatomes*,[1] and in the conscious patient assess movements in both upper and lower limbs. For example, the spinal centers for elbow movements are C5/C6/C7 and C8 levels, with C5/C6 supplying the flexor movement of that joint and C7/C8 essentially the extensor movement. In the lower limbs the hip movements are controlled by L2/L3/L4 and L5 spinal cord centers with the more distal knee joint controlled mainly by L3/L4/L5 and S1. Figures 7.6–7.8 show these levels and their relationship to joint movement. Reflexes, when present, identify the viability of corresponding levels in the spinal cord. To find normal resting muscle tone and normal reflex activity are reassuring signs and even with apparent loss of motor power, *a degree of guarded reassurance can be given to the patient.*

In First Aid

1 Always consider the possibility of spinal cord injury in both the conscious and unconscious patient.
2 Avoid further damage to the spinal column and spinal cord with extrication and transportation of the patient from the scene
3 At the scene of the injury check the airway as the first priority.
4 If the accident victim is not in further immediate danger avoid unnecessary movement of the patient.
5 Apply the ABC rules of first aid, maintain:

- **A** airway
- **B** breathing
- **C** circulation

Keep the injured cervical spine in the 'mid position' particularly avoiding flexion and rotation. If a cervical injury is suspected apply a cervical collar. Lateral tilt and rotation of the head and neck must be avoided. If necessary, use a makeshift pillow under the side of the head. If a collar is not available, use a jacket or jumper which can be rolled-up and the long sleeves of the garment tied in front to form a supportive collar. A rolled-up towel or newspaper can also be a useful temporary substitute.

The patient must be observed at all times. If a lone attendant has to leave the patient to seek help, then the patient should be left in the lateral coma position with the underside leg bent and back supported to reduce the danger or inhalation should vomiting occur. In the conscious patient, roll the patient gently into the supine position provided there is no increase in the patient's symptoms or aggravation of pain with this movement. In the unconscious patient, roll the patient to the supine position and transfer to an appropriate frame or stretcher with constant observation of the airway. The 'first-aider' must be prepared to move the patient to the lateral coma position immediately if vomiting occurs.

Transportation of the spinal patient to a specialized unit for further assessment and treatment should be arranged as soon as possible and a skilled attendant must accompany the injured person during transfer. A patient with a higher level cervical spinal cord lesion

---

1 RJ Last Anatomy, regional and applied

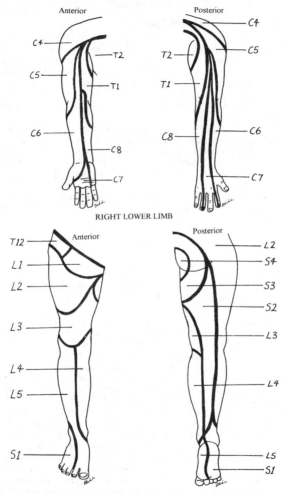

Fig. 7.6 Dermatomes

requires oxygen by mask or intranasal catheter and, if possible, *in all patients*, the stomach aspirated by an intragastric tube before transfer to reduce the danger of inhalation of gastric contents.

Early treatment and investigations

Early treatment of the spinal-injured patient will frequently include IV infusion avoiding fluid overload and the development of pulmonary oedema. Assessing cardiovascular efficiency is important since the hypotension following spinal cord injury is the result of the profound paralysis below the level of the lesion, loss of the 'peripheral pump' and the bradycardia as a result of loss of sympathetic activity to the heart. In addition, there may be the added complication of surgical shock from multiple injuries.

In the patient with a spinal cord injury, an infusion of less than 3L of an appropriate IV fluid should be given over the first 24h, and the patient carefully assessed. Radiological investigations will be necessary to clarify the lesion involving the spinal column. Directly identifying the damage to the spinal cord will necessitate the use of CT and MRI scans.

Damage to the spinal cord is classified under the headings of:

1 *Concussion* where there is a transitory loss of function without permanent sequelae.

2 *Contusion* with bruising—mild, moderate or severe

3 *Laceration* which is equivalent to severe bruising and will have a poor prognosis.

There are now an increasing number of spinal injuries where there is partial damage to the spinal cord. Within recent years, the proportion of the incomplete spinal cord lesions now approaches almost 50% of patients admitted to specialized spinal units and these patients will have useful recovery. There will always be a degree of associated soft tissue injury, and ligaments, muscles, disks, and joint capsules will all require an appropriate period of time to heal adequately and for the scar tissue to develop a degree of elasticity and allow return of 'pain-free' range of movement.

The patient will be assessed by the spinal surgeon and frequently internal fixation, with or without traction, will be required for cervical fracture/dislocations. The patient with suspected spinal cord injury should be nursed in the spinal unit with specialized nursing staff and with the assistance of mechanized beds and special mattresses to avoid trophic skin ulceration, which develops rapidly if patients are left immobile. Regular turning on lifting of the patient requires a skilled nursing team. Physiotherapy services will also be required constantly, more frequently for patients with higher lesions, where there is the danger of sputum retention and pulmonary collapse. The paralyzed neurogenic bladder requires drainage with an indwelling urethral catheter or suprapubic drainage during the period of spinal shock. Later, this is usually replaced with intermittent catheterization or use of reflex stimulation to promote intermittent emptying of the bladder. Urodynamic studies will assist in identifying which type of neurogenic bladder is present after the period of spinal shock and investigations with IV pyelograms and cystograms will assess the dangers of reflux and the development of hydronephrosis from chronic overdistention of the bladder.

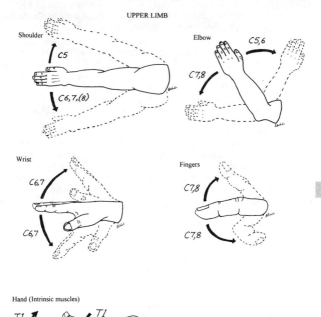

Fig. 7.7 Segmental innervation of movement

The paralyzed neurogenic bowel will require specialized nursing procedures to ensure adequate emptying and later with the introduction of appropriate medications and enemas or suppositories.

- *The continuing monitoring of respiratory function is* important since even a detailed clinical examination may overlook the development of progressive pulmonary congestion and consolidation. Diminishing vital capacity measurements will alert the clinician to the development of these serious problems and necessitate intensifying chest physiotherapy and posturing of the patient. Tracheostomy may be necessary, particularly if the measured vital capacity remains below 600ml.

- *Repeated neurological assessment is essential* in the patient with spinal injuries where spinal cord damage is susceptible and should be repeated daily during the first 10 days. Any sudden loss of motor power or sensation at or above the level of the lesion will alert the spinal surgeon to the possibility of continuing displacement or instability of the injured spinal column. Further compression may occur on the injured spinal cord with extradural hematoma which will require urgent evacuation.

- *Always consider the additional complications of associated injuries.* In a review of a series of 330 patients admitted to 2 major spinal units in Sydney, 36 patients had associated significant abdominal injuries. Laparotomy was necessary in 50% of these patients with the indication for exploration being:

1 Position peritoneal lavage for blood
2 Free gas on plain x-ray
3 Persistence of unexplained abdominal tenderness (12 patients)

Always consider the possibility of associated intraabdominal and intrathoracic injuries, particularly in thorac.lumbar spinal lesions. Consider splenic rupture, liver laceration, diaphragmatic rupture, traumatic pancreatitis, intestinal injury, renal injury, hemothorax, pneumothorax, and hemopericardium. Retroperitoneal hemorrhage associated with fractures and fracture dislocations of the lumbar spine frequently produce prolonged paralytic ileus persisting for up to 18 days. Although the loss of neural pathways below the level of the spinal cord injury results in diminished generalized rigidity and rebound tenderness, intact vagal afference and spared sympathetic afference still allow localization of pain and tenderness with a modified guarding response in patients with significant spinal cord injury.

X-rays

Plain radiographs

Are an appropriate initial investigation to identify vertebral alignment, fractures, and the possibility of ligamentous injury. Adequate views of the cervical spine must include the C1 vertebra down to the T1 vertebra. Spinal canal narrowing and congenital fusions/abnormalities or old injuries may be identified. Careful flexion and extension views in the conscious patient will assist in determining whether there is instability present by identifying shift in the vertebral alignment and/or abnormal increase in the interspinous space. A unilateral cervical facet dislocation may only be confirmed by oblique views—a single lateral view may not be sufficient.

LOWER LIMB

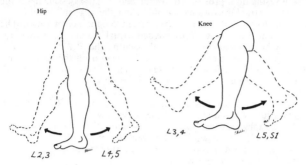

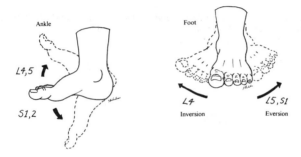

Fig. 7.8 Segmental innervation of movement (note EHL=L5)

Computed Tomography (CT)

This investigation provides a useful additional assessment of the fracture or fracture dislocation including the size and position of bony fragments and their encroachment on the spinal canal. The spinal canal contents are only vaguely visualized and CT myelography may be necessary to adequately identify the presence of significant disk prolapse causing further compression on the spinal cord. Magnetic resonance imaging (MRI) can identify disk protrusion with a clearer assessment of spinal cord or nerve root compression.

Bone scans are not usually recommended in the 'acute lesion' but may be of assistance in assessing progress or the possibility that an apparent injury to bone is old rather than new.

Myelography may be of assistance particularly in the lumbar spinal injury where the damaged intervertebral disk may bulge significantly in the upright position rather than in the supine position.

In all patients with spinal injuries:

- *Soft tissue injuries* which include damage to ligaments, muscles, capsules of joints, and disks, as well as nerve root neuropraxia are present.
- *Fracture and fracture dislocations* and subluxations of the vertebrae of the spinal column, which will require more detailed assessment and complicated treatment.

Soft tissue injuries

- *Treatment of soft tissue injury* will require initially an appropriate period of rest with gradual introduction of controlled pain free range of movements at the effected level. The patient with suspected damage to the vertebral column and/or spinal cord will be assessed by the spinal surgeon and frequently internal fixation, with or without traction, will be indicated.

- *Torn ligaments and muscles* will require at least 10 days for healing and a further 10 days where the scar tissue formed will 'mature' with return of some degree of elasticity. The application of cold pads assists in the reduction of the initial oedema and associated pain from tissue tension—improvement in blood flow should then be encouraged after 8h with applications of heat, gentle massage, and vibration. Improving blood flow assists the healing process and the subsequent period of tissue maturation.

- *Persistence of pain* despite controlled mobilization necessitates detailed review of the underlying pathology and if necessary repeating the appropriate x-ray investigations.

- *Nerve root irritation* can occur with narrowing of the intervertebral exit foramen or lateral disk protrusion. Traction injury to the brachial plexus (stinger/burner) from falling in water skiing or in contact sports such as football cause severe nerve root pain. Nerve root pain is identified by a specific distribution of pain often subsequent loss of sensation in the appropriate dermatome distribution and weakness in the corresponding myotome segments. Injury to peripheral nerves nay lead to nerve 'sheath' repair.

- *Intervertebral disk lesions* are most commonly seen in the lumbar spine, particularly at the L4/5 and L5/S1 levels. Occasionally, cervical disk lesions are associated with cervical spinal cord (e.g. injury from diving into shallow water). Thoracic disk lesions are rare and when they occur produce unusual clinical syndromes (e.g. loss of posterior column with a severe functional impairment due to loss of proprioception). The injured thoracic frequently calcifies.

- *A central disk protrusion* or rupture may produce bilateral signs. The lateral disk protrusion causes unilateral symptoms and signs. Apart from direct injury to the nerve roots, compressions may also produce ischemia in the spinal cord and cauda equina due to obstruction of the normal blood flow. The anterior spinal artery lies superficially in the anterior spinal sulcus and is particularly at risk when there is congenital narrowing of the spinal canal or cervical spondylosis with osteophyte formation allowing direct pressure on the vulnerable anterior spinal artery. Compressive injuries to the vertebral column can occur in weight lifting and in contact sport (e.g. 'spear tackling' in football). *Spear tackler's spine* occurs when the head/neck is used to tackle opponents. Axial loading occurs. There is a high risk of quadriplegia. X-rays show congenital narrowing of the canal, reversal of cervical lordosis, and torticollis (such athletes should not play contact sport). Fractures of the pars interarticularis occur in cricket (e.g. fast bowlers) usually at the L5 level as well as in gymnastics, running, golf, and tennis. Ligament and muscle strain, as well as recurrent tearing of pre-existing scar tissue from earlier injuries can be associated with the identified bony injuries.

- *Transient quadriplegia* is an acute transient neurological event of the cervical cord with motor/sensory charges in both arms and legs. Lhermitte's symptoms may be present. Also, congenitally narrow canal, disk otaophyte compression of the cord.

- *Indications for urgent surgery* to remove a damaged disk include **canda equina (surgical emergency)**. (1) the development of progressive major neurological deficit, (2) presence of a foot drop, and (3) disturbance of bladder control. Where there is a diffuse distribution of limb pain and less specific loss of sensation or motor power in the lower limbs then a non-operative approach should be seriously considered.

- *A short period of immobilization* in order to control pain is more appropriate than controlled mobility in a pain-free range, to encourage repair and improve muscle efficiency. Use analgesic medication sparingly in order to assess the level and distribution of pain and provide a guide to the patient's response to treatment. Antiinflammatory medication should be avoided immediately following injury.

- *Hydrotherapy* with gravity controlled or eliminated allows total body activity and will assist in improving movements of the spinal column while not exposing the paraspinal soft tissue to undue stress and strain during the healing period. Persisting radicular pain will necessitate further clinical assessment and radiological studies to identify whether diskectomy, with or without fusion, is necessary.

- *Rehabilitation programs to prepare the athlete for return to sport.* Consider a period of 2–3 weeks as appropriate for adequate healing of torn paraspinal ligaments, muscles, and joint capsules before returning to sport. Damage to bones of the vertebral column will necessitate a period of at least 3 months absence from sport, particularly when there is a degree of uncertainty to unexpected impact and degree of repetitive effort.

  Patients with damage to the vertebrae with or without involvement of the spinal cord should not return to play competitive contact sport, such as football, even if there is only a single level cervical fusion involved. The initial damage to produce bony disruption will inevitably cause ligament and capsule damage and expose the patient to undue risk in the future. Where there has been damage only to ligaments, muscles, or disks, and an appropriate period of preparation without any recurrence of transient symptoms or signs has passed and on radiological evidence of instability or canal stenosis is present, then the player should be considered suitable to return to contact sport within 3–6 months of the initial injury. Where there have been no neurological signs and only soft tissue injury to the spine then return to playing contact sport can be considered at an earlier stage when the player continues to be symptom-free.

- *Other conditions* which may be identified in the patient complaining of persistent symptoms after spinal injury include: *vertebral apophysitis*, where mechanical pain is worse with activity and relieved by rest and confirmed by radiological evidence; *Scheuermann's disease* affecting the spine at multiple levels in the thoracic spine can contribute to a thoracic kyphosis and a compensatory lumbar lordosis, symptoms precipitated by rowing and butterfly swimming;

Schmorl's nodes are associated with intravertebral disk herniation. Treatment emphasizes paraspinal muscle strengthening exercises with particular attention to posture. Surgery is infrequently indicated. *Congenital abnormality* may be found with single or multiple levels of fusion within the vertebrae of the spine (e.g. Klippel–Feil anomaly which involves multiple levels of the cervical spine), and athletes should not play contact sports, as there may be incidence of spinal canal narrowing and risk of quadriplegia.

Players who have had treatment for spinal injuries and return to sport should be encouraged to report any recurrence of symptoms relating to the previous injury; or the development of further symptoms relating to the previous injury; or the development of further symptoms not necessarily related to the spine.

Prevention

Primary: avoiding injury

- *Awareness* of high risk sports by participants. Diving into shallow water, Rugby football, and horse riding are activities associated with spinal injury
- *Prepare for the sport*. Enjoy the play and being involved. Be comfortable in the position for which you are chosen. In contact sport prepare with specific exercising to protect vulnerable regions (e.g. head and neck in scrummaging, and tackles in the various codes of football).
- *Neck exercises* will help to strengthen the paraspinal cervical muscles and assist with the transmission of impact from the head to the shoulders without unduly exposing the small cervical vertebrae, particularly in flexion and rotation.
- *Prepare for play* with an adequate period of warm up which includes repetitive movements and gradually developing into the full range for each major joint in limbs and spine. Avoid over-stretching, particularly in the cold weather where active muscle relaxation may be limited. *Remember*: (1) muscle not only *actively* contracts but *actively* relaxes, (2) muscles work as members of a group of muscles, either as a 'protagonist' or 'antagonist', and (3) input is as important as output to achieve efficient and balanced co-ordinated limb and trunk function.
- *Obey the rules and report injury.*
- *Avoiding returning to the field of play while there is still pain*, as this suggests that continuing healing and repair are necessary.
- *Use protective equipment as necessary*. For example: (1) the approved full face helmet in motor cycling and professional motor car racing to assist in the transmission of force from impact that can occur to the head, and to the shoulders often avoiding damage to the cervical spine and spinal cord; and (2) be appropriately restrained in a motor vehicle whether participating in a competitive sporting event or traveling to or from the sporting event.

Secondary: avoiding further damage to spine or spinal cord after initial injury

- Accurate diagnosis of the injured person at the site of the accident.
- Careful extrication and transportation from the scene of injury.
- Intensive care with control of fluid balance, support of respiration, and avoidance of inhalation of gastric contents.
- Differentiate between surgical shock with hypotension and tachycardia and the hypotension in spinal cord injury, where there is usually bradycardia in the patients with high level lesions above T6.
- Identify associated complications of long bone fractures, intraabdominal pathology, particularly hemorrhage or intrathoracic damage with pneumothorax and hemothorax.
- Be prepared to review the patient's (player's) clinical condition.

Table 7.3 Sports associated with spinal injuries

High frequency (>10 cases)		Medium frequency (>2 and <10)		Low frequency (<3 cases)	
Diving	(147)	Trailbike/		Water slide	(2)
Rugby football	(127)	Pro-motorbike	(9)	Scuba diving	(2)
Equestrian	(52)	Swimming	(6)	Motor boat	(2)
Water skiing	(18)	Para/Hang-gliding	(5)	Rodeo	(2)
Bicycle	(17)	Soccer	(5)	Soft/Baseball	(2)
Surfing	(14)	Fishing	(5)	Glider plane	(2)
Snow skiing	(11)	Gymnastics	(5)	Trampoline	(2)
		Rock climbing/		Wrestling	(2)
		Abseiling	(4)	Cricket	(1)
		Parachuting	(4)	Basketball	(1)
		Bodyboard	(4)	Bushwalking	(1)
		Touch football	(3)	Australian Rules	(1)
				Netball	(1)
				Flying fox	(1)
				Swing	(1)
				Judo	(1)
				Golf	(1)
				Hockey	(1)
				Snowboard	(1)
				Dune buggy	(1)
				Slippery dip	(1)

[1] Sports and recreations which resulted in acute admissions to spinal injuries units and the associated frequences of these admissions, 1984–1994.

Based on review of log book records of acute admissions to the spinal units of Royal North Shore Hospital, and Prince Henry Hospital, Sydney. The count included those admissions with and without neurological deficits.

1 J Lawson, S Wilson *et al* Report *Head and neck injuries in Sport, NSW Government Sporting Injuries Committee, Sydney.*

8 Shoulder[1]

EUGENE SHERRY

1 D Bokor 1997 In E Sherry, D Bokor (ed) *Manual of sports medicine* Ch10 p125–44. GMM, London

Introduction

Because of its great mobility and intrinsic instability the shoulder is the most vulnerable joint to injury in the body. It is required to provide a large range of movement with speed and force so the athlete can deliver a top performance. Humans were never intended to be involved in above-shoulder activity and it is therefore of little surprise that this joint is prone to a variety of injuries from the stresses being applied to the bones, chondral surfaces, and soft tissues—8–13 per cent of injuries sustained by athletes involve the shoulder.

Anatomy and biomechanics

The shoulder function consists of four separate joints: the glenohumeral joint (the main one), the acromioclavicular, sternoclavicular joints, and scapulothoracic. Disorders of any one of these may manifest as a dysfunction of the glenohumeral joint.

The **glenohumeral joint (GHJ)** is a ball and socket joint. The humeral head comprises about one-third of a sphere. The articular surface has a medial angulation of 45° to the shaft and is retroverted about 30°. The glenoid fossa is pear-shaped (radius of curvature is half that of the humeral head and so the area of bony contact is small). The glenoid labrum increases the depth of the fossa and increases the contact area of the humeral head and the glenoid. Ligamentous stability is supplied by the superior (major stabilizer) middle, and inferior glenohumeral ligaments and the capsule. (Further stability derives from negative intraarticular joint pressures, the rotator cuff muscles, and the coracohumeral ligament (Fig. 8.1)).

The **acromioclavicular joint (ACJ)** is a diarthrodial joint which links the arm to the axial skeleton. There is little inherent bony stability. It has a variable fibrocartilaginous disk/meniscus. The capsule and the superior acromioclavicular ligaments stabilizes at physiological loads, along with the coracoclavicular ligaments., the conoid and trapezoid.

The **sternoclavicular joint (SCJ)** has two incongruent articular surfaces with a fibrocartilaginous disk forming two independent joints. It is stabilized by the interclavicular, anterior and posterior sternoclavicular ligaments, and the costoclavicular ligament (rhomboid ligaments). The joint has three planes of motion. (The fulcrum is the rhomboid ligament, not the SCJ articulation.)

Despite the low weight of the arm (5% of bodyweight, i.e. 3.6 in a 72kg man) *high torque forces* are generated by its long lever arm. The rotator cuff and other shoulder muscles generate movement and glenohumeral control. In throwing, all the muscles of the trunk and upper limb work in a synchronized balanced manner to propel an object forward. Throwing action is divided into: cocking (or wind-up), acceleration, and follow-through phases. Imbalance, fatigue, or damage to these structures may result in pain, tendinitis, and/or instability (Fig. 8.2).

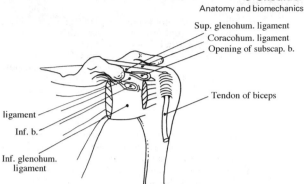

Sup. glenohum. ligament
Coracohum. ligament
Opening of subscap. b.

Tendon of biceps

ligament
Inf. b.

Inf. glenohum.
ligament

Fig. 8.1 Anatomy of the shoulder ligaments

247

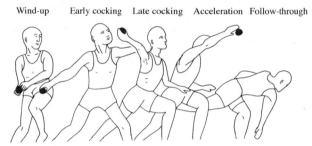

Wind-up   Early cocking   Late cocking   Acceleration   Follow-through

Fig. 8.2 Phases of throwing

Instability

Shoulder instability is common in sport. Apart from a frank dislocation, a wide range of symptoms result from variable degrees of slipping of the shoulder. Partial dislocation is referred to as subluxation. This is not an insignificant injury to the GHJ, severe injuries occur from subluxed joints. These are *instability events* (and potentially damaging to the joint), (95%) of shoulder instability is anterior/anterior-inferior direction (other directions include posterior/multi-directional.)

Anterior instability

This occurs when the arm is in abduction/external rotation and an anterior force applied on the shoulder joint (falling on the outstretched hand or tackling a player with the arm out from the side, e.g. rugby). May occur without an obvious traumatic event. Overhead sports (baseball or tennis), cause a gradual stretch of the anterior capsule and symptoms of the shoulder slipping. *Note*: hierarchy of support mechanisms controling glenohumeral stability and thus cascade of injury (Table 8.1).

Symptoms of instability include frank dislocation; slipping; pain with the arm in abduction/external rotation; apprehension when using the arm overhead or a 'dead arm' feeling with a tackle or overhead action. **Clinical examination** check ROM, strength, increased anteroposterior translation of the humeral head (Fig. 8.3), apprehension (Fig. 8.4), and relocation signs, note coincident tendinitis or labral tears, and also signs of ligament laxity. (Hyperextend knee, elbow, MCP joints hand; flex wrist so hand touches forearm.)

The natural history[1] of the first acute anterior shoulder instability is now known. Recurrence in *young patients* (under 22 years) is 62% (if a participant in contact sports repeat instability is over 90%; recurrence in *older patients* (30-40 years) is 25%. Over a 10-year period there is a 12% chance of a contralateral instability and a 20% incidence of arthritic changes on x-ray (9% moderate or severe). This arthropathy is thought not to be influenced by the number of dislocations or whether surgery has been performed.

Acute dislocation

Assess for any nerve or vascular injury x-ray the shoulder (AP + lateral in plane of scapula). Closed reduction can be performed in the emergency room using either pethidine (50-100mg IVI), diaepam (5mg IVI), nitrous oxide (Entinox: 50% N_2O/O_2),[2] or with an intraarticular injection of lignocaine 1% (5cc). General anesthesia may be required where there is excessive muscle spasm (or young male with huge shoulder muscle girdle).

Techniques for closed reduction of the dislocated shoulder are described in (Table 8.2). The arm should be placed in a sling, and physiotherapy started after 1–3 weeks. Younger patients have a high risk of recurrence; so for special sporting requirements consider an acute arthroscopic assessment and capsular/labral repair.

1 L Hovelius 1987 *JBJS* **69a** 393–9   2 E Sherry *et al* 1989 Comparison of midazolam and diazepam for the reduction of shoulder dislocations and Colles' fractures in skiers on an outpatient basis. *Austal J Sci Med Sport*

Table 3.1 Glenohumeral stability:
hierarchy of support mechanisms

Minimal loads
- Joint concavity
- Finite joint volume
- Adhesion/Cohesion
- Joint forces

Moderate loads
- Active coordinated
- Cuff contraction

Massive loads
- Capsuloligamentous structures
- Bony supports

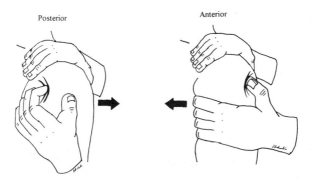

Posterior

Anterior

Fig. 8.3 Assessing instability of shoulder, whether anterior or posterior

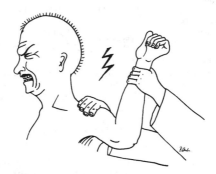

Fig. 8.4 Apprehension test

Instability (cont)

Recurrent dislocation

If *recurrent* instability becomes a problem, options include: modification or avoidance of the precipitation event, a physiotherapy rehabilitation program to strengthen the shoulder, or surgical reconstruction of the shoulder. Several surgical techniques are used including those that tighten or use bone blocks to avoid dislocation. *Correction of the pathology* (i.e. anatomical reonstruction) includes repairing the avulsed inferior glenohumeral ligament (*Bankart lesion*) and correcting any associated capsular redundancy (*capsular shift*) (*preferred option* in surgical management of the unstable shoulder). The success rate for surgery is 95%. Procedures that correct the pathology (anatomical reconstruction) are more likely to restore full range of motion. Especially for those involved in upper limb sports requiring a throwing action (e.g. baseball). Many of the non-anatomical reconstructions restrict external rotation and so restrict athletes. Types of shoulder reconstruction are described in Table 8.3.

Multidirectional instability (MDI)

Most shoulders show a variable degree of laxity (and is normal) where there is marked laxity this may become a problem. This may be insidious in onset or be related to a trauma. Important to differentiate *laxity* from *stability. Laxity* is a physical finding, whereas *instability* is the combination of symptoms and signs. The diagnosis of MDI is based on finding least two directions (**inferior** plus either/or both *anterior and posterior.)* Patients have pain and weakness associated with a shoulder that subluxes inferiorly as well as anteriorly and posteriorly.

Take care in the evaluation of these patients. A small subgroup of MDI patients demonstrate a *habitual/voluntary aspect to their problem.* This group of patients should be evaluated for associated psychological problems and potential secondary gains. *Surgical procedure will fail in this group.*

Treatment focuses around **rehabilitation**: strengthening of rotator cuff and scapula stabilizers, proprioceptive/biofeedback techniques, and modification of activities. Most will respond to physiotherapy. If necessary, surgery will include an inferior capsular shift with closure of the rotator capsular interval and tightening of the superior glenohumeral ligament. The results of surgery are 80-90% successful.

Posterior instability

Posterior dislocation is uncommon (4% of all dislocations). Occurs from a fall; or violent muscle contractions as in an electrocution or grand mal convulsion. **The diagnosis is often delayed or missed**. There is pain and the arm is locked in internal rotation. The (anteroposterior) x-ray may look normal *but beware*, check the axillary view (is diagnostic). *If there is any doubt then a CT scan should be performed.*

Posterior subluxation

Can occur from sports such as baseball. Suspect when the athlete experiences symptoms with the arm in front of the trunk. May then be associated with multidirectional instability. Clinical examination may reveal increased posterior glide, and symptoms reproduced on posterior load of the shoulder in 90° forward flexion. The x-rays are often normal.

Table 8.2 Techniques for closed reduction of the dislocated shoulder

Technique	Details/Comment
Longitudinal traction	Patient lies supine and the affected arm is slightly abducted. Traction is applied to the arm with a sheet around chest, or foot (minus shoe) in the axilla, or applying counter traction (Fig. 8.5). Simple, classic, and *effective*
Scapular rotation maneuver	Patient lies prone on table with injured arm hanging off the edge of the table (Fig 8.5). The scapula is manipulated to open the front aspect of the joint so allowing congruence of the humeral head and the glenoid to be restored (inferior tip scapula pushed toward the spine). *Elegant and effective*
Stimson's technique	The patient lies prone. Weight is applied to the arm with the affected should hanging off the edge of the table. *Simple but lacks style*
Forward elevation maneuver	The patient lies supine. The arm is gently elevated in the plane of the scapula up to about 160°. Traction is applied in elevation with outward pressure on the humeral head. *Simple and possibly effective*
Kocher maneuver	The patient is supine. A sheet is applied around the patient's chest. Traction is placed on the arm in slight abduction while the arm is externally rotated, adducted, and then internally rotated. Old technique. Painful. May fracture or displace the neck of the humerus. *Avoid*

Table 8.3 Types of shoulder reconstructions

Type	Surgical details
Anatomical	
Bankart repair	The anterior detached capsule and labrum are repaired back on to the glenoid neck
Capsuloraphy	Stretched or redundant capsule is tightened by plication.
Inferior capsular shift	Similar to a capsuloraphy but mobilization of the capsule extends inferiorly to take up redundant inferior pouch. Done in patients with very lax shoulders
Non-anatomical	
Putti-Plan	The anterior capsule and subscapularis muscles are divided, overlapped, and tightened (similar to converting a single-breasted coat to a double-breasted coat). Decreases external rotation of the arm
Bristows' procedure	The coracoid process is detached from the scapula and screwed on to the antero-inferior glenoid neck to give extra support to the shoulder.
Magnusen–Stack procedure	The subscapularis, capsule, and a portion of the lesser tuberosity is detached and fixed more laterally on to the humeral head. This tightens the anterior should structures decrease external rotation.

WJ Mallon 1993 In Frymoyer (ed) *OKU 4* p297–302 AAOS, Rosemont, IL

If there is a *locked posterior dislocation*, early recognition and reduction is essential. If the dislocation is longstanding or a large portion of the humeral head damaged then open reduction with surgical reconstruction of the humeral head defect (by autograft, allograft, or tuberosity transfer) is required. Where chondral damage has occurred, total shoulder replacement may be necessary.

In patients with posterior *subluxations and associated multidirectional laxity,* an intensive physiotherapy rehabilitation program is required. Most patients will respond to this. If stability continues then surgical reconstruction is necessary (performed from an anterior or posterior approach). Anterior surgery consists of an inferior capsular shift and tightening of the superior glenohumeral ligament. Posterior reconstruction undertakes an inferior capsular shift only. In both cases, the patient is immobilized in a neutral rotation brace for 6-8 weeks then placed on a graded rehabilitation program extending over 12 months. No return to sport for at least 12 months.

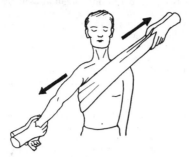

Longitudinal traction

253

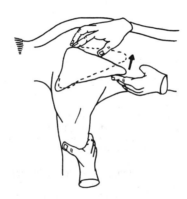

Fig. 8.5 Shoulder reduction techniques for anterior dislocation

Tendinitis and impingement

The supraspinatus is vulnerable to inflammation as it passes under the coracoacromial arch in the crowded space between the arch and the greater tuberosity. Tendinitis of the rotator cuff may occur from overload/fatigue of the cuff tendons, trauma, age-related degenerative changes. The acromion may have a shape which increases the crowding of the cuff tendons here which leads to impingement. *Note*: tendinitis may occur in patients with very lax shoulders (the muscles are overworked to stabilize the humeral head). Therefore, it is important to beware of tendinitis in these patients (younger than 25 years) as this may be secondary to subtle (unrecognized) instability.

Typically, there is pain over the anterior aspect of the *shoulder* with radiation into the deltoid (minimal at rest and *rarely* radiates down the arm or into the neck; aggravated with overhead and rotation activities). Night pain with waking indicates severe cases. **Examination**: tenderness is located over the greater tuberosity. Impingement signs are present (Fig. 8.6). Biceps (tendinitis) provocation test may also be positive. (*Speeds test*–pain with resisted forward elevation of strength arm; *Yergason test*—pain with resisted supination of flexed elbow). The acromioclavicular joint may be involved. Range of motion and strength are often normal, but wasting occurs early. There is pain on loading the rotator cuff muscles. Weakness is due to inhibition from pain. Exclude cervical conditions which may refer pain into the shoulder (where there is cervical irritation the shoulder posture is in a depressed or elevated position).

The diagnosis of tendinitis is a clinical diagnosis. A plain x-ray is essential (include a supraspinatus outlet view). The next investigation is the *impingement test*: 5–10ml of lignocaine is injected into the subacromial bursa, wait 5 minutes, there should be a significant decrease in pain on forward elevation of the arm in order to perform this test (Fig. 8.6). Ultrasound (in *experienced* hands) is accurate in diagnosing full-thickness tears and impingement. Note all shoulders that are stiff, as in adhesive capsulitis, they will show impingement on ultrasound due to tightness of the posterior capsule limiting the inferior glide to the humeral head. Therefore, investigations should be considered in their clinical context. Arthrography will show cuff tears.

Treatment includes activity modification, NSAIDs, and physiotherapy (consisting of stretching and strengthening of the rotator and scapular muscles). Most cases respond. If pain persists inject corticosteroid and local anesthetic (half ampoule Celestone with 5ml 0.5% Marcain plain) into the subacromial space; both diagnostic and therapeutic. If conservative treatment does not help after 6 months, then acromioplasty (open or arthroscopic) is successful in 90%.

Rotator cuff tears

Normal tendons seldom tear. In young patients, a violent injury is required to tear the cuff. For older patients, there are underlying degenerative changes in the rotator cuff so less trauma is required to disrupt it. With repetitive overhead use of the arm (tennis or baseball), microdamage to the cuff can progress to a full-thickness tear. The **symptoms** are similar to tendinitis. Pain is worsened by overhead activities, and at *night*. Weakness is present (however, with full-thickness tears there is often a normal active range of motion). Only *massive* rotator cuff tears lose active range of motion. The long head of the biceps may also be torn.

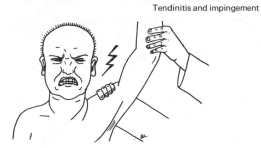

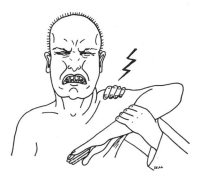

Fig. 8.6 The impingement test

Perform x-rays (may show an acromial spur and narrowing of the acromiohumeral gap where the tear is large), may need an arthrogram, ultrasound, or MRI to confirm the diagnosis, extent of damage, atrophy of muscles, and associated joint disease (note ultrasound is usually sufficient and cost-effective).

Treatment in young patients (under 50 years)—surgery (with acromioplasty and rotator cuff repair) is required as there is a risk of increase in tear size and deterioration of shoulder function. In older patients, a short trial of activity modification, NSAIDs, physiotherapy, and corticosteroid injection is reasonable. If pain, then surgery with acromioplasty and rotator cuff repair is indicated.

Internal derangements within the glenohumeral joint

Labral tears, SLAP (superior labral anterior/posterior) lesions, loose bodies

Are caused by trauma, direct or in association with instability. The *labrum*, most developed in the upper part of the shoulder joint tears here and may extend into the biceps anchor. *SLAP lesions*—four types (frayed labrum/also detached biceps/detached superior labrum/ also into biceps anchor). *Loose bodies* arise from trauma or synovial disease (synovial chondrometaplasia).

There is pain with sudden motion, clicking, or catching (with rotation). Pain is worse with resisted elevation of the arm while forward flexed (90° and slightly adducted with the hand in internal rotation). When the hand is externally rotated in the same position the pain decreases. Also, there may be associated features of instability. **Diagnosis** is *difficult*[1] and requires **investigation** (e.g. MRI with gadolinium enhancement, or arthroscopy). **Treatment** is often arthroscopic with either resection or repair of the torn labrum and removal of loose bodies. Also important to treat the underlying cause (e.g. instability).

1 CA Rockwood, FR Lyons 1993 *JBJS* **75A** 409–24

Acromioclavicular joint injuries

The acromioclavicular joint (ACJ) is commonly injured from a fall on to the point of the shoulder.[1] The injury is chondral or meniscal. More severe injuries result in subluxation or dislocation of the joint. Classified as sprain, subluxed (coracoclavicular ligament intact), or dislocated (coracoclavicular ligament torn).

On **examination**, localized tenderness and swelling is seen. In dislocations, the outer clavicle appears superiorly displaced (in fact, it is the shoulder that sags below the clavicle). Forced cross body adduction provokes discomfort.

X-rays of the joint should include standing weighted views of the ACJ with the weight to the wrists of the patient. **Treatment**: for *undisplaced* injury ice packs, rest, and then gradual return to activity over a 2–6 week period is required (note that seemingly minor ACJ injuries may give rise to grumbling discomfort for up to 6 months). *Major dislocations may require surgical stabilization* in athletes if their dominant arm is involved, and if they participate in upper limb sports or are workers who use their arms above their shoulders.

1 RR Richards 1993 Acromioclavicular joint injuries. *Instr Course Lecture* **42** 259–69

Clavicle fractures

Common injury, occurs from a fall on to the outstretched hand. Fractures occurs in the mid shaft, (also medial or lateral possible). There is pain, swelling, and deformity over the site of the fracture. Neurological lesions are rare (brachial plexus) as are vascular injuries.

The *majority* will go *on to union with little morbidity,* even when moderate shortening or angulation (the bone ends only need to be in the same room). Some may develop symptoms with cross body actions if the clavicle is too shortened. (If the fractures are lateral and involve the coracoclavicular ligaments or ACJ, treatment may require surgical fixation of the outer clavicle.) Most fractures are treated with a sling for elbow support. (Clavicle rings to pull shoulders back may help and stabilize the fracture ends.) Take care to avoid skin pressure problems and axillary neurovascular compression. *With marked displacement or shortening*, early open reduction and internal fixation may be considered (but rarely).

Outer clavicular osteolysis[1]

Occurs from a *direct blow or fall,* may develop in athletes who work-out in the gymnasium on overhead machines or in overhead sports. Probable pathology is a chondral or minor osteochondral fracture which triggers an inflammatory response, leading to resorption of the outer clavicle.

There is pain over the ACJ (radiates to the deltoid or base of neck). Examination reveals localized tenderness and swelling over the ACJ, in advanced cases a palpable gap is present at the ACJ. X-rays show irregularity of the outer clavicle with osteolysis ('suck-candy' appearance). A bone scan (not always necessary) will be hot.

Treatment is rest, activity modification, and NSAIDs. If the pain is severe then surgical excision of the outer clavicle is required.

1 M Scarenius, BF Iverson 1992 *Am J Sports Med* **29** 463–7

Medical clavicular sclerosis (osteitis condensans)

A rare disorder where there is osteosclerosis of the medial end of the clavicle. Etiology is unknown (low grade osteonecrosis or osteomyelitis proposed, but never proven). Occurs in middle aged women with a long insidious onset of pain and discomfort (with elevating the arm).

X-rays show mild enlargement and sclerosis of the medial end of the clavicle (no bone destruction or periosteal reaction). Confirmation by CT scan (although MRI useful). **Treatment** is non-operative (analgesics and NSAIDs). May be symptomatic for many years. Condition is rarely painful enough to warrant surgical excision.

Sternoclavicular dislocation

Although limited ligamentous support of the inner end of the clavicle exists, dislocations are rare. May be anterior or posterior. Usually occurs from a fall on to the side and from compression of the shoulder from another player falling on top.

Anterior dislocation displays a painful prominence of the medial end of the clavicle. **Treatment**: closed reduction in the acute situation (many surgeons prefer to leave the dislocation and treat the patient symptomatically). The **diagnosis is confirmed** with a CT scan as x-rays of this region are difficult to read.

Posterior dislocation may cause pressure on vital structures in the neck with dysphagia, dyspnea or great vessel compression. A **surgical emergency. Posterior dislocations should be reduced urgently if there is compromise of the thoracic outlet mediastinal structures**. Place a bolster between the shoulder blades and apply posterior pressure to the shoulders. If the clavicle does not so reduce around the clavicle and pulls forward to reduce hook a sterile surgical towel clip.

Muscle ruptures

A number of muscles may rupture around the shoulder, including *pectoralis major*, *long head of biceps*, and *subscapularis*. A muscle tears when there is contraction against an unexpected resistance. Weight lifters (bench pressing, large weights) incur such injuries. When the arm is in 90° of abduction and in extension the subscapularis may tear.

There is severe pain and a tearing sensation (at the time of rupture), followed by swelling and bruising. The torn pectoralis major bunches on contraction. Long head of biceps rupture may be associated with rotator cuff disease. Subscapularis rupture is to pick (*Note*: weakness on the posterior lift-off test—not able to move back of hand off sacrum.)

For the ruptured pectoralis muscle surgical repair is necessary, as the athlete will notice deformity and weakness. A subscapularis tear may cause long-term changes in rotator cuff balance and function; so repair is recommended.[1]

1 BL Berson 1979 *Am J Sports Med* 7 348–51

271

Biceps tendon injuries

The biceps may be injured with anterior instability or inflamed with impingement and rotator cuff tears; 95% biceps tendonitis secondary. There is pain over the anterior shoulder. **Examination** pinpoints tenderness in the biceps groove. A click from subluxation of the tendon may occur with rotation of the arm. **Treatment** is rest, NSAIDs, and steroid injections in the biceps groove. If pain persists or there is dislocation of the biceps then surgical tenodesis is required. If the long head of biceps ruptures the pain often subsides. The rupture is treated symptomatically and surgery is rarely required.

Nerve injuries

Around the shoulder occur from direct trauma, traction, compression, or instability. The nerves may sustain a neuropraxia or division. Nerves involved include the axillary, suprascapular, musculocutaneous, long thoracic (in swimmers—scapula winging; thoracolumbar brace with scapular pad may help), and radial nerve. A brachial plexus palsy (partial or complete) occurs with high energy trauma (burners/stingers, transient, football; root avulsions carry poor prognosis). Thoracic outlet is compression of nerves/vessels between scalenes and first rib, abnormal scalenes or cervical rib. C8–T1 signs. Wright test (arm is extended/abducted/externally rotated; head turned away), postitive. Treat symptoms/no pulse. Improve posture. Surgery is rarely neessary.

There is pain related to the injury and weakness. Careful neurological examination is required to localize the injury.

Usually, the injury is a neuropraxia and will recover. EMG studies may ascertain whether the lesion is complete and/or recovering. Exploration and repair of the nerves is indicated if the lesion does not recover within 6 months. If suprascapular nerve compression is evident then an MRI scan may reveal a spinoglenoid notch ganglion cyst pressing on the nerve. (Surgical excision/release transverse suprascapular ligament.)

275

Other conditions

- *Scrapping scapula* from irritation of periscapular bursae, may be voluntary, difficult to treat, NSAIDs, inject, or partial distal scapular resection.
- Adhesive capsulitis (frozen shoulder synovitis with capsular contraction), painful shoulder with global ROM (end stage inflammation; exclude post dislocation shoulder/OA neck), autoimmune problem, after trauma or immobilization onset in stages; x-ray shows osteopenia. Needs NSAIDs, physiotherapy, steroid injection, and MUA.
- *Calcific tendinitis*—deposition of calcium in supraspinatus tendon in middle aged women, pain in the resorptive phase, localized deposit on x-ray, may benefit from needling/steroid injection, or surgical excision (including bursoscopy).

Prevention of injury to the shoulder

Very important to have a *general condition program*. In upper limb activity sports, this includes muscle strengthening and stretching around the shoulder and scapula. Resulting appropriate strength and muscle length allows for optimal muscle function.

Prior to exercising, *warm-up* is the first step. Stretching of the rotator cuff and posterior capsule and then gentle strengthening exercises focused on the rotator cuff and scapular stabilizers is important.

Technique of throwing needs to be developed carefully under supervision to optimize performance without excessive undue strain on the shoulder capsule or muscles. At the first sign of fatigue or discomfort the athlete should rest to prevent any injury progressing to a more serious level. After activity, the athlete should cool down the affected area and then go through a gentle stretching program before rest.

It is important to realize that *high level performance* at sport places *an extreme demand* on the body's tissues and the sport off-season is essential for allowing any microdamage to heal. (Appropriate complementary exercises are also important during this period.) Such exercise should not place the same strain on tissues but should be directed at maintaining aerobic fitness in preparation for the next season.

By following these points, all athletes should be able to enjoy their sport for many seasons with a minimal risk of injury.

9 Elbow[1]

EUGENE SHERRY

1 D Bokor, D Duckworth1997 In E Sherry, D Bokor (ed) *Manual of sports medicine*, Ch11, p145–60. GMM, London

Introduction

The elbow is a difficult joint to examine, diagnose, and treat (not a frequent site of trauma and injury). Nevertheless, the elbow is becoming better understood as more participate in throwing or overhead sports, resulting in an increasing number of elbow problems requiring treatment.

Overuse injuries in throwing or catching sports create most chronic elbow problems (may involve the ligaments, capsule, muscles, or articular surfaces of the joint to impair function). Certain sports cause specific injuries around the elbow (see Table 9.1).

Table 9.1 Sports specific elbow problems

Sport	Condition
Golf	Medial epicondylitis
Tennis	Lateral epicondylitis
Baseball	Medial collateral (ulnar) ligament injuries (MCL) injuries
	Valgus extension overload
	Little leaguers elbow
	Osteochondritis dissecans (OCD), Panner's disease
	Ulnar neuritis/cubital tunnel
	Acute rupture MCL
	Medial epicondylitis
Gymnastics	OCD
Javelin	Acute rupture MCL
	Partial rupture MCL
	Epicondylitis

Anatomy and biomechanics

The elbow is a highly constrained hinge joint (its stability is maintained by ligamentous, osseous and capsular structures) with a slight degree of varus/valgus and rotational laxity (3–5°) throughout the flexion–extension arc. The elbow has three articulations see also (Fig. 9.1):

1 Ulnohumeral joint: allows 0–150° flexion
2 Radiocapitellar joint
- Proximal radioulnar joints (radiocapitellar allows 75° pronation and 85° supination).

  Note: most daily activity is carried out through a 100° arc of flexion and extension (usually *30–130°*). Forearm rotation occurs in an arc of *100°*degrees, (usually 50° supination and 50° pronation). Any loss of this arc of movement may limit one's function.

- *Elbow stability.* Ligamentous *stability* is provided by the medial and lateral ligamentous complex. (The relative importance of these ligaments depends on the position of the arm.)
- *Medial collateral ligament* has three parts. The *anterior oblique ligament* is the most important of these bands, originating from the medial epicondyle and inserting on to the medial aspect of the coronoid process. The anterior band is the primary constraint to Valgus instability and the radial head is of secondary importance (clinically, this is noted in throwing as the repetitive valgus stress can result in microtrauma and attenuation of the anterior oblique ligament).
- *Lateral collateral ligament* has three parts and offers varus stability (rarely stressed in the athlete). The lateral ulnar collateral, the most important of these ligaments, plays an important role in rotational instability, it originates from the lateral epicondyle and inserts on to the tubercle of the supinator crest of the ulna. Its function is to prevent *varus* and *posterolateral* rotatory instability of the elbow. The capsule serves as an important constraint to instability in full extension.
- *Neurological anatomy.* Neurological compression syndromes are common here due to the close proximity of the nerves. The ulnar nerve is vulnerable within the cubital tunnel, posterior to the medial epicondyle. The median nerve is anterior, deep within the cubital fossa, the radial nerve is lateral and branches in the cubital fossa.

284

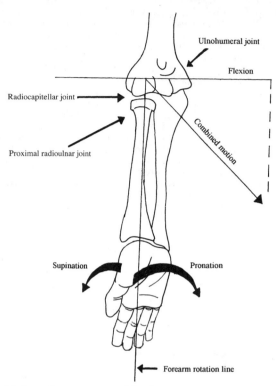

Fig. 9.1 Axes of movement around the elbow

Ligament injuries and instability

Medial (ulnar) collateral ligament injuries (MCL)

From *throwing sports* where repetitive valgus stress results in small tears in the anterior band of the MCL and subsequent rupture. Occurs in javelin throwers and baseball pitchers (in throwing there is an enormous valgus stress on the elbow during the late-cocking (wind-up) phase so overloading the ligament leading to attenuation and rupture). Occasionally, there is a single acute painful throw or a fall on to the outstretched hand.

Examination reveals swelling and pain (localized to the medial side) and occasionally paresthesia in the ulnar nerve distribution. Valgus deformity and elbow contracture may follow. Valgus stress testing with the elbow at 30° of flexion displays increased laxity and pain. Incongruity develops between the olecranon process and its fossa with loose body formation at the medial side of the olecranon. X-rays may show osseous bodies in the MCL or fluffy calcification at the tip of the olecranon. **Treatment** is rest, activity modification, NSAIDs, and physiotherapy. If posteromedial pain continues then arthroscopy is necessary to debride the osteophytes. If there is chronic MCL laxity or instability then surgical reconstruction (primary repair or use palmaris longus, is necessary).

Acute rupture of the MCL

Isolated tears of the anterior oblique ligament may occur in javelin throwers. The mechanism is almost pure valgus stress with the elbow flexed at 60–90°. There is severe pain and a 'pop' on the medial side of the elbow. Ulnar nerve symptoms may occur with ecchymosis around the elbow (48h later). If the diagnosis is in doubt stress tests or stress x-rays are useful. Acute repair of the ligament is necessary.

Valgus extension overload

Seen in *pitchers* during the acceleration phase. (In the early phase of acceleration excessive valgus stress is applied to the elbow causing impingement.) This results in osteophyte formation posteriorly and posteromedially, which can cause chondromalacia with loose body formation.

The pitcher presents with pain on pitching (early in the game) and is not able to let go of the ball. Pain over the olecranon fossa occurs in valgus and extension. X-rays show a posterior osteophyte at the tip of the olecranon (on lateral views). **Treatment** (should be started early) by increasing functional strength, and using heat and ultrasound. An osteophyte needs surgical excision.

Posterolateral rotatory instability[1]

Differentiate from a frank elbow dislocation. Caused by a laxity or disruption of the ulnar part of the lateral collateral ligament which then allows a transient rotatory subluxation of the ulnohumeral joint (and secondary dislocation of the radio-humeral joint). There may be preceding trauma (dislocation or sprain from a fall on an outstretched hand). Previous surgery, radial head excision, or lateral release for a tennis elbow, may be the cause of instability.

1 SW O'Driscoll *et al* 1991 *JBJS* **73A** 440

Ligament injuries and instability (*cont*)

There is a history of a recurring click, snap, clunking, locking of the elbow, and a sense of instability that the elbow is about to dislocate. Such stability episodes occur with a loaded extended elbow and supinated forearm. **Examination**, often unremarkable, should include the *lateral pivot shift test* (posterolateral rotatory apprehension test; see Fig. 8.2—performed with patient supine, preferably under general anesthesia. The elbow is extended overhead and the forearm fully supinated; a valgus and supination force is then slowly applied to the elbow going from the extended to flexed position; this results in subluxation of the ulnohumeral joint and radio-humeral joint).

On x-ray, the joint will look normal (unless taken with the joint subluxed) so the diagnosis is made from the history and after the above test. When symptomatic surgery is required (reattach the avulsed lateral ulnar collateral ligament or reconstruct it, with a tendon graft).

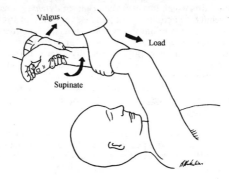

Fig. 9.2 The lateral pivotal shift test

28

Tennis elbow (lateral epicondylitis)

A lateral tendinitis which involves the origin of *extensor carpi radialis brevis*. It is related to activities that increase tension and stress on the wrist extensors and supinator muscles (not all activities include tennis). It occurs between the ages of 35 and 55 years, with pain localized to the lateral epicondyle especially after a period of unaccustomed activity (such as tennis 3–4 times a week). The pain is worsened by movements such as turning a door handle or shaking hands. **Examination** reveals pain localized to the lateral epicondyle and distally. Typically aggravated by passive stretching the wrist extensors or actively extending the wrist with the elbow straight (Fig. 9.3).

X-rays are often normal (to exclude OA, LB, or tumor). A bone scan will show increased uptake about the lateral epicondyle. An ultrasound or MRI will show degeneration within the belly of ECRB. The **differential diagnosis** includes: posterior interosseus nerve entrapment (has a more distal localization of the pain and associated weakness); radial tunnel syndrome (pain distal and exacerbated by resisted extension of long digit, i.e. ECRB); OA/LB/tumor.

It will resolve over a 10–12 month period but there is a 30% recurrence, *therefore* **treat comprehensively**[1] with rest, progressive resisted exercise (Chapter 19), activity modification, NSAIDs, heat, ultrasound, phonophoresis with 10% hydrocortisone cream, brace (counterforce effect), eccentric muscle strengthening, modify tennis handle (usually too large), or tennis stroke (occurs in back hand stroke). Injection of corticosteroids (no more than 3 times, just below ECRB, anterior and distal to the epicondyle), and then surgery (symptoms >12 months, release and excise ECRB, note Nirschl scratch effect). Return to sport when strength 80% back or after 4–6 months.

1 CC Teitz *et al* 1997. *JBJS* **79A** p138–52

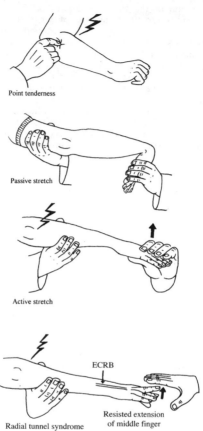

Point tenderness

Passive stretch

Active stretch

ECRB

Radial tunnel syndrome

Resisted extension of middle finger

Fig. 9.3 Tennis elbow (lateral epicondylitis)

Golfer's elbow (medial epicondylitis)

An inflammation of the flexor tendinous origin from the medial epicondyle. From repetitive activity of wrist flexion and active pronation (e.g. baseball pitching or occasionally golf and tennis). The pathology is at the interface of pronator teres and FCR. **Presents** with tenderness over the medial epicondyle radiating down the forearm, exacerbated by resisted palmer flexion and pronation. Ulnar nerve symptoms are present in 60% of cases. **Treatment** is very similar to lateral epicondylitis. Exclude other ulnar neuropraxia, joint stability, or cervical pathology. Treatment is rest, progressive resisted exercise (Chapter 19), activity modification, NSAIDs, and physiotherapy. Avoid repeated steroid injections (so close to ulnar nerve). Only rarely is surgical release needed (release the common flexor origin with occasionally a medial epicondylectomy).

Osteochondritis dissecans (OCD)

This is a spontaneous necrosis and fragmentation of the capitellar ossific nucleus (thought to be from compression forces at the radio-capitellar joint producing focal arterial injury and bone death). Occurs in gymnastics and throwing sports (baseball pitchers).

There is lateral elbow pain post activity, occurs in the 10 to 15-year-old group, and involves the dominant arm. **Examination** shows an inability to fully extend the elbow and pain on forced extension. Panner's disease is a similar condition; the major difference being the x-ray appearance (fragmentation of entire capitellar ossific nucleus vs island of subchondral bone in OCD) and age of onset (under 10 years). Initially the x-rays may be normal and if clinically suspected a bone CT scan is needed. **Treatment** is rest for 6 weeks. However, if pain and contracture persist fragmentation may have occurred. Arthroscopy is then performed and the fragment is separately removed (occasionally reattached if large).

Panner's disease

An 'osteochondrosis' which affects the growth centers in children resulting in necrosis followed by regeneration. Here, it involves the capitellum resulting in fragmentation and then regeneration. **Commonly confused with OCD** due to similar presentation of dull aching elbow pain aggravated by use, loss of full elbow extension, and lateral swelling. X-rays show fragmentation, irregularity, and a smaller capitellum (compared to OCD) (as growth progresses the capitellum returns to normal) A self-limiting condition, **no specific treatment** is necessary apart from rest during the acute period.

Little leaguer's elbow

A medial epicondylar stress lesion or acute valgus stress syndrome which occurs in children. Results from repetitive valgus stress in a young throwing athlete which causes a flexor forearm muscle pull on the medial epicondyle epiphysis (Fig. 9.4). **Presents** with medial-sided elbow pain with decreased throwing effectiveness and throwing distance. Examination reveals medial epicondylar tenderness and pain on loading the flexor muscles. An elbow flexion contracture may be present.

X-ray shows separation and fragmentation of the epiphyseal lines. **Treatmen**: a benign injury that responds to rest and activity modification. Return to throwing after 6 weeks, and only occasionally (if a large fragment separated) surgical fixation.

1. <u>Separation.</u> Widened epiphysis secondary to repetitive valgus stress.

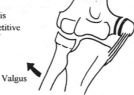

Valgus

2. <u>Displacement.</u> Fall resulting in displace medial epicondyle fracture.

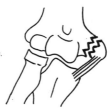

299

3. <u>Entrapment.</u> Occasionally the fragment is caught in the joint.

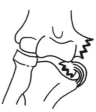

Fig. 9.4 'Little leaguer's elbow'

Medial epicondylar fractures

A substantial acute valgus stress (fall or violent muscle contracture while throwing) can produce a fracture through the epiphyseal plate seen in adolescents and throwers. **Presentation**: there is pain and localized tenderness over the medial epicondyle. A 15° flexion contracture is present.

X-rays may show a minimal to markedly displacement (with the fragment sometimes caught in the joint). **Treatment** depends on the degree of displacement. If the fragment is undisplaced or displaced less than 1cm, then immobilize for 3–4 weeks. If grossly displaced or caught in the joint or if ulnar nerve symptoms are present then open reduction is necessary.

Olecranon bursitis

Acute

An inflammation of the superficial olecranon bursa (from direct trauma or repetitive stress around the elbow). Non-traumatic causes are gout or rheumatoid arthritis. **Presentation**: there is an enlarged, non-tender bursa with normal ROM. Exclude a septic bursitis (the bursa is inflamed and tender; the patient septic with fever and malaise). If worried about sepsis then aspirate under aseptic conditions.

For recurrent bursitis x-ray to look for an *olecranon spur* or *calcification as seen in gout*. If the bursitis is associated with an inflammatory condition then control the underlying condition. On **first presentation** use NSAIDs, and treat cause. **Treatment**: rest, activity modification, and NSAIDs will usually relieve the bursitis (over a few months).

Chronic

Severe persistent olecranon bursitis will require operative intervention (a posterior incision with excision of the burial sac).

Septic

Note: infection of the bursa does not mean elbow joint infection (as it does not communicate with joint); one-third of patients give a history of a previous non-infected bursitis.

Symptoms are either acute onset of cellulitis to a low grade process of 2 or more weeks. The bursa is erythematous and tender and there are signs of generalized sepsis. Diagnosis is confirmed by aspiration (look for organisms) and an increased white cell count (consistent with infection). The presence of crystals in the aspirate indicates gout or pseudogout. **Treatment** is aspiration and antibiotics. However, if this fails surgical drainage is required.

Tendinous ruptures

Tendon injuries around the elbow[1]

Apart from epicondylitis, injuries to the tendons around the elbow are uncommon. The tendons that can rupture are the distal biceps (from the radial tuberosity) or the distal triceps (from its insertion into the olecranon).

Distal biceps rupture

3–10% of all biceps ruptures occur in the dominant arm of a well-developed male (in his 40s–50s). The result of a single traumatic event (sudden extension force while flexing—contracting—the biceps). There is sudden sharp pain and discomfort in the antecubital fossa. *Note* weakness of the elbow flexion and supination (with the elbow flexed). The muscle contracts proximally and a defect is noticeable.

Surgical treatment is (difficult, suggest anterior approach with anchor suture to bicipital tuberosity) almost always recommended (conservative management leads to moderate weakness especially in manual workers). Complications of surgery include cross union between the radius and ulna or a posterior interosseous nerve palsy.

Rupture of the triceps tendon

May occur spontaneously or after injury (from a decelerating force on the arm in extension during a fall). It can also result from sudden forced flexion while the elbow is being extended. Sudden pain and local swelling with a corresponding defect in the triceps tendon. X-ray may show a small bony fragment (avulsion of the tendon from the olecranon). Some loss of extension power is present.

1 RP Nirschl 1993 In BF Morrey BF (ed) *The elbow and its disorders* 2nd edn p537–52. Saunders, Philadelphia

Fractures and dislocations

Supracondylar fractures

The worrisome fracture. These occur in children with 97% being posteriorly displaced or angulated (from an extension injury due to a fall on an outstretched hand, causing the distal lower humerus to be pushed backwards).

There is a painful, swollen elbow and S-deformity. *Check the pulse (and circulation)* which may be compromised from swelling and fracture configuration. *Check the nerves* as 10–15% have a neuropraxia of radial, anterior interosseous, median nerve, ulnar—in that order. **Treat** undisplaced fractures in a collar and cuff for 3 weeks (monitor the position with serial x-rays). Displaced fractures require at least a closed reduction and (occasionally) percutaneous K-wires if unstable.

Complications include cubitus varus (gun-stock deformity, cosmetic) or neurological. Vascular insufficiency resulting in Volkmann's ischemia and later myositis ossifications can occur (*a disaster*). Adult supracondylar and intercondylar fractures are not nearly as common (generally require open reduction and internal fixation).

Lateral condylar fractures

The lateral condyle epiphysis begins to ossify by 1 year and fuses to the shaft by 12–14 years of age. During this period (4–10 years) fracture separations may occur. It is important to look out for such a fracture as it may lead to growth plate damage, and as it involves the joint accurate reduction is critical. Later problems include cubitus valgus with tardy ulnar nerve palsy. If undisplaced, splint the arm in a backslab at 90°; if displaced, accurate reduction is needed and fixation with K-wires.

Fractures of the radial head

More common in adults than children, result from a fall on the outstretched hand thus pushing the elbow into valgus and compressing the radial head. If undisplaced, treat in a backslab; if displaced, requires open reduction (if possible); excision (if grossly comminuted).

Fractures of the neck of the radius

Same mechanism as radial head fractures. (In adult, fracture of the radial head; children, due to the cartilaginous epiphysis, fracture through the radial neck). Up to 20° of radial tilt is acceptable, beyond 20°, closed reduction and occasionally open reduction (if difficult). Monteggia fractures result from a fall on an outstretched hand resulting in a fracture of the ulna with dislocation of the radius (often missed). This fracture requires a closed reduction and immobilization, closely monitoring the position of the radial head (on x-ray line down the middle of the radial shaft should bisect radial head in all views).

Elbow dislocations

More common in adults. Without fracture, are called simple, and classified according to the direction of the displacement of the olecranon (79% are posterior or posterolateral). Result from a fall on the outstretched hand (with the elbow in extension); the anterior capsule brachialis. The surrounding ligaments may stretch or rupture depending on the direction of the dislocation. There may be a fracture. There is obvious deformity, pain, and swelling. There may be vessel and neurological damage. (Neuropraxia seen in 20% of cases; involves the ulnar or median nerves, and transient). X-rays are necessary.

Treatment: closed reduction is performed (apply longitudinal traction, with the free hand move the olecranon back on to the trochlea, ideally under general anesthetic so as to assess the elbow stability post reduction). If stable, can return to protected motion as soon as possible although may lose the last few degrees of extension and supination.

Associated injuries and complications (*do note*) include fractures (or avulsion of the medial of epicondyle), head of radius, or olecranon process; heterotopic ossification, recurrent dislocations, and vascular or neural injury.

Nerve compression syndromes

Numerous nerves may be compressed around the elbow. These include:

- *Ulnar nerve*—cubital tunnel, Guyon's canal.
- *Radial nerve*—radial tunnel/arcade of Frohse (posterior interosseous nerve)/Wartenburg syndrome.
- *Median nerve*—pronator syndrome/anterior interosseous syndrome/carpal tunnel.

Compression may occur from fracture or gradual onset (no injury) from degenerative changes about the joint, a space-occupying lesion (ganglion or bursa), or musculotendinous anomalies. *Clinically localized* sensory and motor changes specific for a particular nerve are seen.

Cubital tunnel syndrome

This is an irritation or compression of the ulnar nerve within the cubital tunnel at the elbow (in the athlete, a response to chronic activity). Chronic valgus strain may cause traction neuritis, scar formation, spurs, calcification in the MCL, or osteophytes (all can compress the ulnar nerve). **Presentation**: pain along the medial side of the forearm which may be proximally or distally. Paresthesia in the little finger and ring finger is seen early and precedes any detectable motor weakness of the hand. *Ulnar paradox* present (claw deformity the of hand is less than if the ulnar nerve is compressed in the hand as flexo digitorum profundus (FDP) to little not working). There is a positive percussion test over the ulnar nerve at the elbow, abnormal mobility of the nerve over the medial epicondyle and a positive provocative test (Fig 9.5: hyperflex elbow; dorsiflex wrist pain, ulnar nerve stretched). Clumsiness of the hand, especially after pitching may be noted.

Diagnosis may require nerve conduction studies. **Differential diagnosis** includes cervical spine pathology, thoracic outlet, or pathology involving the ulnar nerve at the wrist. **Treatment** is initially an elbow splint and correction of the underlying pathology. If this fails, then surgical decompression with transposition of the ulnar nerve (or medial epicondylectomy).

Radial nerve (radial tunnel)

May be compressed along its path from the lateral head of triceps to mid forearm (where it branches into the posterior interosseous nerve) from trauma. There is lateral elbow pain (similar to lateral epicondylitis pain). Neurological **symptoms and signs** including weakness of wrist and finger extension and paresthesia dorsally over the base of the thumb (exacerbated by resisted extension of the middle finger; which differentiates from tennis elbow). Surgical decompression is often required.

Median nerve

The median nerve is vulnerable to compression from: supracondyloid process (ligament struthers), fibrosus lacertus, pronator teres, or flexor superficialis arch. Such compression may produce the *pronator syndrome*—not uncommon in athletes. **Symptoms** are vague (discomfort in the forearm) with numbness of the hand in the median nerve distribution secondary. Repetitive activities such as in factory work,

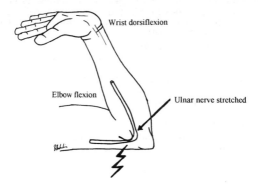

Fig. 9.5 The positive provocative test

weight training, or driving will provoke symptoms. **Signs** include tenderness over pronator muscle, proximal forearm pain on resisted pronation, elbow flexion, and wrist flexion. **Test**: tesisted flexion of the middle or ring finger PIP will reproduce symptoms.

Anterior interosseous syndrome. Where the anterior interosseous branch of the median is compressed between the two heads of the pronator muscle. Pain in proximal forearm, weakness of end pinch with FPL, and index finger FDP (difficulty forming the 'OK' sign with flexion of DIPJ index finger and IPJ of thumb; see Fig. 10.8). **Treatment** requires surgical release.

Musculocutaneous nerve

May be compressed between biceps and brachialis by lateral epicondyle. **Surgical release** is sometimes necessary.

Intraarticular derangements

Loose bodies

In the elbow from old trauma, OA, OCD, and synovial chondromatosis. Extension is reduced and there is pain and locking (intermittent) or grating. X-rays are useful. If troublesome, then remove surgically (arthroscopically, or if multiple loose bodies, then via an arthrotomy). Synovectomy may be necessary for synovial chondromatosis.

Osteoarthritis of the elbow

OA of the elbow joint from trauma, OCD, or synovial disease (chondrometaplasia). Pain with loss of range of motion, locking, localized tenderness, joint thickening, crepitus, and flexion contracture often with associated ulnar nerve irritation. **Treatment**: rest, physiotherapy, and NSAIDs with modification of activity. Later, arthroscopic debridement, radial head excision, or arthroplasty may be required.

10 Hand and wrist[1]

EUGENE SHERRY

314

1 B Dilley *et al* 1997 In E Sherry, D Bokor (ed) *Manual of sports medicine*. Ch12, p161–79. GMM, London

Introduction

The hand and wrist are frequently injured in sport. Careful assessment and investigation will improve diagnosis and management. The essential functions of the hand are touch and, firm and precise grip (the thumb opposes the fingers and provides this precision grip). The wrist is the stable platform for the hand and so fine-tunes grasp. Hunter, tool-maker[1], surgeon, and athlete all depend on their hands.

1 Were our big-brained ancestors the first tool-makers or were they some distant, dead end, small—brained vegetarian cousins? It's not that clear. Ann Gibbons 1997 Tracing the identity of the first tool-makers. *Science* **276**, p32

Biomechanics

Biomechanics and function are inextricably linked. (This interplay is nowhere more evident than in the hand.) Tendons, intrinsic muscles, nerves, and vessels form an intricate, yet robust unit capable of delivering a knock-out punch or putting the ball to the cup. A knowledge of surface anatomy is important (Fig. 10.1). (*Note*: learn about other more common anatomic variations, e.g. flexor digitorum superficialis to the small finger is absent in a significant number of people, an extensor digitorum manus brevis may be confused with a ganglion.)

Note that a relatively small amount of oedema in the finger is enough to significantly restrict movement (especially at the PIP joint, see Fig. 10.2).

Normal   With oedema

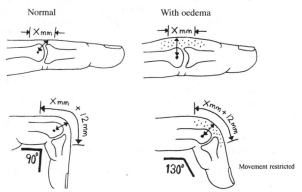

Fig. 10.1 Surface anatomy of the hand

Normal   With oedema

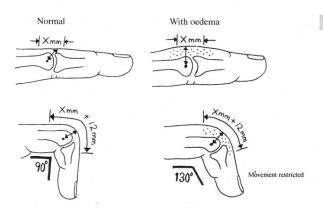

Fig. 10.2 Effect of oedema on movement of finger

Assessment of injury

What is the *chief complaint*? Either '*It doesn't feel right; it doesn't work right; it doesn't look right.*' What was the position of the hands and fingers at the *time of injury*? Such an understanding of the *mechanism of injury* with the chief complaint will be enough to secure the diagnosis (confirmed by examination and x-ray). The sports doctor may have witnessed the injury as it occurred.

Check the skin and nails, each joint (ligaments for stability, mobility of joints). Nerves (check sensation and motor supply), vessels (pulses, branching of nail bed) and bones (provide stability). Ask the patient to localize ('point with *one* finger, to *one* spot!') the site of the problem. (The site of *maximal tenderness.*) The **examination** should proceed in an orderly sequence. *Look, feel, move. Always compare sides.*

- *Look.* Inspect the dorsal and palmar surfaces. Look from the side, above, and end on. Note the position of wrists, hands, and fingers. (Any abnormal posture suggestive of a fracture, ligament, or tendon injury). *Note* swelling, lacerations, bruises, and sweat patterns.
- *Feel.* Palpate the area of concern, seek sites of tenderness, instability, masses, etc. Assess sensation and circulation. Perform the relevant provocative maneuvers. Assess grip and pinch strengths.
- *Move.* Ask the patient to make a complete fist and fully extend, abduct and adduct all fingers and both thumbs. Check wrist dorsiflexion, palmarflexion, radial and ulnar deviation, pronation, and supination.
- *X-rays* (specify views and sites, a minimum of two views at right angles). Special views are useful in assessing wrist injury (PA clenched fist for scapholunate gap, carpal tunnel for (hook and hamate fracture and pisotriquetral views). At the very least: PA views a neutral, ulnar and radial deviation, and direct lateral are necessary.
- *CT scanning* will provide additional anatomic information in trauma to the wrist (where difficult or unusual fractures, fracture/dislocations around the base of the metacarpals and carpus).
- *Bone scans* (where, but not what) are useful in the assessment of chronic wrist pain.
- *Ultrasound* ('operator-dependent') can localize non-radioopaque foreign bodies, and give much valuable information about soft tissue masses, tendons and ligaments.
- *MRI* may be of value in assessing the triangular fibrocartilage complex (TFCC).

Management of an isolated hand injury

Initial priorities
- stop bleeding (direct pressure)
- relieve pain (digital/wrist block)
- assess injury (and splint)

Path of recovery
- pain relief
- protection
- physiotherapy

A digital, or wrist block is the best way of relieving pain (lignocaine 2%, without adrenaline, in doses not exceeding 5mg/kg, any nerve injury must have been assessed and documented prior to the nerve block.)

Splinting the injured part is a simple (sadly often forgotten) way of providing effective and rapid pain relief. Splint as it lies or in the '*safe*' position (the wrist in about 30° extension, metacarpophalangeal joints 70–90° flexed, and the interphalangeal joints fully extended. The thumb, if included, is held parallel to the index finger). In this position, the collateral ligaments are at their longest.

The coach can correct faulty technique and advise the medical team on the demands of the sport. *But the patient is primarily responsible for his/her recovery. Only the patient can do and carry out the given advice.*

Pain relief, *protection*, and *physiotherapy* are the three Ps on the path to recovery:

- *Pain relief.* Use ice pack, elastic bandages, and elevation (to reduce pain and swelling). Analgesics are used. Ice pack, heat, laser, and TENS will also reduce pain. *Steroids.* (Betamethasone (Celestone) or methylprednisolone (Depomedrol) have no place in acute injury. *But* useful in chronic inflammatory conditions (only 2 or 3 injections be given in one area). Complications with prolonged use include skin atrophy, fat necroses, infection, and tendon rupture.

  Athletes (under pressure to get back into competition) may request a '*pain-killing injection*'. Injection of local anesthetic is not indicated. If the hand is too painful to stand up to the demand of competition it is not 'ready for them'.

- *Protection.* Continue splinting from acute phase of injury if necessary to stabilize and protect (allows protected movement— 'buddy taping' to a healthy digit is easy and useful, apply tape so as not to interfere with joint movement, be careful when 'buddying' an injured small finger to the right ring finger as a deforming rotatory force may be applied to the injured digit). *Dynamic* splinting is best and often used in combination with static splints (at night). (S-Thumb will protect thumb or wrist, see Fig. 10.3). Surgery may be necessary to get stability and protection.

- *Physiotherapy.* Early active movement should begin as soon as possible. When pain settles, stability is established, and movement returns, stretching and strengthening are started. Any impediment to movement should be removed—pain, instability, and oedema.

Oedema is reduced by movement, elevation, ice pack, and pressure from elastic bandages (Coban or similar) or tailor-made gloves. Massage, laser, and intermittent positive pressure (Masman pump) will help.

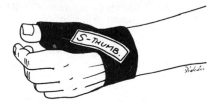

Fig. 10.3 S-Thumb splint

Fractures

The biology and biomechanics of fracture and soft tissue healing are no different in the athlete. (Athletes do not heal any quicker because they seek the advice and treatment of a sports doctor.) In general, fracture union in the upper limb occurs in about 6 weeks (in the adult, and about 3 weeks in a child, fracture consolidation takes twice as long). What is different is the *attitude to injury*. The demands of competition (especially at the élite level) may result in the athlete returning to training and competition too early (so running the risk of further injury). Financial concerns may bear on this decision to return. The athlete will make the ultimate decision. It is the role of the sports medical team to advise what the risks are and how they can be minimized.

The **clinical signs** of fracture are important (pain, swelling, deformity, and loss of function). **Diagnosis** is confirmed by x-ray. Early movement is the key for a swift return to full function (so the fracture must be of a stable pattern, or be rendered stable by splinting or surgical fixation). Outcomes deteriorate if active range of motion is delayed beyond 3 weeks.

A fracture is reduced under appropriate anesthetic by closed or open means and rendered stable. (Confirm by x-ray and repeat 1 week post injury and later as necessary.) If the fracture cannot be made stable by splinting, surgical fixation is necessary. In general, displaced fractures involving joint surfaces will require reduction and surgical fixation. *Note* the so-called 'clip' or 'avulsion' fractures, the bony equivalent of a tendon or ligament rupture, will usually require surgical repair.

Distal phalanx fractures

These result from a direct blow, often with the finger being 'crushed' between the bat and ball. The hallmark is a *subungual hematoma*. The nail plate maybe lifted out of the nail fold, suggesting that the fracture was displaced and that a significant injury to the nail bed has occurred. A painful subungual hematoma under pressure may be relieved by drilling the nail plate with a sterile 19-gauge needle, x-rays should then be taken (surgical cleaning of the fracture site, with accurate repair of the nail bed, magnification, and fracture fixation where appropriate, give the best result). Some surgeons feel a hematoma involving more than 25% of the nail plate is an indication for its removal to allow nail bed repair.

Bony mallet

Catching a finger on the ground ball or an opponent may result in avulsion fractures of the extensor tendon (*bony mallet*) or less commonly avulsion of the flexor tendon (the latter is more serious and usually less recognized). Almost always requires surgical treatment. *Note*: occasionally the tendon will pull away from the bone chip and be found in the palm.

The bony mallet (if no more that 30% of the joint surface is involved and no joint subluxation) is treated in a hyperextension splint (maintain for at least 6–8 weeks.) Instruct patient in skin care and changing splints.

Middle and proximal phalanges, metacarpals

Transverse fractures of the middle phalanx (distal to the insertion of flexor superficialis) result in extension of the distal fragment, those proximal to its insertion are flexed. Transverse fractures of the proximal phalanx usually result in the interossei flexing the proximal fragment. Transverse fractures of metacarpals tend to have the distal fragment flexed by the long flexors. Reduction and neutralization of the deforming forces may be possible using 'buddy taping' and extension block splinting.

However, short oblique, and spiral fractures of the phalanges and metacarpals may shorten/rotate and so require surgical fixation. *Rotation is assessed with the fingers in flexion.* The fingers should not cross and the tips should individually point to the tubercle of the scaphoid.

'Boxer's fracture'

A fracture of the neck of the small finger metacarpal and can be a result of bar-room brawling, is usually best treated in a resting splint with the hand in a safe position until pain and swelling subside (7–10 days) followed by active mobilization. Such fractures generally do not require fixation despite what appears to be marked x-ray deformity.

Dislocations and collateral ligament injuries

Dorsal dislocation of the PIPJ is common. Closed reduction (direct traction) is possible immediately, on the field, or later, under digital block. Following reduction joint, gauge stability. (The volar plate is avulsed from the middle phalanx, possibly with a bony fragment.) Splinting straight for 7–10 days then 'buddy taping' (or dorsal block splint) for 3 weeks is recommended, and during strenuous activity (for a further 6–8 weeks).

If a dislocation will not reduce easily because of *soft tissue interposition* or entrapment of the dislocated phalangeal metacarpal head. Then open reduction required.

For partial collateral ligament ruptures, start immediate motion, protect with 'buddy taping' for 6–8 weeks (depending on residual tenderness). Complete ruptures (controversial) either splint or surgically repair.

Metacarpophalangeal joint dislocations (rare) require open reduction as are thumb and collateral ligament injuries.

Skier's thumb (gamekeeper's thumb)[1]

This common injury occurs from sudden forced radial deviation (with/without hyperextension) of the thumb phalanx on the metacarpal with disruption, partial or complete, of the UCL/MCP (ulnar collateral ligament of the MCP) of the thumb; often seen in skiers (the ski pole handle does not give protection) and football. **Presents** with ulnar-sided pain, swelling and instability. X-rays may show a bony avulsion. Graded as type I (sprain: splint for 6 weeks in S-Thumb, Johnson and Johnson, and then when return to vigorous sports), II (partial tear, same splint) and III (complete tear, >30 abduction possible, needs surgical repair and protection postoperatively in S-Thumb for 6 weeks and in vigorous sport) (Fig. 10.3). Athletes seem reluctant to seek treatment for such 'minor' injuries. Rupture of UCL/MCP (type III) thumb often requires open exploration and repair as it is almost impossible to tell whether or not the avulsed ligament has come to lie superficial to the adductor aponeurosis (Stener lesion). However, most surgeons will not explore where stable (<30 abduction). Investigation of previous injuries similarly shows the ligament folded back on itself beneath the adductor aponeurosis.)

Mallet/baseball finger[2]

Closed rupture of the distal extensor tendon results in the 'mallet', or 'baseball' finger (Fig. 10.4). Provided no joint subluxation, or fracture one-third or less of the articular surface, splint the DIPJ in slight hyperextension for 6–8 weeks (even if present after 7–19 days). In supple fingers, if a swan neck deformity develops at the PIPJ include this joint in the splint for 3–4 weeks (in slight flexion). Commercial splints are available.

Rupture middle slip

Of the extensor mechanism over the PIPJ is commonly missed and results in a boutonniere deformity (difficult to correct). Suspect in a 'jammed' PIPJ, when the joint is swollen, and tender over its dorsum.

1 CS Campbell 1995 *JBJS* **37B** 148–9   **2** EB Kaplan 1940 *Surgery* **7**, 784–91

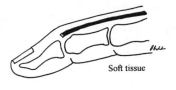

Soft tissue

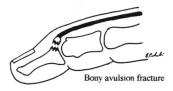

Bony avulsion fracture

Fig. 10.4 Mallet finger injury

Specific tests: inability to extend actively the last 10–15° at the PIPJ, and the Elson test (flex the PIPJ to a right angle 'over the edge of a table', ask the patient to extend the PIPJ, a central slip rupture will display no movement of the middle phalanx and the distal phalanx will tend to extend). Lack of full extension, although full passive extension of the PIPJ by tenodesis when the wrist and metacarpo-phalangeal joints are fully passively flexed, indicates rupture. Later signs are fixed flexion of the PIPJ with decreased passive DIPJ flexion with PIPJ fully extended. **Splinting** is the most effective treatment. First correct PIPJ flexion and then DIP flexion (may take a minimum of 8 weeks or more to achieve the desired results).

Ruptures of the extensor mechanism at the level of the MPJ may occur (a ruptured sagittal band, on the radial side of the middle finger). There is localized pain, swelling and an inability to extend actively the MPJ. *Note* that the patient can maintain full extension of the joint if it is passively extended. Triggering (extensor tendon subluxing between the metacarpal heads) of the finger at MPJ rather than PIPJ level may later present. If seen early these injuries respond to splinting the MPJ in extension for 3 weeks. Other joints are left free. If seen late the tear is best repaired.

May see rarely at MPJ level a longitudinal split in the extensor tendon and rupture of the dorsal MPJ capsule (result of a direct blow, as in boxing or martial arts). Surgical repair is indicated.

Flexor tendon avulsion ('jersey' finger)[1]

Is not common and not well recognized (from an attempt to grab the jersey or equipment of an opposing player. Not able to flex, DIPJ bruising is present and a tender lump in the palm. The ring finger commonly affected. Players of 'Oztag', a variation of touch football in which a 'tackle' is effected by ripping a velcro fastened tag from the shorts of an opponent, cause this injury.

Early repair is best. Later, repair is difficult because of swelling and collapse of the flexor sheath. If there is no pain and little functional deficit leave. Hyperextension of the DIPJ with or without 'weakness' in the finger may be treated by DIPJ fusion. Two-stage tendon reconstruction is difficult.

32

Wrist fracture

Scaphoid fracture

The most common carpal fracture. Volumes have been written about the appropriate management of this fracture. Suspected after a fall on to the hand and tenderness over the scaphoid or in the anatomic 'snuff box' (scaphoid impaction test, SIT, is positive, Fig. 10.5). Swelling and 'thickening' in the AP length of the wrist may be seen. Resisted pinch is painful. The x-rays should include a 'scaphoid view' (PA in ulnar deviation).

X-rays may be negative. Place the patients in a 'scaphoid cast' and x-ray again at 2 weeks. If still pain with negative x-rays, consider a truly 'occult' fracture, or a scaphoid–lunate ligament injury and obtain stress x-rays and a bone scan.

The median time for union of a scaphoid fracture is 12 weeks. (The more proximal the fracture is, the more likely avascular necrosis and/or non-union.)

Treatment: immobilize tubercle or non-displaced (*no displacement*) wrist fractures in a short arm cast (including the thumb up to, but not including the IPJ) with the thumb pulp opposed to the pulp of the middle finger for 6 weeks. If no evidence of union progressing fix the fracture with a Herbert screw. *Displaced waist and proximal third fractures* are fixed immediately with a Herbert screw. If early mobilization is desired, as with athletes, the fracture is also fixed immediately. Return to sport 3 weeks after surgery in *non*-contact sports (contact and collision are not permitted until union has occurred and not before 6–8 weeks post fracture).

Other carpal fractures

Fractures of the triquetrum are the second or third most common carpal fracture (usually avulsions from the dorsum of the bone). Immobilize in a splint for 3–4 weeks to allow pain to settle for resumption of activity (occasionally becomes source of ongoing pain and fragment excision, and ligament repair may be required).

Fracture of the hook of hamate

Accounts for 2% of carpal fractures and are common in 'club' or 'racquet' sports (hockey, golf, baseball, cricket, tennis). The mechanism of injury is an impact between the base of the club, bat, or racquet and hypothenar eminence. (The handle of a cricket bat is sprung to absorb impact and so a 'batsman' is less likely than a 'batter' to incur fracture.) The golfer implodes the ground on the swing.

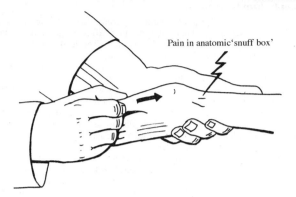

Fig. 10.5 Pain in the anatomic 'snuff box': the SIT test

33

Carpal instabilities and ligamentous injuries

Scapholunate ligament

Commonly injured (presents like a scaphoid fracture) from a fall on the outstretched hand. There may be 'pop' after a back hand volley. Pain is over the dorsal aspect of the ligament. Tenderness located over the ligament (distal to Lister's tubercle) may be the only sign. *Kirk Watson* has a provocative maneuver to assess the stability of the scaphoid: radially deviate the hand while stabilizing the scaphoid with volar pressure—pain results. X-rays show a scapholunate gap (the Terry Thomas sign). Clenched fist PA views (compare with the non-injured side) are helpful. Arthrography will show the tear. MRI is still unreliable. Arthroscopy will indicate diagnosis and treatment. **Treatment** is difficult, recovery long, and controversial: whether limited intercarpal fusion or capsulodesis.

Chronic tears may lead to a dorsal intercalated segment instability (DISI) with eventual degenerative change throughout the carpus.

Tears of the lunotriquetral ligament may present with ulnar wrist pain. Test this joint by balloting the bones with respect to each other, pain and symptoms are reproduced. X-rays may show a step off in the curve formed by scaphoid, lunate and triquetrum at mid carpal level. Later changes may result in a volar intercalated instability (VISI). Assess the midcarpal joint and triangular fibrocartilage complex (TFCC) as these injuries may be associated with, or mimic, each other. Arthroscopic debridement, reduction, and pinning of the joint has been tried with small numbers of patients with some success.

Midcarpal instabilities may present with a painful 'clunk' and this can be reproduced by *Lichtman's maneuver* (patient makes a tight fist and moves the wrist from radial to ulnar direction).

333

Triangular fibrocartilage complex (TFCC) tears

These injuries cause ulnar-sided wrist pain. Tenderness is just distal to the tip of the ulna. 'Grinding' of the TFCC by compressing the dorsiflexed and ulnar deviated carpus against the complex will reproduce symptoms. Degenerative tears of the TFCC increases with age. 'Congenital tears' have been described.

If pain is aggravated by pronation and supination the **distal radio-ulnar joint** (DRUJ) may be injured (compress the joint as the patient pronates and supinates the forearm). *Stability* of the DRUJ is assessed by stressing the dorsal and volar radioulnar ligaments in neutral, full pronation, and supination. (In full supination the volar ligaments are taut and there should be no volar translation of the ulna; and the converse.)

Arthroscopy is a good way of **investigating** these problems and will allow debridement or suture of tears.

Soft tissue wrist pain

A cause of chronic wrist pain in the athlete, **diagnosable** by arthroscopy, is injury to the chondral surfaces. Good relief of symptoms has been reported with debridement of isolated lesions, occult ganglion may be present where diagnosis is difficult (detected by ultrasound or MRI).

De Quervain's tenosynovitis

Not uncommon in tennis, squash, racketball players, and weight lifters, there is tenderness over the first extensor compartment of the wrist. *Finkelstein's sign* is positive (flex thumb and ulnar deviation of wrist causes pain over 1st extensor compartment). **Treatment** is rest, splinting, and 1 or 2 injections of steroids and local anesthetic into the compartment. If this management fails, operative release (open 1st extensor compartment, care with dorsal radial) gives good results cutaneous nerve).

Wartenberg's syndrome[1]

This is neuritis of the radial sensory nerve and may be confused with De Quervain's tenosynovitis (or be associated with it). Seen in weight lifters with tight wrist bands. Typically, forearm pronation worsens; symptoms with paresthesia in the distribution of the radial sensory nerve. Responds to steroids and splinting, or (rarely required) a neurolysis.

Extensor pollicis longus may become inflamed. But note steroid injection is *contraindicated* (as ruptured of the tendon here is not uncommon). Surgical release of the tendon sheath is better.

1 MB Woods, JH Dobyns 1986 *Clin Orthop* **202** 93–102

Intersection syndrome

This is inflammation at the crossover between the first and second extensor compartments (where APL/EPB tendons cross the ECRL/ECRB tendons) may occur in rowers, weight lifters and, skiers. Splint the wrist extension, surgical 'release' seldom required.

Scaphoid impaction syndrome

Is seen in weight lifters and gymnasts. This **presents** with dorsal wrist pain (reproduced by forced dorsiflexion). It is caused by impingement of the scaphoid against the radius. X-rays show an osteophyte on the dorsoradial aspect of the scaphoid. **Treatment**: splinting for 6 weeks, or remove osteophyte.

Injury to the growth plate (*physis*) of the distal radius may occur in young, élite, female gymnasts with premature closure in severe cases. **Treatment** is modification of activities that aggravate the pain (up to 6 months may be necessary).

Other causes of ulnar-sided wrist pain include ulnar abutment syndrome, subluxing extensor carpi ulnaris tendon, extensor carpi ulnaris tendinitis, and acute calcific 'tendinitis'.

34

Ulnar abutment pain

Is caused by forced ulnar deviation. X-ray shows an ulnar *plus* variant. Later changes seen in the lunate (chondral lesions often noted at arthroscopy). **Surgical treatment** is arthroscopic excision of the ulnar head and debridement of chondral flaps, or ulnar shortening.

Subluxation of ECU is demonstrated on pronation and supination of the forearm. **Surgical reconstruction** is required. Tendinitis is treated with splinting, NSAIDs, and local infiltration of steroids. Acute calcific tendinitis needs to be distinguished from with infection and acute rheumatic conditions. Usually settles with splinting and NSAIDs.

Nerve compressions

The median nerve

May be compressed at several levels in the arm: by the ligament of Struthers, in the forearm at the level of the lacertus fibrosus, pronator teres, or at the origin of the flexor digitorum superficialis. There is activity-related discomfort in the forearm and median nerve paresthesia. Forced repetitive pronation in weight training may be a cause. The '*true*' *Tinel's sign* (sustained pressure directly over the nerve) reproduces paresthesia; what is now called Tinel's sign will be positive at the site of compression and so define the exact level of compression. **Symptoms** will be reproduced by resisted elbow and wrist flexion (compression *at lacertus*), resisted pronation (*at pronator*), or resisted long and ring finger PIPJ flexion (*at superficialis arch*). Nerve conduction studies are unreliable. **Treatment** is rest and modification of aggravating factors. Surgical release is occasionally needed.

Carpal tunnel syndrome

Is no different in the athlete (Fig. 10.6). Mild symptoms are treated with splinting the wrist (in neutral). Surgical release gives excellent relief, but be warned of the persistence of 'pillar pain' at the incision site associated with forcible grip for about 3 months. Note that *Kienböck's disease* (avascular necrosis of the lunate) can sometimes present as carpal tunnel syndrome.

Ulnar nerve (handlebar palsy)

May be compressed in Guyon's canal in cyclists as a result of wrist hyperextension and direct pressure from handlebars (Fig. 10.7). Numbness in the ulnar two and a half fingers is the usually presentation. Motor signs are often present. Avoid prolonged riding (for a time); use padded gloves and modify handlebars (may persist for several months), otherwise the most common cause of ulnar nerve compression at this level is a ganglion (seen on ultrasound).

Anterior interosseous nerve compression

May **present** with vague forearm pain and occasionally weakness of flexor pollicis longus, index profundus, and pronator quadratus (not able to make 'OK' sign Fig. 10.8). Possible causes: Anatomic variations in vessels, muscle origins, or nerves; space-occupying lumps such as ganglia and lipoma. **Management** as for pronator syndrome.

Radial nerve (radial tunnel syndrome, RTS)

Radial nerve compression may be confused with or be associated with lateral epicondylitis. Provocative tests for lateral epicondylitis (with straight elbow passive flex wrist, or ask patient to hold wrist dorsiflexed against resistance) produces pain over the extensors a few centimeters distal to the lateral epicondyle. **Test for RTS**: arm straight resisted compression long digit, tenses ECRB, and reproduces symptoms. Rested and splinting the forearm in neutral generally resolve symptoms. Numbness in the radial sensory nerve is rarely seen in runners who maintain marked elbow flexion throughout their gait cycle. Technique modification is usually all that is required.

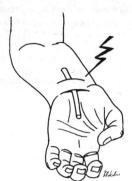

Fig. 10.6 Carpal tunnel syndrome

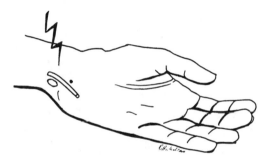

Fig. 10.7 Guyon's canal syndrome

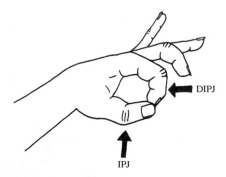

DIPJ

IPJ

Fig. 10.8 The 'OK' sign is normal (no nerve palsy)

Distal posterior interosseous nerve syndrome

An unusual cause of dorsal wrist pain. **Diagnosis** is secured if injection of local anesthetic into the fourth dorsal compartment eliminates symptoms. Transaction of the nerve may be needed.

Repetitive trauma to the *ulnar digital nerve* of the thumb occurs in ten-pin bowlers, and racquet sports. Equipment and technique modification are necessary to avoid permanent damage. Neurolysis is necessary for more severe cases.

Chronic compartment syndrome

Exertional pain over the first dorsal interosseous muscle and flexor forearm compartments may be due to a chronic compartment syndrome. **Diagnosis** is made by careful examination and compartment pressure studies. Fasciotomy may be necessary.

11 Hip, thigh, and pelvis[1]

EUGENE SHERRY

1 J Ireland 1997 In E Sherry, D Bokor (ed) *Manual of sports medicine*, Ch 13, p181–97, GMM, London

Introduction

Injuries of the hip, thigh, and pelvis are not that common in sport. They may be subtle in presentation and diagnosis is difficult or catastrophic with serious immediate and long-term consequences (e.g. hip fracture or pelvic fracture with shock).

Biomechanics

The hip is a ball-and-socket joint with simultaneous motion in all 3 planes (up to 120° of flexion, 20° of abduction, and 20° of external rotation). The joint reactive forces are 3–6 times bodyweight due to contraction of the large muscle groups around it; and this is increased with jumping or running.

The acetabulum has a fibrocartilaginous rim (labrum) to deepen it and so add further stability. The posterosuperior surface of the acetabulum is thickest to accommodate weight bearing. the neck forms an angle of about 125° with the shaft and is 20° anteverted. The hip capsule drops down across the front of the neck but only part way at the back. It is reinforced by three ligaments (the iliofemoral ligament of Bigelow is the strongest). The major blood supply to the head is from the medial circumflex branch (of the profunda femoris) which is at risk from fractures of the neck of femur and dislocations.

Contusion of quadriceps (cork thigh, Charley Horse)

The result of a direct blow during contact which varies from mild to severe. Often worse when the muscle is relaxed and occurs in the musculotendinous junction of the rectus femoris (central position of the quadriceps). **Clinical features** There is pain, stiffness, a limp, and progressive swelling with bruising. The pain is increased by resisted knee extension and hip flexion. Due to bleeding into the soft tissues symptoms become worse over the subsequent 48h. Classified according to that of Jackson and Feagin[1] (see also Table 11.1).

Treatment: there are three phases in the treatment.[2] Measure thigh diameter and follow to exclude small chance of compartment syndrome developing.

The *first* is limitation of motion to minimize hemorrhage (with Rest, Ice, Compression, and Elevation—RICE). The leg is maintained in extension and quadriceps isometric exercises are allowed. Do for 24h in mild contusions, 48h in severe. A more recent study suggests an alternative of keeping hip and knee flexed (probably as effective).

The *second* is the restoration of movement. This depends on the condition of the quadriceps stabilizing and the patient being pain-free at rest. Use continuous passive motion and gravity assisted motion. Supine and prone inactive knee flexion is encouraged along with isometric quadriceps exercises. Once a pain-free passive range of motion of 0–90° is achieved, and good quadriceps control, proceed to static cycling with increasing resistance. Eventually, there is ROM >90° and normal free gait (without a crutch).

The *third* is functional rehabilitation with progressive increasing resistance exercises that builds strength and endurance. **Must always be pain-free**.

1 DW Jackson, JA Feagin 1973. *JBJS* **55A** 95-105   2 B Rooger *et al* 1991 *J Orthop Trauma* **5** 57-59

Table 1 Classification of contusion quadriceps

Mild	Localized tenderness in the quadriceps, knee motion of 90° or more, no alteration of gait. The athlete is able to do a deep knee bend
Moderate	Swollen tender muscle mass, less than 90° of knee motion and antalgic gait. The athlete is able to do knee bends, climb stairs, or arise from a chair without pain
Severe	Thigh is markedly tender and swollen and the contours of the muscle cannot be defined. Knee motion is less than 45° and there is severe limp. The athlete prefers to walk with crutches and frequently has an effusion in the ipsilateral knee

Myositis ossificans traumatica

A severe contusion or tear in the quadriceps with hematoma followed by acute inflammation. Fibroblasts then form osteoid. Specific risk factors have been identified:[1]

- Knee motion <120°
- Injury from football
- Previous quadriceps injury
- Delay in treatment (>3 days)
- Ipsilateral knee effusion

Clinical features: pain is over the front of the thigh along with a fluctuant mass which forms into a hard mass at 2–4 weeks. (May resolve after 6 months if the injury is low grade and in the musculotendinous region.) **Treatment** as for contusion of the quadriceps. Aspiration or open drainage of the hematoma may be necessary. Femoral nerve blocks, NSAIDs, and radiotherapy have been used.

Quadriceps strain and ruptures[1]

The result of a severe contraction when either accelerating or kicking (usually the rectus femoris and distal in the thigh). **Clinical features** are localized tenderness or a palpable defect (Fig. 11.1). The pain is exacerbated by resistance of hip flexion in extension and full knee flexion in a prone position. MRIs show a high signal on a T2 weighted image.

Differentiate from an L3 nerve root lesion (pain is in both midlumbar back and leg; made worse by straight leg raising). **Treatment** as for quadriceps contusions.

364

1 JB Ryan *et al* 1991 *Am J Sports Med* **19** 299-304

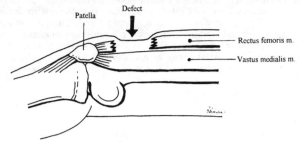

Fig. 11.1 Defect in rectus femoris (quads); patient may still be able to raise straight leg

Avulsions of the iliac spines

The mechanism of injury is a sudden violent contracture of the rectus femoris muscle (occasionally the sartorius muscle seen in soccer players). Players tend to be in their mid teens. **Clinical features**: include severe pain point tenderness and bruising (sometimes dramatic). **Treatment** includes RICE. If there is persisting functional impairment then **surgery may be necessary** to fix the apophysis or avulsed fragment. Sometimes the bone fragment needs to be excised (at later date).

Hamstring strains

In the late swing phase of the gait cycle, hamstrings decelerate the limb, with sudden acceleration from the stabilizing flexion to active extension, strain is put on the hamstring muscles. This injury is most likely to occur with sudden hamstring contraction in athletes when they are cold or have not done adequate stretching. Common situations are at the starting blocks, sprinters at take off, (or high jumpers and long jumpers), an sudden acceleration, or resisted extension by football players (Fig. 11.2). The short head of the biceps femoris is most commonly affected. Occasionally, dystrophic calcification is seen.

The patient may describe a twinge or a snap and localize an area (e.g. the short head of the biceps). Swelling and a palpable defect are common. **Treatment** includes RICE and physiotherapy (local cryotherapy and ultrasound). A stretching program to be commenced once pain has subsided. Recovery is from days to weeks (depending on the severity).

The **key to treatment is to remedy poor training techniques and improve flexibility.** The athlete must carry out an adequate warm-up and stretching program prior to a return to sporting activities. The significant imbalance between quadriceps and hamstrings needs to be overcome, and adequate return hamstring strength before returning to sport. A firm elasticized support is useful.

Reinjury may occur with longer recovery; therefore exercise good judgment about when to return to sport.

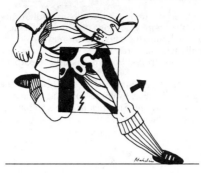

Fig. 11.2 Starting or acceleration maneuvers may avulse/tear hamstrings

Ischial apophysitis (weaver's bottom, ischial bursitis) and avulsions

The result of excessive running (especially in adolescents). Repetitive strain is put on the apophysis; worsened by tight hamstrings. Severe contracture of the hamstring musculature may avulse the tuberosity. There is a dull ache and tenderness in the area and associated tightness of the hamstrings. Ecchymosis and a palpable defect are present.

X-ray will show fragmentation or avulsion of the apophysis. **Treatment** includes RICE, physiotherapy, and a flexibility program as for a hamstring strain. Significant displacement or functional disability may necessitate surgical fixation.

Groin strains (adductor strain)

The groin is an *ill-defined area* and most injuries here involve the adductor muscles. **Important**: exclude fractures, avulsions, hip joint injuries, inflammation of the pelvic joints, bursitis around the hip, snapping hip, nerve entrapment, and various forms of referred groin pain from hernias, prostatitis, urinary infections, gynecological disorders, rheumatological diseases, bone infections, and tumors.

Occurs in sports where cutting, side stepping, or pivoting are required (as in soccer and rugby). There is a violent external rotation with the leg in a widely abducted position. Occurs at the musculotendinous junction. Injuries are often acute-on-chronic disruptions due to increased collagen at the musculotendinous junction, and therefore reduced extensibility. **Symptoms**: the athlete describes a sudden knife-like pain in the groin area. Bruising and swelling are noted and tenderness is well localized. The pain is exacerbated by adduction against resistance. In chronic cases the symptoms are more vague and diffuse. Renstrom[1] described pain with exercise as most common but also at rest often associated with stiffness in the morning, and some weakness.

MRI identifies adductor longus as the sole affected muscle. **Treatment** includes RICE. After the initial 24–48h hemorrhage should have ceased and physiotherapy modalities (cryotherapy and ultrasound) started. Antiinflammatory medication is useful for short periods in chronic cases. A stretching program is then started with isometrics, without resistance, followed by the gradual introduction of resistance (within the limits of pain). Attention should be directed to a lack of flexibility and to improving training techniques. Use of an elasticized tape for support is useful. Steroids occasionally are of benefit in chronic cases.

Surgery is only contemplated after conservative management for 6–12 months. A release of the adductor longus tendon is carried out with the hip in a flexed and abducted position. Any degenerate nodule should be debrided, failing this a tenotomy is often useful. Inguinal and femoral hernias may need repair (return to sport in 6–8 weeks).

A grade III complete rupture is very uncommon (it occurs at the femoral attachment). In selected cases surgical repair is undertaken.

1 PAHF Renstrom 1992 *Clin Sports Med* **11** 815-31

Hip pointer and fracture iliac crest

The result of a direct blow to the iliac crest resulting in bruising (muscle or bone) or fracture. From contact sports after a tackle or fall on to the iliac crest. **Clinical features** include maximum tenderness usually over the mid point of the iliac crest corresponding to the divergence of abdominal and lumbar musculature (the muscle fiber separation). Otherwise, the area of tenderness is at the point of contact. Swelling and ecchymosis are seen over 24h.

X-rays needed to rule out a fracture and subsequent x-rays may show periostitis or exostosis formation. **Treatment** includes RICE (first 24h). Occasionally, aspiration and injection of local anesthetic needed. After bleeding has ceased, ultrasound and other physical therapy modalities useful. Protective padding when returning to contact sports. Surgical fixation is rarely required for displaced iliac crest fractures (where skin tenting).

Iliac crest apophysitis and avulsion

May result from repetitive stress in adolescents especially running with a crossover style of arm swing. Severe contraction or a direct blow may also avulse the iliac crest. **Clinical features** are tenderness (anteriorly or posteriorly) on the iliac crest depending on whether tensor fascia lata, gluteus medius, or oblique abdominal muscles are involved. Resistance to abduction and contralateral flexion of the trunk frequently exacerbates the pain.

X-rays are needed to exclude avulsion of the iliac apophysis. **Treatment** includes RICE and physicotherapy. It may be necessary to change the athletes running style; gradually reintroduce activities. Occasionally, surgery is necessary to reduce the avulsed iliac crest.

Trochanteric bursitis and snapping hip

An inflammation of the bursa over the greater trochanter region as a result of increased shear stress caused by the iliotibial band over the trochanter. Often, a broad pelvis and large quadriceps angle (Q-angle). Leg length discrepancies, pelvic tilt or crossover type running style may be present.

A snapping hip is due to thickening of the posterior part of the iliotibial band which produces a painless snapping sensation (*snapping iliotibial band syndrome*). **Clinical features** are pain over the lateral aspect of the thigh when lying on the affected side (in the posterior and lateral aspect of the trochanter). Abducting against resistance in an internally rotated position will exacerbate the pain. A snapping sensation may be noted with the patient standing on the extended knee and pushing the hip into an adducted and flexed position.

Other snapping hip is seen with repetitive rubbing of the capsule in running or ballet (involves the iliopsoas tendon), so-called iliopsoas bursitis.[1] **Clinical features** include pain around the medial aspect of the groin which occurs with rotation of the hip. Resistance to flexion of the hip from 90° of flexion leads to increased pain and tenderness in the groin. Clicking is reproducible and *note* that pain may be referred from the lumbosacral spine or sacroiliac joint.

Treatment includes RICE followed by ultrasound (low frequency pulsed) and stretching of the iliotibial band and iliopsoas to overcome contractures. Correct any leg length discrepancy or abnormal running style; orthotics can help. Steroid injections and antiinflammatories may be useful in an acute bursitis. Surgery has a limited place and only after a prolonged period of conservative management (technique involves Z-plasty of the iliotibial band or lengthening of iliopsoas in iliopsoas bursitis).

Bursitis iliopectioneal: pain over anterior hip with antalgic gait. **Treatment**: RICE, NSAIDs, stretching, and flexibility program.

1 M Jacob, B Young 1973 *Am Correct Ther J* **32** 92

Hip strain (pericapsulitis, synovitis, irritable hip)

The result of a direct blow, twisting injury, or from overuse of the hip. Inflammation of the lining or a strain of capsular ligaments occurs and may be cause of hip pain in young athletes. **Symptoms**: there is pain in the groin, radiating into the thigh. Athlete comfortable in flexion, abduction, and external rotation (increases volume of joint capsule so decompressing). Pain is worsened by extension and internal rotation. Antalgic gain may be noted.

Exclude infection (especially in children and in slip of the upper femoral epiphysis, SUFE). X-rays may show joint widening. Bone scan is often useful (positive). **Treatment** includes RICE and non-weight bearing exercise. (In children, bedrest, with springs and slings, until complete resolution of symptoms.) If capsular tightening occurs then a flexibility program is required. Arthroscopy is rarely necessary.

Conjoint tendon strain

Results from stress on the abdominal musculature (from a mark in football or heading in soccer). **Symptoms**: pain and tenderness over the superior pubic ramus. Hip movements are full. X-rays are normal. The bone scan is occasionally positive. **Treatment**: RICE, physicotherapy, and a flexibility program. Only occasionally surgery.

Osteitis pubis

A self-limiting necrosis in the bone of the pubis and synchondrosis.[1]
Results from repetitive shear stress across the symphysis in running
and kicking sports (subacute periostitis). **Clinical features** are a
gradual onset of groin pain worsened by activity. Severe pain when
jumping. Tenderness is maximal over the symphysis, the body, and
rami of the pubis; aggravated by pelvic compression, full flexion, wide
abduction of the hips, and even sit-ups. Exclude hernias, groin strains,
and prostatitis in males.

X-rays changes are delayed for at least a month but show a
periosteal reaction and demineralization of the subchondral bone
leading to a 'moth-eaten' appearance around the symphysis. (In
severe cases erosion can lead to instability; detected in single leg
weight bearing views of the pelvis.) Bone scans are often positive in
the early stages (gallium scans to exclude an infection). **Treatment**
includes rest, NSAIDs, and occasionally steroid injections. Then
gradual reintroduction of a flexibility program and increased weight
bearing. May take up to 12 months to recover.

1 JM Cochrand 1971 *Br J Sports Med* **5** 233.

Nerve entrapment

The nerves usually involved are the ilioinguinal nerve, obturator nerve, genitofemoral nerve, and lateral cutaneous nerve of the thigh. Hypertrophy of muscles (hypertrophied abdominal muscles may entrap theilioinguinal nerve; enlarged hip adductors in skaters may entrap the obturator nerve) or scarring, are the most likely causes. *Meralgia paresthetica* is caused by compression of the lateral femoral cutaneous nerve. A knowledge of the distribution of the nerves will help to make a diagnosis. These areas are likely to exhibit pain and paresthesia. Tenderness may be experienced over the subcutaneous emergence of the nerve Tine positive EMG. **Treatment**: NSAIDs, stretches, and local steroid injections are the first tried, but if symptoms persist then surgical release is necessary. Make sure the athlete is not wearing tight braces, pads, etc. nor carrying out long periods of hip flexion.

Labral tears

Typically seen in dysplastic hips where there are abnormal loads (shear and strain) on the labrum. Also from excessive twisting action. **Symptoms**: a sharp pain or a catching sensation on a background of a dull ache. (Aggravated by flexion and internal rotation of the hip.) X-rays may show acetabular dysplasia. Tears are confirmed by arthrography or arthroscopy (usually in the posterior aspect of the hip joint). **Treatment** is rest and surgical excision/repair (difficult).

38

Stress fractures

First described by Briethaupt in 1855 in German soldiers (Stechow noted stress fractures on x-rays in 1897). Stress fractures of the neck of femur were described by Blecher in 1905. Much of the early literature on stress fractures was from the military. Now, stress fractures are seen in athletes; the highly motivated athletes in peak condition and at maximal performance. Risk factors are endocrine disorders especially in amenorrhoeic female athletes (see Chapter 23); clearly an overuse injury. The mechanism is a partial or complete fracture of bone due to an inability to withstand non-violent stress applied in a rhythmic/repeated submaximal mode.

Controversy exists as to whether they are due to fatigue of muscles leading to increased load or (as Stanitski believes)[1] an increased muscular force plus increased rate of remodeling leading to resorption and rarefaction and ultimately to stress fractures. This will manifest as a periosteal or endosteal response giving an appearance of a stress fracture which may ultimately progress to a linear fracture and, in time, displace.

The **clinical and x-ray criteria** for diagnosis of a stress fracture are:
- premorbid normal bone
- no direct trauma/inciting activity
- pain and tenderness (on percussion and antalgic limp) prior to x-ray changes—useful clinical sign
- subsequent x-rays show resolution and modeling
- positive bone scan

Assess the opposite limb clinically and by x-ray to exclude a stress fracture (as not always symptomatic). Differential diagnosis includes tumor (particularly osteosarcoma and Ewing's tumor), osteomyelitis, or periostitis from TB or syphilis. Jumping often injures the femur and pelvis but stress fractures have been noticed among hikers and fencers (especially in the pelvis). Typically classified into those of the femoral neck or shaft:

Femoral neck (Hajeck)[2]

Compressive of inferior cortex—young patients/early internal callus/sclerosis, may complete/non-weight bearing/modify training.
Transverse of superior cortex—older patients/initial crack in superior/cortex may displace.

Femoral shaft (Blickenstaff)[3]

- medial proximal femur
- displaced spiral oblique
- transverse distal

Crutches (4 to 8 weeks), may complete, often need to operate.

In general: Treatment involves decreased weight bearing and modified training. May be all that is required in early femoral shaft stress fractures and compressive type of femoral neck fractures. In the older patient it is wise to pin at an early stage (there is a risk of progression). Be alert to ensure that both élite athletes and amateurs do not suffer significant stress fractures. Finite element analysis evidence suggests that a maximum of 160km (100 miles) over a 3-month period is the limit for a first time jogger.

1 CL Stanitski *et al* 1978 *Am J Sports Med* **6** 391   2 MR Hajec K, HB Noble 1982 *Am J Sports Med* **10** 112   3 LD Blicken Staff, JM Morris 1966 *JBJS* **48A** 1031

Fractured hip; acute slip of the upper femoral epiphysis (SUFE)

These occur from a severe force applied while the foot is planted and the hip twisted. (Seen in cross country and downhill skiers from a low velocity fall; 'skier's hip'.) Hip fracture may occur or SUFE in a child (Fig. 11.3). **Clinical features**: there is severe pain and an inability to weight bear, with shortening and external rotation in the hip. Exclude a past history of ache or an antalgic gait with an acute or chronic slipped upper femoral epiphysis. **Treatment** is immediate immobilization and then immediate operative stabilization and drainage of the capsular hematoma.

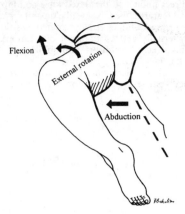

Fig. 11.3 SUFE: external rotation with flexion of the hip

Dislocation of the hip

Results from a direct impact to the flexed knee and hip (anterior or posterior). **Clinical features**: there is severe pain and typical deformity with the leg in a flexed and internally rotated position (posterior dislocation) or externally rotated (anterior dislocation). The sciatic nerve may be involved. **Treatment**: immobilize the athlete, give analgesia, and plan *immediate* reduction (open if necessary) of the hip to reduce the likely development of AVN and later OA. This is a **surgical emergency** with serious long-term consequences for a young athlete.

Fractured femur and pelvis

High velocity injuries. Significant pain and deformity occurs. Exclude neurological or vascular compromise. There often are associated head, neck, chest (pneumothorax), and abdominal life-threatening injuries (splenic/hepatic/renal/bladder/urethralrupture) which must be found and treated urgently. **Treatment**: apply MAST suit immediately. Note blood at tip penis (indicates urethral rupture).[1] Resuscitate, with special attention to head injury, immobilize the neck, exclude need for chest tube peritoneal lavage/exploratory laparotomy. Optimize volume replacement (up to 40 Units of blood can disappear into a fractured pelvis) and give adequate analgesia. Surgery is almost always required to reduce and hold fractures of the femur (neck/shaft) and quite often for the pelvis (external fixateur to tamponade bleeding in displaced and unstable pelvic fracture). Consider applying pelvic clamp in emergency room (if >10min to get to operating room, and BP is low). Such athletes have high chance of long-term back pain, leg length discrepancy, pelvic pain, and impotence.

Hip arthroscopy. Bowman first reported hip arthroscopy in 1937. It has recently become more widely used but the uses, apart from diagnostic, are fairly limited. It is a difficult, technique-dependant procedure. Possibly useful where there is unexplained hip pain, synovitis, early osteoarthrosis (can be used for lavage), for treatment of labral tears, and removal of loose bodies (from fractures, osteo-chondromatosis and villonodular synovitis). Several techniques have been described.

1 E Sherry 1993 MD thesis UNSW

397

Avascular necrosis femoral head

A partial or complete disruption of the blood supply to the femoral head resulting in necrosis of a segment which may then undergo collapse before revascularization has occurred. A catastrophe for a young athlete.

Most commonly follows a fracture of the head or femoral neck or dislocation/subluxation (especially if associated with *delay* in reduction). Posterior dislocations, in particular, disrupt the superior retinacular vessels). *Perthe's disease* results from an increased intracapsular pressure following a synovitis which compromises the vascular supply to the femoral head. AVN is classified according to that of Ficat,[1] with diagnostic and surgical intervention noted (Table 11.2).

1 RP Ficat, J Arlet 1980 *Ischaemia and necrosis of bone.* Williams & Wilkins, Baltimore

Table 11.2 Ficat's classification of AVN

Stage	Pain	Exam	XR	Bone scan	MRI	Treatment
0	None	Normal	Normal	Normal	Normal	Normal
1	Minimal	↓I.rot	Normal	No help	Some changes	?Core decompression
2	Moderate	↓ROM	Porosis/ sclerosis	Positive	Positive	Graft
3	Advanced	↓ROM	Flat, crescent sign	Positive	Positive	Joint replacement
4	Severe	Pain	Acetabular changes	Positive	Positive	Joint replacement

Osteoarthritis

High correlation with high impact sports especially track and field and racquet sports. Work performed by Radin shows that compression of the joint with oscillating repetitive high impact loads leads to microfractures. Conditions associated with avascular necrosis will advance the onset of osteoarthrosis. Athletes with extensive sports participation have a 4 to 5 fold increased incidence of OA[2] (up to 8.5 if *also* involved in an occupational risk of OA). Patients who have had hip replacements should not play impact.

1 E Vingard *et al* 1993 *Am J Sports Med* **21** 195-200

12 Knee[1]

EUGENE SHERRY

1 J Sullivan 1997 In E Sherry, D Bokor (ed) *Sports medicine problems and practical management* Ch 14. GMM, London

Introduction

The size, lack, of stability and forward prominence of the knee make it prone to injury.

Biomechanics

The knee is a complex hinge joint which allows free flexion, and some rotation in flexion. With progressive flexion there is roll-back of the femur on the tibial surface, limited by tension in the posterior cruciate ligament.

The articular surfaces of the knee have poor congruity and thus little inherent stability (check some dried bones). Articular congruity is improved by the menisci, but stability depends on ligaments, capsule and muscle control.

The knee is injured from high torsional and deceleration forces (in running and contact sports). Diagnosis rests with history and clinical examination. The mechanism of injury often gives a useful clue to diagnosis (a knee which dislocates or slips with pain and a 'pop' suggests an isolated rupture of the anterior-cruciate ligament (ACL)).

407

Ligament injury

The four main ligaments are the medial and lateral collateral ligaments, the anterior and posterior cruciate ligaments. A useful (and conceptually new way) of looking at the knee is to view the ACL as proving a stable platform for the action of the quadriceps; conversely, the PCL for the hamstrings (Fig. 12.1). Integrity of these ligaments is crucial for stability and kinematics. Altered kinematics may lead to OA of the knee in the long term although there is no convincing evidence that an ACL-deficient knee is prone to OA as is a medial or lateral meniscal tear.

Medial collateral ligament (MCL)[1]

Extends from the medial femoral epicondyle, widens and inserts on to the tibia 8–10cm below the joint line. Orientated in a posterior to anterior direction it is taut in extension. It is susceptible to contact and non-contact injuries when a valgus force with external rotational force is applied and is twice the tensile strength of the ACL. **Clinical features**: there is swelling over the medial knee, and later bruising. The knee is *typically held flexed* with a *painful soft end point-limiting extension* (pseudolocking). There is tenderness along the ligament, most marked at the femoral insertion; the integrity of the MCL is checked at 30° of flexion; apply a valgus force—Fig. 12.2—watch the patient's face: severe pain means partial tear (grades I, II), mild pain complete tear (grade III); stay out of range of angry footballer's left hook!). Grade III injury has >1cm opening of the medial joint line. If knee opens up in extension there is a more complex ligamentous disruption (± ACL/PCL).

X-rays are usually normal (an avulsion fragment is rarely seen). Large calcification seen at the site of femoral insertion is the Pellegrini–Stieda lesion. **Treatment**: isolated MCL injuries (grades I–III) can be treated in a knee brace for 4–6 weeks: start with RICE and graded quadriceps strengthening. Realize that in normal gait there is a closing force on the medial joint line, and so early weight bearing can be allowed and bracing may not be necessary for grades I–II MCLs. *Brace* grade III injuries and where the patient feels instability on weight bearing. Recovery from grades I–II injury takes 3–4 weeks; grade III, 6–8 weeks.

Lateral collateral ligament (LCL)

The LCL extends from the lateral femoral epicondyle to the head of the fibula. Isolated tears are rare. More commonly injured with disruption of the posterolateral corner. Usually requires surgical reconstruction (along with other ruptured ligaments).

Anterior cruciate ligament (ACL)

Structure

The ACL is the commonest major ligament knee injury in sport. It runs from the posterosuperior aspect of the lateral wall of the intercondylar notch in the femur to the tibial spines. (Average 12mm thickness with 2 major bundles, the anteromedial and the posterolateral: it is a primary stabilizer to anterior tibial translation and controls the rotational screw-home mechanism in terminal knee extension.) Tensile strength is 2160N.

1 DM Daniel *et al* (ed) 1990 *Knee ligaments: Structure, function, injury and repair.* Raven Press, New York

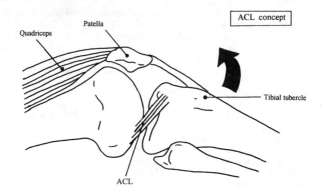

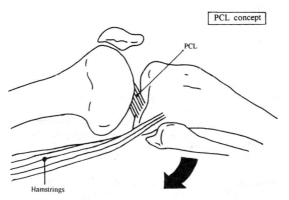

Fig. 12.1 The ACL and PCL concepts

Mechanism of injury[1]

80% of ruptures result from non-contact injury. Where there is internal rotation and anterior translation force of the tibia caused by pivoting cutting or landing awkwardly from a jump. (Also ruptured by hyperextension of the knee and will fail with progressive valgus in combination with a medial collateral ligament tear.)

In isolated non-contact injuries the patient 'steps-off' the knee at speed, feels pain. There is a characteristic 'pop' and a fall (giving way). *Pivot shift* test is accurate but possibly painful and better performed in post acute phase (for right knee: hold leg straight and with your other hand push posterolateral corner forward as knee is slowly flexed, when the ACL is ruptured the tibia moves far forward and then clonks back). *Lachman's test* is accurate and easy to perform in acute phase (Fig. 12.3: flex knee 30°, if tibia moves forward on lower end of femur with no firm end point, then positive; the dynamic Lachman's test is performed by allowing patient to extend actively knee and the tibia is seen to move (too) far forward).

Swelling is almost immediate, from a *hemarthrosis.* **Note**: in the absence of fracture 80% of acute knee hemarthroses are due to rupture of the ACL. **Examination** reveals a tight *effusion* in a flexed knee (increases capsule volume) with tenderness over the anterolateral joint line from a commonly associated capsular injury. The Lachman test is performed.

X-ray may show an avulsion fracture involving the tibial spine (especially in younger patients). Note avulsion fracture from the anterolateral tibia (Segond fracture). An MRI will accurately show the ruptured ligament (too expensive and not necessary when careful examination made). **Treatment** is *determined by associated injuries* (meniscal, ligamentous), degree of instability, and patient expectation. Initially, manage conservatively with RICE and muscle-strengthening program. Where persistent joint line symptoms or locking may have meniscal tear and need arthroscopy. (Patients who have an associated grade III rupture of the MCL better served by early ACL reconstruction.) Otherwise, ACL reconstruction is for patients who want to return to high demand sports where ongoing instability.

Chronic ACL insufficiency

After an isolated rupture of the ACL most knees settle down over 6–12 weeks. The ligament does not heal. One-third of patients are asymptomatic, some are only symptomatic with jumping or other sports (e.g. netball, football, skiing); a small group is significantly symptomatic with all activities. Symptoms include giving way (with pain) and recurrent swelling (repeated giving way may injure the menisci and cause osteochondral trauma with the later development of OA).

Examination may show good muscle tone and no effusion (range of motion is preserved). The Lachman, pivot shift, and anterior draw tests (ADT) are positive (ADT: hyperflex knee, sit on foot, pull tibia forward—excessive, >1cm, motion indicates ACL tear). *McMurray's test* will indicate associated meniscal tear (put thumb and index finger across joint lines and fully flex knee rotating internally then externally; abnormal click suggests meniscal tear). **Treatment**: occasional instability with high demand sports requires modification of activity

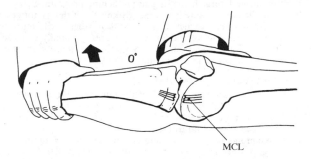

Valgus load with knee in 30° flexion to check integrity of MCL

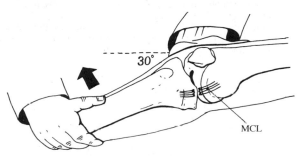

Fig. 12.2 Checking integrity of the MCL after injury

Comparison and frequency of the 5 most common injuries in adults compared			
Injuries in adults	%	Injuries in children	%
Knee sprain	25.0	Knee sprain	28.0
Shoulder dislocation	5.0	Shoulder dislocation	12.0
Shoulder sprain	4.5	Shoulder sprain	9.0
Fractured wrist	3.5	Fractured wrist	5.0
Sprained wrist	3.5	Sprained wrist	5.0
Remainder	58.5	Remainder	41.0

411

Ligament injury (*cont*)

and an intensive lateral hamstring-strengthening program. Symptomatic instability will require knee brace (S-knee) or if that is not good enough then ACL reconstruction (up to 85% of patients will return to their pre-injury level of sports; laxity of the graft gradually increases but patients remain asymptomatic). No strong evidence exists that reconstruction lessens the development of OA.[1]

Posterior cruciate ligament (PCL)

Runs from the anterior medial wall of the intercondylar notch of the femur to the central posterior tibia (1cm below the joint line). Comprises of anterolateral and posteromedial bands. Primary restraint to posterior tibial translation.

Early symptoms may be mild and isolated ruptures. Examination will show a posterior sag with tibial drop back (hyperflex knee and note posterior sag; otherwise note posterior sag with push on tibia— Fig. 12.4).

X-rays may show an avulsion fracture involving the tibial insertion (treat operatively). An MRI scan will slow the ligament tear. **Treatment** of midsubstance ruptures is non-operative; intensive quadriceps strengthening needed. A PCL-deficient knee will develop (due to the altered kinematics, patellofemoral pain with OA of the patellofemoral and medial compartments). Early reconstruction is probably better for young patients.

412

1 DW Jackson 1996 *Indications, contra indications, and treatment decision-making ACL reconstruction* San Diego, AAOS Summer Institute

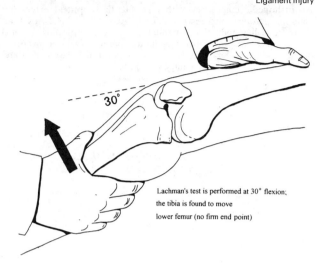

Lachman's test is performed at 30° flexion;
the tibia is found to move
lower femur (no firm end point)

Fig. 12.3 Lachman's test

413

Knee dislocation[1]

An orthopedic emergency with injury to the popliteal artery and common peroneal nerve (when lateral) (ACL, PCL, MCL, LCL are torn). **Immediate reduction** is mandatory and then immobilize (splint). Check pedal pulses and organize an angiogram. (Delayed occlusion of the popliteal artery may occur due to an intimal flap tear.) Later, surgical reconstruction is almost always required.

1 JC Kennedy 1963 *JBJS* **45A** 889–904

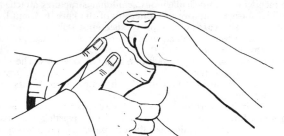

Posterior sag (passive or active) indicates rupture of PCL

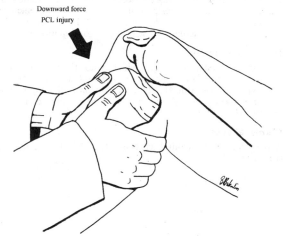

Downward force
PCL injury

Fig. 12.4 Assessing integrity of PCL after injury

Meniscal tears

The menisci are fibrocartilaginous semilunar structures attached to the tibial surface (improve the congruity of the knee, transmit load, act as shock absorbers, and improve knee joint stability). *Note* that after meniscectomy contact area is reduced, contact pressures increase by more than 350%.

Shock-absorbing capacity reduced, and OA develops. The blood supply is limited to the peripheral one-quarter to one-third (tears in the vascular region have potential for healing). Medial tears are 5 times more common than lateral.

The meniscus is torn when *trapped* between the two bone surfaces as a rotary force is applied to the loaded knee (twisting when rising from a full squat). **Examination**: there is *pain, delayed effusion, and locked knee with a bucket handle tear*). Smaller tears cause recurrent clicking, catching, and joint line pain. There is an effusion, wasting of the quadriceps, pain on forced extension, pain on forced flexion, and a positive McMurray's test.

MRI will exclude other pathology. **Treatment**: arthroscopy affords good visualization and partial meniscectomy. Peripheral bucket handle, and incomplete bucket handle tears (in young patients) should be repaired /sutured. Reconstruct an associated anterior cruciate ligament rupture, prevent recurrence of the meniscal tear. (Unhappy 'triad' is: medial, some say the LCL, collateral/anterior cruciate ligament/medial meniscal injury combination.)

416

Discoid meniscus[1]

A meniscus, usually the lateral, which is not the usual C-shaped, but nearly covers the whole plateau (3 types: incomplete/complete/Wrisberg-type; no posterior attachment). Mechanical symptoms of joint line pain and 'clunking'. Partial menisectomy may be required (i.e. reshape) (Fig. 12.5).

Meniscal cyst

Arises from a horizontal cleavage tear of the lateral meniscus (Fig. 12.6).

1 PM Aichroth *et al* 1991 *JBJS* **73B** 932–6.

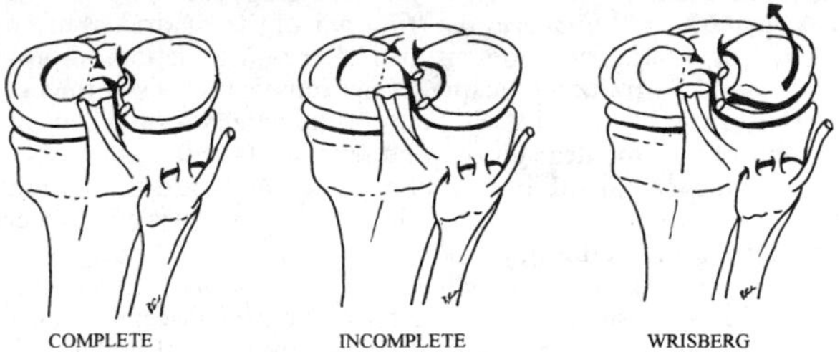

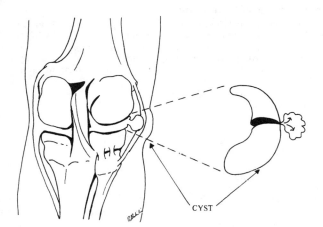

Fig. 12.5 Types of discoid meniscus

COMPLETE   INCOMPLETE   WRISBERG

CYST

Fig. 12.6 Lateral meniscal cyst

417

Patellofemoral joint problems

The patellar is a *sesamoid bone* in the quadriceps tendon (present at $7\frac{1}{2}$ weeks gestation). It *improves the efficiency* of the quadriceps mechanism by lengthening the moment arm, decreasing friction, improving stability, and centralizing the quadriceps muscle pull, also protects the anterior aspect of the joint. Stability of the patella is provided by the anatomy of the trochlear groove and patella, static tension in the soft tissues of the medial and lateral retinaculum, and the dynamic control of the quadriceps. The vastus medialis obliquus muscle is especially important in maintaining patellofemoral balance and normal tracking. *Acute injuries* to the patellofemoral joint *include* direct trauma, subluxation or dislocation, patellar fracture, quadriceps tendon, or patellar ligament rupture. Many patients present with anterior knee pain with no injury.

Anterior knee pain syndrome

The commonest sports knee complaint. Pain may be well localized (patellar tendinitis), but usually vaguel anterior; aggravated by loading a flexed knee (climbing stairs or inclines) or after sitting for prolonged periods. There is crepitus, catching, weakness, giving way, and an effusion. Causes are many and physical examination unremarkable apart from retropatellar crepitus:

- *Trauma* (osteochondral injury)
- *Mal-alignment*
  - anatomical predisposition
  - muscle imbalance
  - patellar subluxation
  - patellar dysplasia
- *Compressive*
  - excessive lateral pressure syndrome
  - hamstrung patella
- *Overuse*
  - patellar tendinitis
  - medial plica syndrome
  - retinacular irritation
  - Osgood–Schlatter's disease
  - bipartite patella
- *Degenerative/Inflammatory*
- *Idiopathic*
  - primary chondromalacia

80% of such patients respond to non-operative measures. Identify precipitating and aggravating activities. A physical program includes quadriceps strengthening and in particular vastus medialis toning (straight leg raise externally rotated leg) with hamstring stretching. Patellar taping or S-knee brace will help . If improvement is not seen within 6–8 weeks, the diagnosis should be reassessed and further investigation undertaken.

Chondromalacia patellae

A softening of the patellar cartilage either from a direct blow or malalignment (with patellar subluxation). Typically seen in young overweight girls with knock-knees. The cartilage damage is classified.

41

Patellofemoral joint problems (*cont*)

Acute dislocation of the patella

Occurs from an *external rotation with a valgus force* with the knee in extension or from a direct blow. The **diagnosis** is obvious and reduction achieved by gentle extension of the knee (spontaneous reduction usually happens). There is hemarthrosis, tender medial patellar retinaculum, positive patellar apprehension test (push patella laterally as knee is flexed and note pain), and patellar instability.

X-ray to exclude a significant osteochondral fracture (arthroscopy and excision of the fragment is required). **Treatment:** drain a tense hemarthrosis for pain relief, immobilize in extension (a removable Zimmer splint). Start isometric quadriceps exercises (no knee bending) and may weight bear as tolerated. As the effusion resolves graduated flexion started and the knee splint discarded (by 3 weeks). Return to sport when regained normal quadriceps muscle tone/bulk and a negative apprehension test present.

Recurrent dislocation of the patella

Clear from history, if no response to an extensive quadriceps-strengthening program, **surgery is required** (a lateral release and repair or advancement of the medial retinacular tissue and vastus medialis; if intraoperatively this does not achieve stability a distal bony realignment required).

Recurrent subluxation of the patella

There is anterior knee pain and giving way. Examination shows increased *Q-angle* (line of pull of the quadriceps), valgus or rotation factors, out-turned patellae or patellar alta (high). The patella tracks in a J-curve (Fig. 12.7). The patella may be subluxable or dislocatable. Lateral retinacular tightness present (not able to lift lateral border of patella >1cm).

X-rays (skyline views) and CT scan may show patellar dysplasia or subluxation. **Treatment**: if there is no improvement with a protracted program, surgery is required (soft tissue or bony realignment).

Patellar tendinitis (jumper's knee)

An *overuse injury* (seen in basketball). There is anterior knee pain (with exertion). With point tenderness over the central insertion of the patellar ligament into the patella, with swelling and crepitus. The hamstrings and gastrocnemiae maybe tight.

MRI scan shows altered signal at the site of the degenerative tendon. A bone scan shows creased uptake. **Treatment** includes rest with modification of activities (jumping); a graduated exercise program to strengthen the quadriceps; and intensive stretches for the hamstrings and gastrocnemii. The overlying bursa may be injected with corticosteroid and local anesthetic ($\frac{1}{3}$ ampoule Celestone with 2mls of 0.5% Marcaine with adrenaline). If symptoms persist surgical debridement of the degenerative tendon with a segment of patellar bone may be necessary.

Patellar fracture

Direct impact on the patella from a fall on a flex knee or a dashboard injury, also following violent resisted contraction of the extensor mechanism. If there is disruption of the extensor mechanism (indicated by *a lag* or inability to straight leg raise; a significant

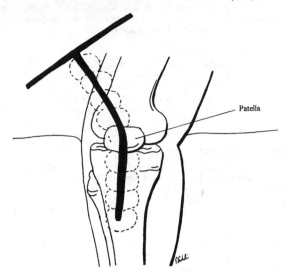

Fig. 12.7 J-curve of subluxing patella

421

gap on x-ray) **surgical** repair is essential. Undisplaced minimally displaced fractures with preservation of the extensor mechanism are treated by splinting in extension for 6 weeks.

Quadriceps rupture

Caused by sudden resistance to a strong quadriceps contraction. Seen in the older patient group (as with other tendon degeneration conditions—President Bill Clinton's knee injury in 1997). There is pain with loss of quadriceps function, a lag, and a palpable gap. When the diagnosis is unclear (rectus femoris only torn and vastus medialis/lateralis intact) and particularly when presentation is delayed MRI is useful. To restore function, operative repair is required.

Patellar ligament rupture

Occurs in younger patients, as insertion on to tibial tubercle, by the same mechanism as quadriceps tendon rupture (also by penetrating injuries, dashboard). In older patients, may avulse from lower pole of patella. There is pain and loss of quadriceps function with a significant lag. The defect is usually palpable. Surgical repair is indicated.

Prepatellar bursitis

The *bursa* over the anterior aspect of the patella is prone to injury and inflammation from repetitive contact (seen in football players and gymnasts). Tendency to become recurrent. Examination shows enlargement of the thickened bursa with crepitus. Acute cases may have secondary infection with cellulitis. **Treatment**: inflammatory bursitis is treated with RICE and NSAIDs. Padding and protecting the area on return to sport is important to minimize the risk of recurrence. Where secondary sepsis use antibiotics and surgical draining. Recurrent or chronic bursitis will eventually require excision of the thickened bursa.

Bipartite patella (accessory ossification center)

Present in <15% of patellae, usually asymptomatic and at the *superiolateral corner*. **Symptoms** may occur after direct contact injury or overuse. Includes anterior knee pain and tenderness (over the site of the pseudarthrosis).

X-rays show the bipartite patella (a bone scan is helpful following significant trauma). **Treatment**: most settle with a conservative program as in the management of anterior knee pain syndrome (p. 418). Rarely is excision of the fragment required.

Plica syndrome

Vestigial synovial plicas are common (either patellofemoral, medial, or over ligamentum mucosum) and often seen at arthroscopy. They may become symptomatic following a direct injury causing thickening and scarring of the plica, or from overuse. There is anterior knee pain syndrome with clicking, snapping, and tenderness over the medial femoral condyle.

Those that do not settle with rest and a conservative program require arthroscopic resection.

Iliotibial band friction syndrome

Seen in joggers and distance runners. There is inflammation over the lateral epicondyle caused by rubbing of the iliotibial band. Examination reveals point tenderness over the lateral epicondyle, reproduced as the iliotibial band passes back and forth over the lateral epicondyle. There may be tightness of the tensor fascia lata and hamstring muscles. **Treatment** involves rest and stretching of the iliotibial band and hamstring muscles. A break of 3 months from distance running is may be necessary.

Semimembranosus tendinitis[1]

This is seen in male athletes and may be difficult to diagnose (posteromedial knee joint pain with hamstring spasm). A cyst may occur which is difficult to excise.

426

1 JM Ray *et al* 1988 *Am J Sports Med* **16** 347–51

427

Loose bodies

Cause mechanical symptoms of locking and recurrent effusions. Occasionally, they can be palpated. They can be due to a meniscal fragment or osteochondral fragment (traumatic, degenerative, osteochondritis dissecans), or synovial chondromatosis. X-rays will demonstrate radioopaque loose bodies. **Treatment** is arthroscopic removal.

Hoffa disease

Old entity, trauma, with bleeding into anterior fat pad around patellar tendon, common in children; or genu recurvatum. **Treat** with activity modification, NSAIDs, knee pad, or arthroscopic minimal resection.

It is his feet which confer upon man his only real distinction and provide his only valid claim to human status[1]

1 WF Jones 1929 *Men's place among the mammals*. Arnold, London.

433

Biomechanics

The foot has evolved from an arboreal grasping organ to an agent for motion (probably over last 1.8 million years). The big toe became aligned with the shortened smaller toes, the subtalar joint became stiffer, the medial arch, and a higher heel developed. The body is now supported on the sustentaculum tali with the calcaneus bowed under the ankle joint (Fig. 13.1). It is easily toppled from this ledge where it is balanced in tension by the lateral ligament complex.

Little wonder then that 25% of all sporting injuries involve the ankle and foot. There are 23,000 new ankle sprains in the USA every day (5000 per day in the UK).

The tibiotalar articulation allows 25 dorsiflexion, 35 plantar flexion, and 5 rotation. The instant center of motion lies on a line along the tips of the malleoli and posterolaterally on the talar dome. Up to 5 times the bodyweight is transmitted across this joint.

Gait has two phases (Fig. 13.2): (1) stance (60% of cycle; foot flat, heel off, toe off), (2) swing (40% of cycle; toe off/toe, clear/heel strike). During walking one foot is always on the ground. In running both feet are off the ground at one point in the stride. The weight is borne from the heel, along the lateral border of the sole, then inward across the metatarsal heads from the 5th to the 1st MTP joint. Stability is gained by the talar mortise and ligament support. The subtalar joint functions like a hinge and allows eversion and inversion. The midfoot permits abduction and adduction. The forefoot provides flexion and extension. Pronation of the foot (5) involves coupled dorsiflexion, eversion, and abduction (sole turned down). Supination (up to 20) involves coupled plantarflexion, inversion and adduction (sole turned up). The foot transmits 3 times the bodyweight during running, through 3 arches (medial, lateral, transverse). The second metatarsal is the keystone of the midfoot in gait; the first metatarsal in the stance phase.

Biomechanical advantage in certain sports may result from *pigeon toes* (sprinters, tennis, squash); *swayback* (increased lumbar lordosis with anterior pelvic tilt, sprinters, jumpers, gymnasts); *duck* (everted) *feet* (breastroke); *inverted feet* (backstroke, butterfly); *double jointedness* (ligamentous laxity; gymnasts).

Susceptibility to injury is increased by: postural defects, muscle weakness/imbalance, lack of flexibility, malalignment problems (pronated feet, LLD with pelvic tilt); training techniques (>64km (40 miles)/week of jogging), playing environment and equipment contribute. Pay particular attention to the athlete's footwear and ankle support. 'Sexy shoes painful feet the women's shoe wear problem'[1]— most of the forefoot problems of women can be traced to undersized, though sexy, fashionable shoes. Make an outline of the patient's bare foot with patient standing on a sheet of paper, and note that it is often 2–3 shoe sizes wider than the sole of their shoe.

Sports-specific injuries often associated with particular sports include: *skiing*, peroneal tendon subluxation, nerve entrapment, plantar fasciitis; *running*, lateral ligament sprains, stress fractures, shin splints; *ballet*, os trigonum/FHL impingement, sesamoiditis, stress fracture, hallux valgus; *football*, turf toe, ankle, and midfoot fractures; *tennis*, gastrocnemius strains, TA injury, stress fractures;

---

1 The title of a very popular Instructional Course lecture at the American Academy of Orthopaedic Surgeons Annual Meeting in Atlanta in 1996 by MJ Coughlin *et al*

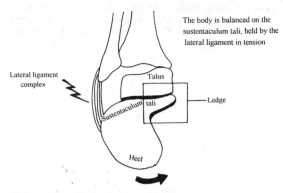

Fig. 13.1 Design problems with the ankle (see text)

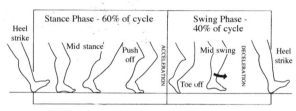

Fig. 13.2 The gait cycle

Biomechanics (*cont*)

soccer, ankle sprains, stress fractures; *basketball*, lateral ligament sprains, plantar fasciitis, Jones' fracture (diaphyseal fracture base 5th metatarsal); *gymnastics*, Severs' disease (traction apophysitis of the calcaneus).

Assessing function

Gait. Video analysis of gait on the track or field provides documentation and allows correction of incorrect posture in many sports. *Footwear*. Examine wear patterns on shoes (excessive wear of the outer heel with tibialis posterior problems, blownout medial shoe with hallux valgus), and/or check the wet footprint. Normal bearing points are centrally under the ball of the foot and posterolaterally at the heel. *Note*: orthotics are more effective for planovalgus foot rather than pes cavus.

History: collect details of the mechanism of injury (high v low velocity, spontaneous onset, rolled over on heel), problems with shoe wear, and athletic performance. Where is the pain: if localized, and other characteristics, is there stiffness of the ankle/subtalar joint (tarsal coalition) or big toe? Any swelling or instability (of ankle joint). Medical history. Previous injury.

Examine the whole patient (exclude other injuries and underlying medical condition, e.g. diabetics, cerebral palsy) and the whole limb (alignment, flexion contractive hip, varus/valgus/flexion contracture knee). Review gait (limp present? antalgic/short-legged/neurological) and whether walk with foot extremely rotated (to avoid pain of roll through). Correlate with examination findings. Test power (heel stand, toe stand, stand on inside/outside foot). Assess medial arch (pes cavus or flat foot). Patient sits on bench, you sit at patient's foot with small stool between. Note extent and area of swelling. Carefully palpate: ankle joint (*note* point tenderness) from tip medial malleolus to tip lateral malleolus and behind ankle to TA insertion, midfoot, and forefoot. Document ROM ankle joint, subtalar joint, midfoot (abduction/adduction), and forefoot (extension / flexion 1st MTPJ) Palpate tibialis anterior (in front medial malleolus) and tibialis post (behind medial malleolus). Assess power of tibialis posterior with single heel rise test: patient stands on small stool, faces wall, lifts other foot; note heel raise of foot in question: hesitation /inability = positive test) (Fig. 13.3). Perform *Windlass test* (dorsiflex big toe, medial arch should rise) (Fig. 13.4).

Perform stability tests on the ankle: anterior draw test (ADT)— hold lower tibia, foot plantarflexed, cradle heel in other hand, and draw forward; no end point is positive for anterior talofibular ligament (ATFL) rupture (Fig. 13.5); inversion test—move heel into inversion, 10 greater than other side is positive for calcaneofibular ligament (CFL) rupture (Fig. 13.6).

Palpate pulses, check sensation, and perform Tinel's test over posterior tibial nerve. Perform Simmond's test (patient prone, squeeze calf, no plantarflexion means TA is ruptured) (Fig. 13.7). Measure calf and midfoot diameters.

Sports shoes

The ideal sports shoe should be comfortable, protect the foot and ankle from injury, and possibly enhance performance. Shoes have caused problems since antiquity and more recently many of the forefoot problems have been related to poor shoe fit (sexy shoes/painful feet).

There has been no convincing reduction in the incidence of injury from the use of athletic footwear. Perhaps we should return to barefeet (Zola Budd and Abebe Bikila preferred this and so do

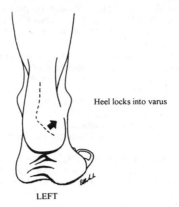

Heel locks into varus

LEFT

Fig. 13.3 Posterior tibial tendon test

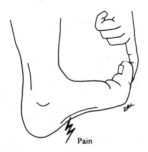

Pain

Fig. 13.4 Windlass test

most schoolchildren) to restore plantar proprioception and reduce stress-related injuries. However, sports shoes are here to stay (market-driven forces have seen to that) and its our job to make them work. Current design concerns are:

- *Shoe fit*—female athletes are stuffing their feet into undersized 'male-designed' sports shoes (female foot has larger forefoot/heel ratio so they need to use smaller heeled male shoe to get hindfoot fit and so cram their forefoot). Manufacturers are responding with 'female-designed' shoes to fix this problem.
- *Cushioning*—transmitted impact forces may damage red blood cells (hemolysis), cause stress fractures (metatarsals), and alter hyaline articular cartilage. It seems that impact-relieving soles will protect the foot and ankle.
- *Control*—hyperpronation of the forefoot is a factor in injury, but this can be prevented with shoe wear (posterior medial arch support), however, the injury location shifts proximally to the knee (or distally to midfoot). It is related to the hindfoot position with take off supination. Better hindfoot control is gained by high-top lace-up boots, or lateral heel flare. Side stepping (or cutting) in sports where there is a rapid change in direction results in the lateral ligament complex. This is reduced with barefeet or with a lateral heel wedge.[1]
- *Flexibility*—Turf toe resulted from excessive flexibility of the American football shoe.
- *Foot/shoe/surface interface.*

There are two interfaces: (1) the foot/shoe, and (2) the shoe/playing surface. Slip inside the shoe should be kept as small as possible (but not much research here). Interaction with the playing surface is easier to study and has received a lot of attention. Injury occurs when the deceleration forces exceed the breaking strength of bone/ligaments (a sudden stop in sludgy snow) or from a slide (on icy snow resulting in collision).

Playing surfaces have changed from grass, clay, wood, concrete, and asphalt to synthetic turf (Astro-turf). The synthetics are easier to maintain, regulate, and probably cause fewer injuries; they are characterized by degree of hardness, ground reaction forces, friction/traction, and energy loss, with loading and compliance. Increased traction (high coefficient of traction with surfaces) may enhance performance but cause injury (as may slip from low coefficient—but probably less likely). The cleating design of football shoes is critical to reduce torque and injury rate (change to soccer-style shoe or Tanel 360 shoe, which has a circular cleat for synthetics and a central forefoot cleat for natural grass).[2]

Sports shoes fall into 5 categories:[3]

1 Hiking/climbing/exercising/running/training/throwing/jumping
2 Court shoes
3 Field shoes—soccer/football—cleated, studded, spiked
4 Winter shoes—skating/skiing
5 Specialty shoes—cycling/golf

1 A Stacoff *et al* 1996 *Med Sci Sports Exerc* 1996 **28** 350–8 **2** JC Delee, D Drez 1994 *Orthopaedic sports medicare* p1666–96. Saunders, London **3** C Frey 1994 In *OKU foot and ankle* p73–84. AAOS

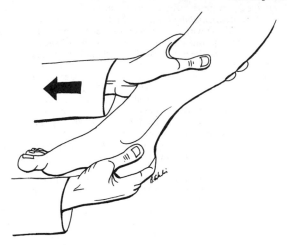

Fig. 13.5 Anterior draw test

441

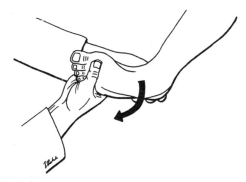

Fig. 13.6 Inversion test

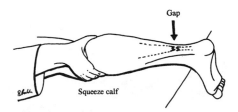

Fig. 13.7 Simmond's test

1 *Hiking boots* need to be rugged, water-resistant, good traction, firm heel counter. *Climbing boots* need inflexible soles. *Exercise shoes* need a light midsole with a firm heel counter, flexible soft upper and good shock absorption. Heel height of 10–15mm. *Running shoes* for short distances: light heel; torsional stability in longer distances from slight wedge (especially curve running), semipointed toebox. Rules for spikes are 6 max for sole, 2 for heel (<2 5mm long and <4 mm wide). Shorter spikes for hurdles, sometimes spikeless or hard surfaces. *Training flats* (road work) need shock absorption, flexibility, and heel counter-stability with torsional stability (designated: light, heavy runners, heel strikers, antipronation, lightweight, rugged terrain); traction variable by variable outsole thickness/tread. *Throwing* events use good grip leather/suede with spikes. *Jumping* events may use spikes but need heel cushioning and have 'jump foot' shoes (right or left).

2 *Court shoes* are subject to heavy use. Tennis requires good lateral support, good tread pattern, ventilation. Basketball needs good ankle support, traction, and a pivot point.

3 *Field shoes*: use studs/spikes. Soccer player needs to feel the ball with soft upper. Football use cleats (but excessive traction may cause knee injuries). Need sturdy toe box and firm heel. Different shoes for different positions in US football (lineman v backs v place kickers). Rugby needs firm toe box.

4 Winter shoes: *skaters* use leather uppers and firm heel counter. Injection moulded models. *Skiing*, one piece injection moulded plastic foot outer shell. Modified for female foot. Crosscountry are soft, lowcut, waterproof, and good ventilation.

5 *Specialty shoes*: cycle shoe similar to running shoe.

Ankle and foot sprains

Acute lateral ligament sprains

Inversion, with supination and plantar/dorsiflexion, causes injury of the lateral ligament complex—the most common sporting injury. Usually (two-thirds of cases) the anterior talofibular ligament (ATFL, the weakest) is involved, sometimes the extraarticular calcaneofibular ligament (CFL), seldom the posterior talofibular ligament (PTFL, the strongest). Those at risk are large athletes, those with pes cavus (high medial arches), and a history of similar injury. Prophylactic (S-ankle) splints (Fig. 13.8) should be worn in high-risk sports (basketball, netball, football). High top boots may help. There is immediate pain and (often marked) swelling with resultant anterior and inversion (tilt) instability. To judge the severity of injury, use the ADT (Fig. 13.5), (easier to perform in acute situation than inversion test (Fig. 13.6) and will give more information). You may specify as grade I, ATFL sprain (two-thirds of cases) (ADT, some laxity); grade II, ATFL and CFL sprains (one-quarter of cases) (ADT and inversion tests, some laxity); grade III, ATFL, CFL, and PTFL tears (both tests positive) *or* simply distinguish *incomplete*—with a firm end point to anterior draw from *complete*—no end point to anterior draw. Careful examination in the post acute phase allows identification of the injured ligaments (after ankle, RICE for 24h). Whether complete or incomplete, treatment is the same—*non-operative*.

X-rays are necessary to exclude fractures. Good talar dome views will exclude osteochondral fractures (ignore bony avulsion of the ligaments). Do not miss a high fibular fracture with syndesmotic injuries (Maisonneuve fracture). Stress x-rays are unreliable but possibly helpful in the chronic phase where the patient does not give a clear history of instability ('going-over' on the ankle). **Treatment**: in the acute stage, RICE, NSAIDs, ankle splint for 6 weeks (S-Ankle; outer strap supports in swing phase and boomerang-shaped heel supports in stance phase with valgus and dorsal tilt), early rehabilitation with peroneal eversion exercises, water jogging, proprioceptive wobble board exercises. Some may become chronic. Elite athletes often elect for early surgical repair of complete ruptures (controversial but not unreasonable where 'wasted' period of 6–9 months conservative rehabilitation).

Note: (downhill) snow boarders may fracture lateral process of talus which may be confused with lateral ligament sprain (often needs ORIF).[1]

Chronic lateral ligamentous laxity

Unsuccessful treatment of acute lateral ligament injury may result in chronic lateral ligament laxity from 'stretched-out' ligaments. There is pain and tenderness over the anterolateral ankle joint extending to the sinus tarsi, exacerbated by repeated inversion injuries on irregular terrain. Distinguish mechanical instability (positive ADT/or inversion test) from functional instability (feels unstable but is mechanically stable; a proprioceptive problem). There is anterior instability and excessive tilt. **Treatment** (peroneal eversion exercises and wobble board) too often forces athletes to persist with months of unsuccessful physiotherapy. A quick effective lateral ligament reconstruction is

1 PJ Abbott 1997 Pers comm. Vail, CO, USA

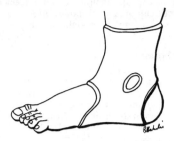

Fig. 13.8 S-Ankle splint

better. (The Brostrom capsularhaphy with reinforcement from the inferior extensor retinaculum, Gould modification, is recommended here. Lateral ligament complex is tightened-up and reinforced. Immobilized for 6 weeks and back to sport in splint in 3 months.)

Medial ligament sprains

Sprains of this type are rare. This is a strong ligament. Injury usually accompanies lateral ligament sprain or fractures, and must be differentiated from lesions of the nearby posterior tibial, FHL and FDL, tendons, and syndesmotic injury. Carefully check for accentuated localized tenderness and consider ultrasound examination (see p00) *Posterior tibial tendon test*, invert plantarflexed foot against resistance; *FDL test*, power of loop flexions toes against resistance; *FHL test*, power of resistance of big toe, (see diagnostic test for syndesmotic injury, p000).

X-rays with bone scan and CT may be necessary to exclude osteochondral fractures when there is severe, localized pain about the talar dome. Weightbearing (WB) x-rays may be useful. An arthrogram in first week may show tear. **Treatment** is splinting and sometimes arthroscopic surgery if chondral damage.

Subtalar instability

This is difficult entity to diagnose. It is really a component of lateral ligament injury (CFL torn) from inversion. There will be increased inversion compared to the other side. Special stress x-rays (Broden— invert heel and 40° caudal tilt) or II may help. **Treatment**: either splint or in chronic cases as above with CFL reconstruction (as part of Brostrom operation).

Syndesmotic ankle injury (high ankle sprain, distal tibiofibular diastasis)

Is a previously unrecognized, ongoing, and painful 'ankle sprain'. In the professional athlete the condition probably results from an external rotation injury. There is marked swelling both sides of the ankle with tenderness over the interosseous membrane. Suspect where an ankle sprain takes a long time to settle down. Perform the squeeze test (compress upper tib/fib and distal pain occurs, Fig. 13.9) or abduction/external rotation tests (hold upper tib/fib and externally rotate/abduct ankle to reproduce pain) and check a mortise view (Fig. 13.10) x-ray (criteria confusing so I suggest <1mm tibiofibular overlap and/or tibiofibular clear space on both AP and mortise talar views as indicative. The clear space is the gap between the medial border of the fibula and the lateral border of the posterior tibia, 1cm above the joint). Late x-rays show calcification of the ligaments. **Treatment** in NWB lasts for 4 weeks. If refractory, use diastasis screw fixation and repair ligament (difficult to suture paint brush to paint brush).

1 TK West 1997 Injuries to the distal lower extremity syndesmosis. *J Am Acad Surg* **5**(3) 174–7

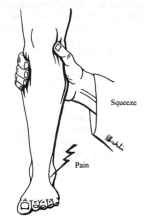

Fig. 13.9 Syndesmotic ankle injury (the squeeze test)

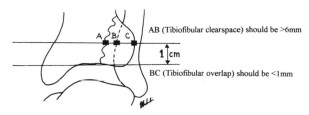

Fig. 13.10 X-ray criteria for diagnosis of syndesmotic ankle injury

Peroneal tendon injuries

The weak peroneal tendons work hard, everting the foot (which wants to revert to gestational equinus) and maintaining the transverse/longitudinal arches of the foot. They are poorly anchored with a weak holding retinaculum. Forced dorsiflexion of the everted ankle in skiing or football can produce tenosynovitis, tendinitis, tear (partial or complete), subluxation, or dislocation of these tendons (especially peroneus brevis which is closer to the bone). There is marked tenderness with reproducible subluxation or dislocation. Turn the foot in and out and note flicking of tendon behind the lateral malleolus. X-rays may show a rim fracture (lateral aspect lateral malleolus) (Fig. 13.11). **Treatment**: strapping may help, otherwise decompression, repair, tenodesis to peroneus longus, or early stabilization in the groove is indicated (because of high recurrence rate). Must be a graduated return to sport over 4–6 weeks, with 'cutting' procedures and sprinting to be avoided for 6 weeks.

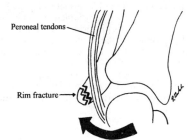

Peroneal tendons

Rim fracture

Rim fracture may be associated with subluxation or dislocation of the peroneal tendons

Fig. 13.11 Rim fracture

449

Posterior tibial tendon injury

Typically occurs especially in middleaged women who are unfit as a result of chronic degeneration, and in older athletes. The pathology is inflammation (tenosynovitis) or partial/complete rupture. There is pain and tenderness along the tibialis posterior tendon, with difficulty lifting the heel off the ground in the single heel raise test (pain/hesitation = tenosynovitis; not able to lift heel = complete tear). The arch is flattened and the foot pronated. Ultrasound examination may secure the diagnosis. **Treatment**: NSAIDs, recommend a medial arch support with heel up for tenosynovitis and partial ruptures. Perform debridement/tenosynovectomy for refractory cases. Reconstruct complete tears (use the FDL).

Anterior tibial tendon injuries

Spontaneous rupture may occur but is unusual. There is localized tenderness and weakened dorsi flexion. **Treatment**: surgical repair is important. Use either direct repair or tendon (extensor) transfer.

Achilles tendon injury

Are common and difficult to treat. Two basic problems of *tendinitis* and *rupture*. Overtraining produces an inflammation around the TA (peritendinitis), in the tendon (tendinitis) or beside it (in front of TA—retrocalcaneal bursitis, behind TA—retroachilles bursitis). The *'painful arc'* sign may help to make the distinction[1] (Fig. 13.12). With tendinitis the site of tenderness moves with the foot, and does not with peritendinitis. Athletes are at risk through excessive training, poor shoe support of the hindfoot, and on cambered surfaces.

A violent contraction of the gastrocnemius-soleus unit may cause partial or complete rupture of the TA. Patients (with complete tear) report having been hit or kicked in the calf during the push off phase of running or racket sports. Partial tears are difficult to diagnose; ultrasound imaging is helpful. Complete tears will invariably lead to pain, swelling, and a palpable gap (prior to swelling). Do not be deceived if the patient is able to plantarflex (through intact long flexors). *Simmonds' test* is easy to perform and is diagnostic. Patient prone, squeeze the calf: if the foot does not move, the TA is ruptured (Fig. 13.7).

Treat *tendinitis/peritendinitis* with rest, NSAIDs, heel raise, low frequency pulsed ultrasound, massage (stretching); rarely by surgery involving debridement. *Retrocalcaneal bursitis* as above, but consider surgery earlier with wide excision of retrocalcaneal exostosis (Haglund's bump). Retroachilles bursitis seldom requires excision of the bursa. *Partial tendon rupture* may require surgical excision of scar and granulation tissue with internal suture splint. *Complete tendon rupture* almost invariably needs surgical repair (open technique); is easier but percutaneous repair is better; if delayed, later repair is difficult and will require fascial or tendon augmentation (with plantaris). Expect slow postoperative recovery, and wound healing takes priority.

Note: avoid steroids. Exclude Reiter's syndrome, infection, gout, tumor.

Gastrocnemius injury A tear of the medial head of the gastrocnemius is common in middleaged tennis players (tennis leg). Patient feels as if he/she has have been hit behind the heel. **Treatment** is symptomatic (NSAIDs, stretching, strengthening) and no surgery.

1 MD Miller *et al* 1995 *Review of sports medicine and arthoscopy*. Saunders, London

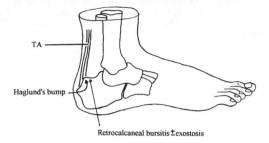

- Area of tenderness does **not** move

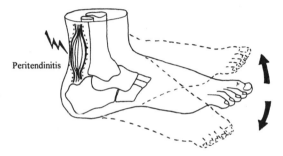

- Area of tenderness moves

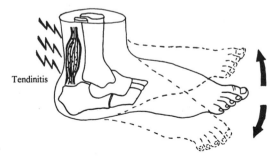

Fig. 13.12 The 'painful arc' sign

Spring ligament sprain

The midfoot is prone to twisting injuries with pain from sprain of the plantar calcaneonavicular (spring) ligament. Pain localized to the medial arch (and proximal to the navicular). It may be associated with posterior tibial tendon problems.

Cuboid syndrome

Involves pain and tenderness over the cuboid in the region of the peroneal (everting) tendons. **Treatment:** S-ankle splint and RICE/NSAIDs.

459

Sinus tarsi syndrome

The tunnel beneath the talar neck and upper calcaneus can be a source of pain from overactivity and inversion injury. It may be related to the strained ligament of tunnel (talocalcaneal ligament). Distinguish from lateral ligament strain by careful point examination. **Treatment**: with NSAIDs, activities for hyperpronation, and possibly steroid injection (0.25ml Celestone). Surgical excision of contents is seldom used.

Fractures

Ankle

Are common and require precise treatment to avoid later osteoarthritis. Displacement of 1mm causes 40% decrease in tibiotalar articulation.

Classification: fractures of the ankle are best classified for practical purposes by position of the *fibular* fracture according to *Weber's scheme* (AO): A, below joint line; B, at joint line; C, above joint line. The *Launge–Hansen scheme* provides a logically based classification according to the direction of the damaging force supination/adduction, supination/external rotation, pronation/abduction, or pronation/external rotation. The simple *Henderson scheme* classifies ankle fracture according to involvement of the lateral, medial, or posterior malleolus, or of a combination of these. Fractures of the ankle usually result from a fall with supination (or pronation) of the forefoot and eversion (or inversion) of the hindfoot. Well-fitting shoes with ankle support will eliminate such injuries (seldom seen in skiers with well fitted boots). The immediate pain, swelling, and deformity are obvious. Never hesitate to x-ray.

Treatment of a *displaced or unstable fracture* almost always involves open reduction and internal fixation. Markedly displaced ankle fractures should be reduced in the emergency room to avoid skin problems (blisters/necrosis and vascular compromise). Exclude a Maisonneuve fracture by careful examination (with x-ray) of upper fibula. Support the ankle postoperatively in a plaster splint for 6 weeks (NWB); permit return to sports at 3–5 months. Rehabilitate aggressively with ROM and strengthening exercises. A *non-displaced fracture* (<2mm) needs 6 weeks in cast with careful follow-up and x-ray review to detect displacement early. An isolated lateral fracture seldom requires ORIF.

Residual ankle pain (not uncommon) after bony union may be residual *traumatic synovitis (Fergel lesions)*. **Treatment**: NSAIDs or arthroscopic excision. Look for other causes of residual pain (p494)

Foot

Tend to be under-appreciated, difficult to detect and sometimes hard to treat. Most can be managed in a below-knee fracture walker orthosis. *Displaced and intraarticular fractures* often require reduction (usually closed) and fixation (usually percutaneous K-wire).

Calcaneus

Can be devastating due to a widened painful heel, nerve entrapment, peroneal tendinitis, and later subtalar OA. **Treatment**: elevate; start foot pump at the admission (to reduce swelling), and operate when skin wrinkles after light stroke (*wrinkle test*). Previously, most of these fractures were treated with closed reduction and sometimes pin fixation. However, better surgical techniques allow a more aggressive approach with ORIF of displaced fractures involving the subtalar joint. Restore Bohler's angle. Extraarticular, anterior process calcaneus, and tuberosity (without TA attachment), may only require closed reduction and immobilization.

Fractures (cont)

Talus

May involve the neck (aviator's astragalus), ORIF when displaced as prone to a vascular necrosis and later OA (above and below), otherwise NWB for 6 weeks) the body/head (accurate reduction to prevent OA), or lateral process (try to leave alone).

Navicular

Can be avulsions (posterior tibial tendon), hairline, comminuted (reconstitute with ORIF and bone graft), or stress types. Treat by reduction and K-wire fixation. Watch for non-union which is painful and difficult to treat. Stress fractures are slow to heal and need 6–8 weeks in NWB cast or bone grafting at 1–2 months if symptomatic.

Subtalar dislocations

The calcaneus and navicular (talonavicular) are dislocated under the talus either laterally (calcaneus lateral, talar head medially and may be entangled in the posterior tibial or long flexions making open reduction necessary) or medially (the converse). *Plan* immediate reduction (open if necessary) to avoid significant soft tissue problems and immobilize for 6 weeks.

Total talar dislocation. The talus is totally dislocated at the ankle and subtalar joints and in big trouble. Immediate reduction (possibly open) and follow closely for AVN and OA.

Midfoot (Lisfranc's) injuries involve the tarsometatarsal joints and in the absence of gross displacement (homolateral, isolated or divergent displacement) can be subtle and easily overlooked with long-term unexplained midfoot pain. Consider both fractures and ligament disruptions. The problem is that the second metatarsal (the keystone of the mid-foot, although recessed between the 1st and 3ird cuneiforms) is still only held by one ligament (Lisfranc's ligament) to the 1st cuneiform. Look carefully at WB x-rays to tell whether the medial border of second metatarsal aligns with medial border middle cuneiform, if not, then ORIF is required otherwise NWB for 6 weeks (Fig. 13.13).

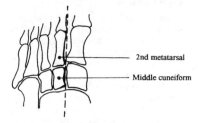

Should align otherwise disruption of midfoot (Lisfranc's)

Fig. 13.13 X-ray criteria for diagnosis of Lisfranc's injuries of the midfoot

Midfoot fractures

Metatarsal fractures

In general, when these fractures are displaced they must be reduced to prevent malunion and abnormal weight bearing over the metatarsal heads (metatarsalgia). The reduction may need to be held with a K-wire or plate. *Fractures of* the *proximal 5th metatarsal* are not uncommon from the significant shear forces applied, especially in long distance runners. Avulsion fractures (peroneus brevis/plantar fascia) can be treated in a NWB cast for 4–6 weeks (differentiate from accessing ossicle which has smooth margins). At the metaphyseal/diaphyseal junctions (Jones' fracture) union may be slow. (Consider ORIF in athlete and definitely when displaced.)

Dislocation of the MTP or PIP joint

Are not uncommonly overlooked. They require prompt reduction to avoid later open reduction and a source of significant pain.

Stress fractures

Should be suspected when an athlete has bone pain with a normal x-ray. There are two types: (1) *fatigue type* due to abnormally increased load on a normal bone; (2) *insufficiency type* resulting from normal loads on deficient bone (as in osteoporosis in ballet dancers/gymnasts who have amenorrhea). Typically such fractures are seen 3–5 weeks into a new and intensive training program as muscles adapt faster than bone. A small cortical crack occurs and spreads by subcortical infarction. Periosteal and endosteal new bone (callus) is seen 2–3 weeks later. X-rays may show the 'dreaded black line' indicative of impending complete fracture. Bone scans are positive early and diagnostic. There is typically localized bone pain and tenderness relieved by rest. The athlete limps. Examine the sports shoes for excessive wear. Common sites are the tibia (mid and distal in runners and basketball), calcaneus, navicular (basketball), metatarsals (recruits and runners) (especially 2nd MT and proximal 5th MT) and sesamoids (1st MTPJ); less commonly the medial or lateral malleolus (basketball), cuboid, talus, and proximal phalanx of big toe.

Treatment should be comprehensive. *Immediate* steps include rest, immobilization (NWB cast for at least 6–8 weeks is critical), RICE, NSAIDs. Recommend crosstraining (e.g. swim/cycle) to keep fit. Long-term treatment involves correction of malalignment, orthotics (for hyperpronation, external tibial torsion), use of sports shoes with better absorptive impact, and alteration of training schedules. Hormone treatment may be necessary for female athletes. *Exclude infection/tumor*. If the 'dreaded black line' of the tibia is still detected at 6 months, surgery may be required (bone graft/drill). Reintroduce activity at 6–12 months. Navicular stress fractures are difficult: slow to heal and may need surgical fixation and bone graft.

466

467

Nerve entrapments

Are common about the foot and ankle but are difficult to diagnose and treat. Many are related to poor sports shoe fit (e.g. ski boots), to training on hard surfaces, and occurs at competition. These include *tarsal tunnel*: the posterior tibial nerve is trapped behind the medial malleolus under the flexor retinaculum, with pain in the medial foot and sole; *anterior tarsal tunnel:* deep peroneal nerve trapped under the inferior extensor retinaculum, with pain in the 1st web space; *jogger's foot:* medial plantar nerve compressed at the knot of Henry (where FDL crosses FHL) pain over medial toes; *sural nerve:* pain along the medial border of the foot; *common peroneal nerve* results from trauma, pain behind the fibula neck; *superficial peroneal nerve:* anterolateral entrapment (12cm from tip of the lateral malleolus where it pierces the deep fascia)—distinguish from compartment syndrome; *saphenous nerve*: injured in thigh (Hunter's canal) or medial knee (post surgical the infrapatellar branch); Baxter's nerve to abductor digiti quinti may be compressed in abductor hallucis and cause of chronic heel pain as part of plantar fascists; *Morton's neuroma:* typically pain between 3rd and 4th metatarsal heads from traumatic entrapment causing neuroma (in runners) of the interdigital nerve. (Here, compression of the metatarsal heads reproduces the symptoms and the patient is aware of 'a mobile pebble' under the ball of the foot.)

All entrapments are **diagnosed** by localized tenderness over the affected nerve at the level of entrapment, decreased sensation after activity, positive Tinel's test and neuralgic pain at rest or at night. Provocative tests may be helpful (s. peroneal nerve: active dorsi flexion and eversion to tighten the peroneal muscles will reproduce the pain). Nerve conduction studies are usually unhelpful.

Treatment: with orthotics (shoe modification), NSAIDs, stretching, massage, Celestone injection. If necessary, surgically release nerve (and excise neuroma but bury nerve end in stable bony tissue bed) at the level of the anatomically located tenderness.

469

Compartment syndrome

Increased pressure within a confined muscle compartment may lead to ischemia, necrosis, contracture, and a useless limb. Early recognition and prompt treatment are essential (Fig). Causes are trauma (with fracture), postoperative crush injuries, and athletic exertion (especially in runners). **Clinical features** of an acute compartment syndrome are severe *pain* (early and reliable index not relieved by immobilization or the usual analgesia), exquisite localized tenderness, pain with movement whether active (usually not possible) or passive, and paresthesia. Pallor, paralysis, and pulselessness are *late* signs where the diagnoses has already been missed. The condition usually involves the lower leg (anterior/extensor/lateral compartments) or the forearm (flexion compartment) when compartmental pressures exceed 30mmHg (or within 10–30mmHg of the diastolic BP). Compartmental pressures can be measured with a Whiteside's infusion technique (Fig. 13.14) or indwelling catheter (or a commercial electronic monitor, e.g. Stryker STIC device) but such measurements are often fraught with problems of accuracy.

Method[1]

Using back-up non-electronic infusion technique. Equipment: mercury/an aeroid manometer, two plastic IV extension tubes, two 18 guage needles, 38mm (1/5 inches) long, one 20ml syringe, one three-way stopcock, one vial N Saline. *Set-up*: prepare limb to be tested. Put 18g needle into top of sterile bottle of saline to break vacuum. Attach 20ml syringe to stopcock, attach IV extension tube to stopcock, attach IV tube with 18g needle to stopcock. Put last needle into top of saline bottle (below fluid level). Aspirate (without bubbles) saline into one-half of this tubing. Turn off stopcock. Attach other extensions tubing from stopcock to manometer. Aspirate 15cc air into syringe (with stopcock closed to saline filled tubing). Insert needle into muscle to be tested/measured. Open system to connect both extension tubes (T-system). Make sure top of column saline in tubing is at same level as needle in patient (to avoid artificially wrong reading). Slightly depress plunger syringe to clear obstruction. Meniscus of fluid is *flat* when system is in equilibrium. Now take readings off mercury column at multiple sites (proximal/distal to fracture—highest pressure is critical measurement for decision making) (Fig. 13.14).

    Caution: the measurement of compartmental pressures *should never* override clinical judgment (even in unconscious patients who are unable to feel, careful examination of a swollen, tight compartment will provoke some response such as ↑BP or ↑intracranial pressure). **Treat externally** by splitting the POP/bandages to the skin (but not through the skin) and elevate to, but not beyond, heart level as may decrease already compromised microcirculation); and internally (if no relieve of symptoms) by surgical release of the compressed compartment (fasciotomy) within 4h to avoid irreversible ischemia. Irreversible nerve injury may occur within 12h. Ischemic/necrotic muscle may need to be debrided.

1 TE Whiteside, MM Heckman 1996 *J Am Acad Orthop Surgery* **4** 1996 p212–14

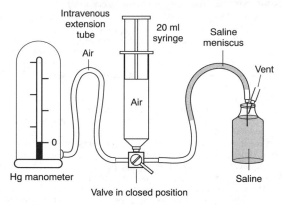

Assemble equipment as above just before placement of needle

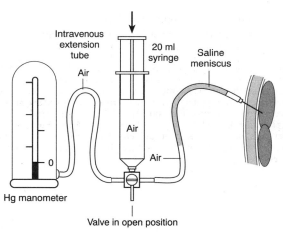

Fig. 13.14 Whiteside's infusion technique for measuring compartment pressures

Compartment syndrome (*cont*)

Chronic compartment syndrome (exertional)

May be subtle in presentation and results from prolonged training (runners, athletes engaged in court sports). The muscles are over-worked, swell and a *vicious cycle* is triggered (Fig. 13.15). The anterior/extensor compartments of the leg are usually involved with *crescendo pain* and tenderness relieved by rest. There may only be paresthesia with exercise. **Differential diagnosis** is essential. Use bone scan to exclude *stress* fracture. Pain over posteromedial distal tibia may be a *compartment problem of posterior tibialis* or periostitis of soleus muscle (*shin splints* see bone scan). Calf claudication with reduced pulses when knee is extended and foot dorsiflexed may result from *popliteal artery entrapment*.

    Treatment of chronic compartment syndrome is by activity mod-ification, massage, exclude footwear (try sports shoes with Poron® impact relieving heels/soles) or surface problems, NSAIDs, orthotics (medial wedge for posterior compartment), use cross training (cycling). Fasciotomy is sometimes necessary (80% successful). First, carefully measure intracompartment pressures before/during/after exercise; look for resting pressure>15mmHg or delay in fall after exercise of >20mmHg over 3 mins.[1] Then consider careful fasciotomy of the compartment involved with mini skin incisions and skin closure/drains.

Plantar fasciitis (overpull of fascia)

Is a common cause of crippling subcalcaneal (usually medial) heel pain. The condition is related to hyperpronation and pes cavus. There is localized tenderness with a positive Windlass effect (dorsiflexing the big toe exacerbates the pain). X-rays may show a heel spur (ignore it).

    Exclude stress fractures, nerve entrapment involving the medial branch of the lateral plantar nerve (Baxter's nerve, with neuralgic component) and Reiter's syndrome. **Treatment**: NSAIDs, stretching (heel cord), cortisone injection (2ml Celestone with 3ml (Marcain) bupivacaine 0.5% plain), and a soft silicone heel cup. **Surgery** (medial heel incision with release of abductor hallucis fascia and excise 3–4mm of plantar fascia, +/− release Baxter's nerve) is sometimes necessary.

1 SA Eirele *et al.* 1993 *Instr Course Lect* **42** 213–17. AAOS, IL

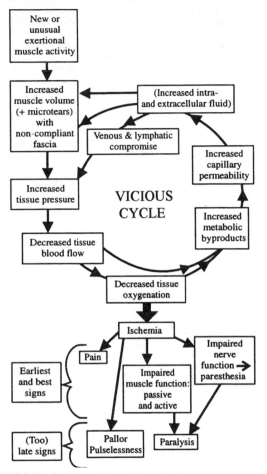

Fig. 13.15 Pathophysiology of chronic (exertional) compartment syndrome

Os trigonum

This ossicle behind the posterior talus (medial tubercle of the posterior process of the talus) may be the cause of pain with plantarflexion in ballet dancers. It can be asymptomatic, fused, fractured, large, or absent.[1]

X-ray to confirm the presence of os trigonum before finalizing diagnosis. **Caution:** do not confuse with FHL tendinitis (where resisted flexion big toe causes medial pain). **Treatment**: injection of 2ml *cortisone* or surgically excise and decompress FHL.

1 R Quirk 1994 *Clin North Am* **25** 127

Turf toe

Is caused by a forceful dorsi flexion of the 1st MTPJ, for instance, in American football, on a hard surface (artificial turf and flexible shoes) (Fig. 13.16). Painful swollen 1st MTPJ. X-rays may show a disruption of the plantar volar plate complex. Exclude stress fracture (proximal phalanx), sesamoiditis, entrapment of FHL. **Treatment:** RICE, taping, custom shoes. Sometimes surgical repair of the disruption is appropriate.

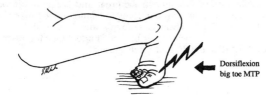

Dorsiflexion
big toe MTP

Fig. 13.16 Turf toe

Sand toe

Is a hyperplantarflexion injury to the great and lesser toes in beach volleyball players (who play barefoot and land on the hyperflexed forefoot)[1] (Fig. 13.17). There is synovitis and loss of dorsiflexion. **Treatment** is taping (in neutral for big toe, 'buddy' tape for lesser toe) exercises, NSAIDs, RICE, and rarely surgery.

1 C Frey *et al* 1996 *Foot and Ankle Internat* **17** 576–81

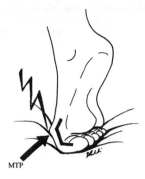

MTP

Fig. 13.17 Sand toe

479

Tibiotalar spurs

May form as osteophytic outgrowths on the adjoining surfaces of the lower anterior tibia and talar neck. Impingement pain will occur with dorsiflexion. **Treatment:** arthroscopic excision is useful (except where OA of ankle joint).

48°

Metatarsalgia

Forefoot pain beneath the metatarsal heads (with callosities) is vague in nature and related to impact sports. Hallux valgus claw toes or pes cavus may be present. It may be a transfer metatarsalgia (from short 1st MT or long 2nd MT). Exclude Morton's neuroma, stress fracture verruca (wart when trimmed will reveal tell tale pinpoint vessels). Freiberg's infraction or simply trimming of callosity. **Treatment**: stretching, NSAIDs, transverse arch supports (HAPADs). Rarely a closing wedge osteotomy (or partial plantar metatarsal head condylectomy) is useful where a single (usually the 2nd) metatarsal is involved.

Freiberg's infraction

Is an osteonecrosis of the 2nd metatarsal head, typically seen in teenage females. The pain is excruciating. X-rays may show increased density or collapse of the metatarsal head. **Treatment**: symptomatic, by debridement, synovectomy, or by limited resection of the distal 2nd MT head.

Hallux valgus (bunions)

Is common in the ballet community (from demi-pointe and rolling in), and results from improper shoe size (and flexibility) in dancers and catchers, as an acute (dislocation of 1st MTP joint) or chronic repetitive injury. Ballet dancers and sprinters are poor surgical candidates due to the debilitating effect of postoperative stiffness. **Treatment**: exhaustive by all available avenues (orthotics, toe spread, shoe box enlargement, NSAID gel to inflamed bunion, HV adduction splint) to delay surgery as long as possible.

Hallux rigidus

Is stiff and painful 1st MTPJ arising from microtrauma, osteonecrosis, or OA. The condition is seen in push off sports (see Fig. 13.2), where the feet are long, narrow, and pronated (long first MT). **Treatment**: by use of stiff sole, HAPADs, or by cheilectomy (excision of painful dorsal osteophytes).

Sesamoiditis

Localized pain usually below the 1st MTPJ which may be part of an FHL/FDB tendinitis or tethering and is seen in dancers.

X-ray (sesamoid views) to exclude fracture. Do not confuse with bipartite sesamoid (usually the tibial and has smooth margins) stress fracture, OA, or dislocation; and consider nerve entrapment. **Treatment**: with metatarsal support, NSAID or, (rarely) shave/excise.

Short leg syndrome

A short leg (>2cm) is prone to injury involving stress fractures, MCL knee sprain, patellar subluxation, plantar fasciitis, and hyperpronation. Other possible problems include equinus foot, postural scoliosis, low back pain, and poor gait. The longer leg is susceptible to iliotibial tendinitis. The shortening may be real or apparent (form tilt of pelvis with tendon contracture—needs stretching). **Treatment**: use partial heel (and midsole) build-up.

493

Persistent painful ankle

It is not uncommon to have an athlete with a persistently painful ankle and no 'apparent' cause. Pinpoint the precise area of tenderness and then image the area by X-ray (mortise view), bone scan (to correlate/confirm area of tenderness with increased update), ultrasound (if well performed will define tendon lesion), CT scan (to define bony lesion such as occult fracture), and possibly MRI (expensive but precise for defining soft tissue and bony lesions). Then work through the list in Table 13.1.

If no solution then consider NSAIDs by local application, S-ankle splint, gentle physiotherapy, low frequency pulsed ultrasound, TENS, WAX., cross training, water jogging, pain clinic, patience, and do not ignore the problem athlete (be prepared to talk, review, and reassess).

Table 13.1 Persistent painful ankle: problems and actions

Problem	Action
'Meniscoid' (Fergel lesion) synovitis ankle	Arthroscopic synovectomy
Avulsion tip of fibula (in children)	Excise
'Asymptomatic' ossicle	Excise
Unrecognized fracture of anterior process of calcaneus	Excise
Peroneal or tibialis postexterior tendon problem (synovitis, partial tendon rupture subluxation)	Surgery
Fracture of lateral process of talus	Fix/excise
Sinus tarsi syndrome	Surgery (debride)
'High ankle sprain' (+/− fracture Tillaux)	See p446
Impingement of inferior band of (syndesmosis) tibiotalar ligament	Excise band
Nerve entrapment	See p468
Tarsal coalition (children)	Excise/fuse
Osteochondral fracture/dissecans	Arthroscopy
Rheumatoid arthritis	Refer
Reflex sympathetic dystrophy (painful ankle, sensitive skin)	Nerve block, physical therapy

14 Gastrointestinal and genitourinary problems

JOHN A CARTMILL

497

Introduction

In sports, gastrointestinal or genitourinary sport trauma are managed identically to gastrointestinal or genitourinary trauma from any cause. As sport covers most human physical endeavor from running to extreme forms of augmented transport, from wrestling to football, and the use of firearms, so the potential range and mechanism of sport injury is enormous.

The injured sportsperson can be physically well conditioned, muscular, and full of 'fight or flight' adrenaline. The physical conditioning can help protect from injury but at the same time can hinder diagnosis by masking the physical signs of injury. Most sportspeople do not conform to this physical ideal, the range of body habitus, physical condition, and underlying medical condition is as broad as the sports people play. A game of rugby football in an area of endemic malaria, for example, has special implications for splenic injury.

499

Basic rules

Despite these potentially confounding factors, the following *basic rules* apply:

- In any injured patient, the trauma **ABC** applies (**A**irway, **B**reathing, **C**irculation).
- The patient should be fasted.
- There is no need to make a precise diagnosis 'in the field'.
- The **only decision** that needs to be made is: 'Does this person need more attention than I (the sports medicine physician) can provide here'. If the answer is 'Yes' then they must be transferred rapidly to an emergency room.
- Intravenous fluids should be started on suspicion of significant injury rather than after confirmation of a problem.
- Narcotic analgesia should be delayed until surgical assessment is complete.
- Any one of the following list of **complaints** is a *cause for concern*:
  - abdominal pain that does not go away
  - pain that is getting worse
  - pain made worse by walking or moving
  - pain that radiates through or around to the back
  - difficulty breathing
  - vomiting or passing blood in the stool or urine
- Any one of the following list of **signs** is a *cause for concern*:
  - increase in pulse rate (tachycardia)
  - increase in breathing rate (tachypynea)
  - abdominal bruising; bruising on the outside may herald bruising (or rupture) of an internal organ
  - penetrating injury
  - involuntary guarding (tensing) of the abdominal muscles
  - abdominal distension
  - the patient looks pale
  - the patient looks unwell

The body has *only a limited number of ways* of reacting to trauma. Bleeding is same whether it is coming from a transected mesentery, the liver, or spleen. The urgency of transfer is the same, and the subtleties of managing one or the other are the responsibility of the admitting surgeon. Do not spend too much time wondering whether the abdominal distension and pulse of 160 is because of liver damage or a splenic injury . . . call the ambulance.

The *trauma protocol* of the receiving institution will be invoked irrespective of the mechanism of injury. Peritoneal lavage, CT scan, or immediate laparotomy, the decision will vary with surgeon, institution, and country.

Laparotomy for trauma

Crossmatched blood is available in the operating room. Reliable intravenous access is ensured by central line and wide-bore cannula. The patient is placed supine on the operating table. If there is blood in the rectum a modified lithotomy position is used with Dan Allan or Lloyd Davies stirrups. The abdomen and chest is prepared and the preparation is carried down to the genitals, perineum, and mid thigh. A Foley catheter is inserted if one is not already in place (see urethral injury, p505). Pneumatic leg compression stockings are used. Experienced assistance is essential and a self-retaining retractor most desirable.

Stand on the right side of the patient. A long midline incision is preferred. Any massive source of bleeding is dealt with directly. Several packs can be held in place to tamponade the bleeding while the wound is extended (xiphisternum to pubis). Retraction. Empty blood by bailing clots and using large packs which absorb blood more rapidly than a sucker. Take the sucker off and use the suction tube alone, protecting it in your cupped hand will make an effective 'sump' sucker able to deal with clots while the loops of bowel are kept at bay. Formal exploration of the entire abdomen is mandatory. If you have a systematic approach, use it. If you need one, start in the upper abdomen where the gastrointestinal tract enters and use this to guide you systematically. Stomach, spleen (reaching high up under the left costal margin and cupping it with the palm), liver (all peritonealized surfaces), duodenum (noting the space lateral to the second part for staining), right kidney while you have the area exposed, pancreas, remainder of duodenum having lifted the mass of small bowel to the right, then every inch of small bowel and its mesentery down to the cecum, around the colon and down into the pelvis, bladder, and rectum. If minor bleeding is encountered, pack the area for later attention; massive bleeding should be dealt with.

Be meticulous with completing the systematic examination of all abdominal organs. Attention can be distracted by the process of repairing an injury and then closing the abdomen leaving an injury further down the checklist undetected.

501

Spleen

Splenic trauma results from a blow or crush to the left side of the abdomen or lower chest. The patient complains of abdominal or left shoulder tip pain (from diaphragmatic irritation). Pallor, tachycardia and hypotension are signs of blood loss and impending shock. The abdomen will be tender or guarded and may be distended. Sportspeople from countries where malaria is endemic are especially prone to splenic injury; bear this in mind as the global sporting community shrinks.

The patient is fasted, intravenous fluids are commenced through a wide-bore cannula, and the patient is transferred urgently to a trauma center. Shock unresponsive to resuscitation or other evidence of ongoing blood loss (progressive abdominal distension, falling hemoglobin, persistent tachycardia) requires emergency laparotomy through a midline incision.

The stable patient can have a CT scan to confirm the diagnosis. The possibility of delayed secondary hemorrhage demands conservative management in hospital with intravenous access, frequent observations, and crossmatched blood available. Surgery will be required for clinical deterioration. Contact sport is prohibited for six months to a year.

Splenic conservation is facilitated by a generous midline incision, capable assistance, and complete, formal mobilization. Operative trauma is avoided. Capsular avulsions may respond to topical hemostatic agents and cautery (the argon beam coagulator is useful).

Subcapsular hematomas may require a polyglycolic acid mesh sac which can also be useful for deep rents although deep suture and even partial splenectomy may be required.

The spleen is an important immunological organ and should be preserved if possible. The splenectomized individual is vulnerable to infection from encapsulated organisms and should be immunized against pneumococcal, meningococcal, and hemophilus organisms.

Liver

A direct blow to the right upper quadrant, epigastrium, or right chest can produce liver trauma although it is uncommon. Crush can produce a more extensive injury. As with splenic trauma the patient complains of abdominal or shoulder tip pain (from diaphragmatic irritation). Pallor, tachycardia, and hypotension are signs of blood loss and impending shock. The abdomen will be tender or guarded and may be distended.

The patient is fasted, intravenous fluids are commenced through a wide-bore cannula, and the patient is transferred urgently to a trauma center. Shock unresponsive to resuscitation or other evidence of ongoing blood loss (progressive abdominal distension, falling hemoglobin, persistent tachycardia) requires emergency laparotomy through a midline incision.

The stable patient can have a CT scan to confirm the diagnosis. Capsular tears, superficial lacerations, and deep hematomas (< 3cm) can usually be managed conservatively (as long as the patient remains stable). However, extensive lacerations, devascularized segments, and large hematomas (> 3cm) will usually require surgery. The liver can be expeditiously mobilized by dividing the falciform, and if necessary the diaphragmatic ligaments. Severe injuries may need to be packed; do not put the packs into the rent as this will keep the vessels open, place the packs above and below the liver so as to force the rent closed, and apply pressure. This may be an opportunity to transfer the patient to a specialized liver unit. Abscess and bile leak are longer-term complications.

Duodenal and pancreatic injuries

Requiring a direct epigastric blow (e.g. the kick of a horse) to compress the pancreas and or duodenum against the spine, this deep, often retroperitoneal injury can remain hidden. Duodenal injuries are usually hard to recognize as the leak can be contained by the retroperitoneum and there need not be any signs until sepsis supervenes. Blunt duodenal injury (the invariable case in sporting accidents) is even harder to recognize. Remain suspicious, delays in diagnosis increase morbidity, and any patient with persistent epigastric pain, usually, but not always, radiating through the back or shoulders must have pancreatic duodenal injury excluded. Duodenal hematoma will present with symptoms of gastric outlet obstruction.

The serum amylase may be elevated with duodenal perforation. The plain abdominal x-ray may have an absent psoas shadow, retroperitoneal air, or a scoliosis. Oral contrast enhanced CT scan may demonstrate a leak and peripancreaticoduodenal edema.

Intraluminal hematoma my be treated conservatively if perforation has been excluded. Total parenteral nutrition may be required.

The duodenum is approached through a long midline incision. Hematoma or bile-stained fluid at any of the lateral margins of the duodenum suggests perforation. The right side of the duodenum is exposed by Kocherizing the second part and carrying this dissection toward the midline in the retropancreaticoduodenal plane. Further exposure requires mobilization of the viscera supplied by the superior mesenteric artery which overlies the third part of the duodenum; small bowel, cecum, and right and transverse parts of the colon. The cecum and right colon are mobilized on their primitive mesentery along with the base of the small bowel mesentery (which represents the left edge of this embryological plane); this plane is carried up to and over the third part of the duodenum.

Simple perforations are debrided and sutured. Segmental resection and anastomosis may be necessary. Patching with a jejunal loop or Roux-en-Y may be used if primary repair is not possible. Duodenal diversion with closure of the pylorus, gastroenterostomy, and decompression for the duodenal loop may be required for rupture. Severe combined duodenal and pancreatic trauma could require a Whipple procedure.

Duodenal decompression, percutaneous, via the stomach, or using a nasoduodenal tube is necessary. Feeding jejunostomy should be considered. The area must be drained adequately. Complications include sepsis and pancreatic or duodenal fistula.

Stomach

Is usually resistant to injury from blunt trauma. The important exception is the full stomach that can burst with a direct blow or crush.

Do not be sidetracked into repairing the stomach until the laparotomy has been completed and the full extent of the injuries determined. If the stomach is leaking gastric contents place a clamp or quick suture to control the contamination before moving on.

The injury is debrided if necessary. If the laceration crosses into the origin of the greater or lesser omentum, clear this meticulously (in the manner of a highly selective vagotomy) to allow seromuscular apposition with the repair. The stomach is repaired with large interrupted absorbable sutures. A two-layer continuous repair is acceptable. Take a larger bite of the seromuscular than the mucosal layer. The repair should be inverted. Decompress the stomach with a nasogastric tube.

Small bowel

Injury includes serosal tear, full thickness rupture and mesenteric injury (hematoma or laceration). Physical signs are indistinguishable from those above. Development of signs can be delayed by days, especially in the case of an isolated small bowel rupture. Developing ileus, progressive distension, and tenderness with a low grade fever are important signs.

Abdominal X-ray may show free air or thickened bowel loops. CT scan will reveal free intraabdominal fluid or thickening of bowel wall or planes.

Serosal tear is usually an incidental finding at laparotomy. Recognition of a full thickness rupture can be delayed by several days as the associated peritonitis can develop slowly. Abdominal wall bruising is an important indicator of possible underlying injury and requires peritoneal lavage or CT. Mesenteric hematoma can extend to the root of the mesentery and cause venous congestion. An expanding mesenteric hematoma must be entered to control the bleeding. A small mesenteric tear can cause a surprisingly large hemoperitoneum.

Resection or repair is carried out with an interrupted or continuous absorbable seromuscular suture. Staples can be used. Run every centimeter (inch) of the small bowel and mesentery.

When repairing an injury, consider the lumen of the small bowel and place a suture line transversely across the bowel where possible. The principles of the successful anastomosis apply to the repair as well as to the formal resection and anastomosis; good blood supply, no tension, no distal obstruction.

Colon

Give broad-spectrum antibiotics to cover the range of colonic organisms. The colon adjacent to the injury is mobilized on its embryological mesentery. Colon may be repaired primarily if there is no risk of subsequent breakdown of the repair. The injury must be less than 12h old, there can be no intraperitoneal contamination, the wall of the colon must be viable with a good blood supply. A diaphragmatic defect is a contraindication to primary repair.

If primary repair is not considered safe the suture line can be exteriorized for early return to the abdomen once sound healing has been confirmed (5–10 days). The defect itself can be brought out as a stoma. Both of these procedures can require extensive mobilization to allow the colon to reach the skin and lie over a colostomy rod *without tension*. An exteriorized repair must lie free of the skin edge so that a breakdown will result in a colostomy rather than a subcutaneous leak.

Note: an injury too low to be exteriorized should be treated as a rectal injury.

Rectum

Rare in sport accidents a rectal injury is suspected with a pelvic crush or penetrating wound in the region of the pelvis (buttocks, hips, perineum). Blood may be found on the examining finger after rectal examination during the secondary survey in the emergency room. The principles of management of rectal injury are well established and require thorough cleansing of the rectum to decrease its potential as a source of contamination during subsequent management:

- Modified lithotomy position using Dan Allan or Lloyd Davies stirrups.
- Exposure by mobilization in the presacral plane
- Rigid sigmoidoscopy with irrigation and a *large bore* sucker.
- Antegrade irrigation via the distal limb of a defunctioning colostomy or through the defect itself before closing if the defect is accessible.
- Drainage of the perirectal fascial planes. The drain is placed in the presacral plane and brought out between anus and coccyx.
- Diversion of the fecal stream by defunctioning colostomy.

Kidney

Suspected with flank bruising, bony injury (lower rib or lumbar vertebrae), and hematuria. *Note* that the absence of hematuria does not exclude renal injury; a devascularized kidney will not cause hematuria, nor will an injury that does not involve the collecting system. A thrombosed and occluded renal artery must be repaired within 3h to save the kidney from acute tubular necrosis.

Expanding retroperitoneal hematoma

- Have proximal vascular control before exploring a hematoma; this may require extensive mobilization of embryological planes.
- Explore central hematomas corresponding in position to the aorta, inferior vena cava, duodenum, and pancreas.
- Explore lateral hematomas suggesting injury to the kidneys, ureters, or mesocolon
- Explore hematomas due to penetrating injury.
- Explore a hematoma in the region of the bladder to rule out bladder injury.
- Do not explore the hematoma due to massive retroperitoneal bleeding of a severe pelvic fracture.

Bladder

More easily injured when full, bladder injury is suspected with hematuria, urinary retention, suprapubic pain, or peritonitis. The rupture may be confined to the retroperitoneum or be free into the peritoneal cavity. **Diagnosed** by contrast study, a simple tear may be managed with Foley catheter drainage alone.

In most cases, the bladder should be opened at laparotomy, the trigone, urethral and ureteric orifices are confirmed to be clear of injury and the injury and operative cystotomy are repaired with two layers of absorbable 2/0 or 3/0 suture. The bladder is drained with a catheter (transurethral or suprapubic) and the extravesical space is drained with penrose drains.

Stent an injury to a ureteric orifice with a ureteric stent.

Male urethra

Caused by a fall astride or severe pelvic fracture. Do not attempt to pass a urinary catheter if blood is seen at the urethral meatus or there is edema and bruising of the penis or perineum, suspect urethral injury and do a urethrogram. Discourage the patient from voiding to minimize extravasation. Passage of a catheter could convert a partial tear to a complete disruption.

Suprapubic catheterization and specialist urological referral are required. If the patient requires urgent laparotomy the suprapubic catheter can be placed with the abdomen open, otherwise a percutaneous technique can be used.

Anterior urethra extends from meatus to urogenital diaphragm. Early exploration is desirable but this should be carried out by a urologist.

Posterior urethra extends from urogenital diaphragm to bladder neck. The prostate will be displaced on digital rectal examination, replaced by a soft boggy mass of hematoma. This injury is invariably associated with a major pelvic fracture.

Perineum

Perineal, urethral, and vaginal injury in the female is best treated with catheterization (suprapubic if necessary) and surgical repair of lacerations to control hemorrhage.

Scrotum and testis

Regrettably, often a deliberate injury associated with contact sport. Ultrasound will confirm the diagnosis. The scrotum should be explored to evacuate hematoma and repair the tunica. Extruding parenchyma is excised to allow the tunica to be approximated with a running 4/0 absorbable suture.

Vulva

Caused by falls astride and the classical water skiing accident this injury is becoming less common as the role of protective clothing is appreciated.

14 Gastrointestinal and genitourinary problems
Basic rules

Abdominal wall

- groin strain
- hernia
- hip pointer (see p374)
- 'stitch'

Groin strain is a non-specific term used to describe injury to the tendons and muscles of the lower abdomen and upper inner thigh.

Musculotendinous injury to the adductor group is often deep but bruising may be visible in an athlete with little fat. Expose the patient from umbilicus to knee; a towel between the legs will preserve some modesty. The patient will be tender over the superior part of the broad tendon that runs from the upper inner thigh down the leg. Diagnosis is based on clinical examination; the role of ultrasound, CT, and MRI imaging has yet to be determined. Management consists of ice, non-steroidal anti-inflammatory drugs, physiotherapy, and rest. Careful stretching may help prevent injury in the future.

After a high energy injury it may be necessary to rule out femoral neck or pelvic fracture. Femoral hernia may mimic groin strain but is uncommon in the athlete. It should be remembered that a lump may not be palpable with a femoral hernia and a 'cough impulse' does not occur. Ultrasound may be helpful. Injury to the hip joint itself may be misdiagnosed as groin strain (see p372).

A more common differential diagnosis is groin hernia. The patient is tender just lateral and superior to the pubic tubercle and/or about half-way between the public tubercle and the anterior superior iliac crest. There is usually a lump or 'cough impulse' but not always. An ultrasound may be helpful. Always examine the scrotum to rule out torsion or testicular injury. A hernia should be repaired.

A group of patients will continue to experience pain in the absence of a demonstrable hernia. Weakness of the posterior wall of the inguinal canal has been postulated as a cause and the role of hernia repair in this group is being evaluated.

Gastrointestinal symptoms associated with sport

Despite their aura of fitness and health, the athlete is susceptible (and in fact predisposed) to common and well-characterized disease processes. The athlete's physical conditioning may obscure signs and delay diagnosis and appropriate referral.

The following is a list of common gastrointestinal symptoms and possible causes. *Those conditions with particular relevance to the sports physician are indicated*:

- *Visceral pain*
  - irritable bowel syndrome
  - peptic ulceration
  - cholelithiasis
  - diverticulitis
- *Heartburn*
  - reflux
  - peptic ulceration
- *Nausea*
  - bowel obstruction
- *Vomiting*
  - gastroenteritis
- *Diarrhoea*
  - infectious diarrhoea
  - runners diarrhea
  - irritable bowel syndrome
  - inflammatory bowel disease

Note: do take stool cultures before commencing therapy

511

512

513

15 Drugs and the athlete

MARK A FREEMAN

Introduction

Athletes are subject to injuries and require medical treatments probably more regularly than their non-athletic counterparts. A wide range of treatments are available for common complaints, but include some specific drugs which are considered to be ergogenic, or performance enhancing. These drugs are banned by sport's governing bodies because they have the potential to give the athlete an unfair artificial advantage over his/her competitors. If a drug test during or outside competition shows evidence of use, an athlete is subject to disqualification or other punishment by their sport's governing body. Consequently, an injured athlete must become knowledgeable about their medications and choose a physician fully *au fait* with their sport's banned and restricted medications.

Athletes who choose to use doping methods and banned drugs contravene the ethics of sport, and physicians complying with their requests are contravening the ethics of medical science. Sport, however, is not fair. Various performance-enhancing techniques have always been employed by athletes seeking to gain an advantage over their rivals. Since Canadian sprinter Ben Johnson's dramatic 1988 Seoul Olympic 100m disqualification for testing positive to the anabolic steroid, stanozolol, the widespread abuse of drugs in sport became patently clear. The International Olympic Committee (IOC) and many individual sports' governing bodies now continually seek to improve their testing methods to try to keep élite athletes 'clean'. The IOC now uses the hypersensitive high resolution mass spectrometer (HRMS), which has detected traces of urine steroid allegedly taken more than 3 months previously. Conversely, athletes seek to remain a step ahead of the detection systems and turn to newer drugs with shorter elimination times so they can continue taking performance-enhancing drugs closer to their competition dates. Testing difficulties obviously exist for the increasingly popular naturally occurring substances such as erythropoietin, blood, insulin-like growth factor-1 (IGF-1) and human growth hormone (hGH), which can all give a competitive edge. Use of performance-enhancing drugs is not limited to the élite, with gyms around the world being a focus of supply to the non-elite athlete.

A major consideration for the athlete and treating physician is the immense impact of a positive test and disqualification. Emotional distress, loss of livelihood, bad press, and loss of respect from peers can follow from even the simple inadvertent use of a banned drug in a cough mixture. It is incumbent, therefore, on the treating physician to be aware of their athlete's sport's drug testing policy and the specific drugs banned. Knowledge of a drug's detection window, detection cut-off dosage and the ability to recognize drug-taking behavior in an athlete are also very useful attributes in a sports medicine practitioner.

Definitions

Doping

The International Olympic Committee has traditionally been the world-wide authority on doping in sport. The governing bodies of most sports generally liaise with and seek direction concerning drugs and doping from the IOC. The IOC's medical commission defines doping, with respect to intent, as:

> the administration to, or the use by a competing athlete, of any substance taken into the body or any physiological substance taken in abnormal quantity or by an abnormal route of entry into the body, with the sole intention of increasing in an artificial and unfair manner his performance in competition.

The IOC's current ban on doping reads:

> **Doping contravenes the ethics of both sport and medical science. The IOC medical commission bans:**
>
> **1 The administration of substances belonging to selected classes of pharmacological agents**: stimulants, narcotics, anabolic agents, diuretics, peptide hormones, and analogues; and
>
> **2 The use of various doping methods**: blood doping, pharmacological, chemical, and physical manipulation.

Explanatory notes detail the classes and methods.[1,2]

Banned substances

Banned classes of drugs may not be used in any sport, for any reason. Even if a substance belonging to a class of banned drugs is not specifically listed in the examples, the term 'and related substances' encompasses all similarly acting drugs, and that substance is also banned.

Restricted substances

Various restrictions apply to some classes of substances. β-blockers, marijuana, and alcohol, for example, are not banned by the IOC, but are banned for some sports. Caffeine is so ubiquitously used in society that it is only banned in higher doses. More complex restrictions apply to corticosteroids, local anesthetics, and β-2 agonists.

Allowed substances

Most prescription drugs have no demonstrable ergogenic effects and are permitted as medical treatments. To assist treating physicians and athletes to identify which drugs are allowed, a 1990 Australian publication, *Drugs and sport*,[2] listed every locally available pharmaceutical product as either allowed, banned, or restricted. Many countries have now produced their own regularly updated and highly useful publications. Classes of allowed drugs include nonsteroidal antiinflammatory drugs (NSAIDs) and benzodiazepines.

The governing bodies of various sports vary in the specific drugs they ban, restrict, and allow, but the principle of banning drugs with potential for performance enhancement in the particular sport always applies.

1 International Olympic Committee Medical Commission Internet site: http://africa.cis.co.za:81/sports/sisa/drugs/doping.html   2 L Badewitz-Dodd (ed) 1992 *Drugs and sport* IMS, Sydney

Cut-off level

Of a certain drug is the urine concentration above which an athlete will be sanctioned. This concept generally applies to classes of restricted drugs since detection of a banned drug at any level is prohibited. Sports differ in the cut-off levels they accept as firm evidence of drug abuse. The testing laboratories can usually detect substances at much lower concentrations than the cut-off level. They have no say in any sanctions applied; leaving judgment of their detection results to the relevant sports authority. The detection limits given in this chapter are guides only, indicating levels all laboratories would detect.

Detection window

The detection window period refers to the length of time following administration of the drug that it can be detected above the cut-off level.

Classes of banned drugs

Stimulants

Common examples: cocaine, amphetamines, caffeine, β-agonists, phenylpropanolamine, ephedrine, pseudoephedrines.

Stimulants arouse the CNS to speed up parts of the brain and body. These are used at competition time (e.g. sprinters and weight lifters) to hasten reflexes, improve confidence, and diminish an athlete's sense of fatigue. Away from major events, their appetite-suppressant effect can be used to help lose weight (e.g. gymnasts, figure skaters, weight class sports). Performance enhancement is questionable with adverse effects including anxiety and psychosis, and in the case of cocaine (especially free-base crack), dependence. (Table 15.1)

This group of IOC-banned substances includes those commonly ingested inadvertently such as caffeine, the ephedrines and pseudoephedrines (in decongestants), and β-2 agonists (asthmatic medications). The IOC has approved some β-agonists for asthmatics as allowed medications (salbutamol and terbutaline by inhalation only), but notice must be given in writing to the relevant medical authority by physicians administering these inhaled β-2 agonists to athletes. The β-2 agonist, clenbuterol, has been specifically banned due to its ergogenic effects. (Table 15.2.)

Anabolic-androgenic steroids

Common examples: stanozolol, methanedienone, nandrolone, clostebol, oxandrolone, testosterone. Anabolic steroids are synthetic analogues of the natural male hormone, testosterone. The chemical modifications are aimed first, at increasing the efficacy of the drug by reducing liver metabolism and secondly, at maximizing the desired anabolic (muscle-building) effects and minimizing the unwanted androgenic (masculinizing) effects of the drug.

Potential benefits of anabolic steroids include increased muscle bulk and an enhanced ability to perform high intensity training. Anecdotal evidence suggests that most strength gains occur when hard training is undertaken concurrently with the steroid 'cycle'. The 'cycling' regimen consists of alternating 6–12 week cycles on/off the drug(s) at 5–100 times physiological male testosterone levels up to 3 times/year and normally away from competition times. 'Stacking' of 1–2 oral and 1–2 transdermally injected anabolic steroids at the one time is perceived by some body builders and athletes to give increased benefit. Human chorionic gonadotrophin (HCG) is sometimes taken concurrently by males to minimize the unwanted side-effects of testicular atrophy and gynecomastia (breast development). (Table 15.3.)

These drugs are widely used by non-elite athletes, often adolescents concerned with the development of a muscular physique. The side-effects are numerous, including the very serious hypertrophic cardiomyopathy and sudden death. More common are increased aggressiveness, acne, facial hair, accelerated baldness, menstrual irregularities, gynecomastia, testicular atrophy, and mandible enlargement. Sperm production remains faulty for up to 2 years.

Advances in testing for steroids (e.g. using HRMS) mean that some athletes are now using tablets and absorbable gel steroids instead of the injectable forms. These preparations are very quickly metabolized and excreted, allowing the athlete to continue taking them up to 2 weeks prior to a competition. Random out-of-competition drug

Table 15.1 Actions of stimulants

Potential benefits	Potential side-effects
Quickened reflexes	CNS: anxiety, agitation, irritability,
Masking of fatigue	headaches, dizziness, seizures, insomnia,
Increased alertness	tolerance, addiction
Appetite suppression	CVS: arrhythmias, tachycardia,
Improved concentration	hypertension, angina pectoris, vasculitis
Increased short-term strength	GIT: anorexia, nausea, vomiting,
Increased short-term endurance	diarrhea
Enhanced feeling of confidence	Other: increased risk of hyperthermia

CNS, central nervous system; CVS, cardiovascula system;
GIT, gastrointestinal system.

Table 15.2 Detection of stimulants

Drug	Detection window (GC/MS)*	Detection limits (GC/MS)
Amphetamines	2–5 days	100ng/ml
Cocaine	5–6 days	50ng/ml
Ephedrines	2–3 days	50ng/ml

*GC/MS: gas chromatography/mass spectrometry, current highest sensitivity
screening method.

Table 15.3 Actions of anabolic-androgenic steroids

Potential benefits	Potential side-effects
Increased muscle bulk	Hypertrophic cardiomyopathy
Increased weight	Sudden death
Increased strength	Aggressiveness
Increased high intensity training capability	Mood swings
Increased acceleration	Depression
Decreased body fat	Psychosis
Enhanced injury repair capability	Accelerated baldness
Reduced recovery time	Uneven bone growth
Improved performance	Acromegaly
	Acne
	Testicular atrophy
	Abnormal sperm production
	Changes in libido
	Gynecomastia
	Facial hair growth
	Menstrual irregularities

testing in most IOC sports is now the biggest deterrent to élite athletes taking anabolic steroids and other banned drugs. (Table 15.4.)

Administration of testosterone is banned but since this is a natural hormone, detection is highly likely. Detection of abuse is based on variation in the normal physiological ratio of testosterone and another biologically related but inactive hormone, epitestosterone. The IOC have declared that in the absence of demonstrable pathology, a urine testosterone to epitestosterone ratio exceeding 6 to 1 is an offence. Further investigations are mandatory where T:E > 6:1, including endocrine investigations, before the responsible authority declares the original sample positive.

β-2 agonists

Common examples: clenbuterol, salbutamol, terbutaline, fenoterol, salmeterol. Although β-2 agonists are also considered to be stimulants; they may have powerful anabolic effects when given systemically. The β-2 agonist, clenbuterol, has been specifically banned due to its ergogenic effects. Clenbuterol has a significant lipolytic effect and stimulates fast-twitch muscle hypertrophy secondary to increased muscle protein aggregation. Clenbuterol is difficult to detect more than 48h after use, and is often used with undetectable hGH as an alternative to anabolic steroids when athletes fear being tested and caught. (Table 15.5.)

Narcotic analgesics

Common examples: morphine, pethidine, buprenorphine, methadone, pentazocine, dextropropoxyphene, dextromoramide, diamorphine. The narcotic analgesics may give an increased pain threshold, feelings of invincibility and euphoria, and a diminished recognition of injury, and as such are IOC-banned substances. Of this group, however, codeine, diphenoxylate, dextromethorphan, pholcodine, and dihydrocodeine are now IOC-approved as a painkiller for athletes. (Table 15.6.)

Peptide and glycopeptide hormones

Common examples: hCG (Human chorionic gonadotropin), ACTH (adrenocorticotropin), hGH (human growth hormone or somatotropin), EPO (erythropoietin or rEPO = recombinant or synthetic EPO), IGF-1 (insulin-like growth factor-1). (Table 15.7.)

Erythropoietin (EPO)

Recombinant human erythropoietin (rEPO) was developed to treat anemia and is almost indistinguishable from the natural kidney hormone. Infusions or subcutaneous injections stimulate erythropoiesis in a sustained manner, giving an athlete elevated red blood cell concentrations for extended periods after the blood concentration has diminished to undetectable levels. The blood profile post rEPO can approximate that due to highaltitude training. *Very serious side-effects* follow from excessive use of rEPO since elevated hemoconcentration and blood viscosity can lead to clotting and intravascular thrombus formation. Many sudden deaths in fit young athletes, especially whilst resting or sleeping, have been attributed to erythropoietin use. *Urinalysis* cannot detect these ergogenic aids so blood sampling of athletes is necessary to detect use of rEPO.

Table 15.4 Detection of anabolic-androgenic steroids

Drug	Detection window
Fat-soluble parenteral steroids	Up to 12 months
Water-soluble oral steroids	1–6 weeks

Table 15.5. Detection of β-2 agonists

Drug	Detection window
Clenbuterol	2 days

Table 15.6 Actions of narcotic analgesics

Potential benefits	Potential side-effects
Increased pain threshold	CNS: mental clouding, dysphoria,
Feelings of invincibility	delirium, seizures, dizziness, parkinsonism,
Euphoria	tolerance, addiction, withdrawal
Diminished injury recognition	syndrome
	Respiratory depression
	GIT: vomiting, nausea, constipation
	Other: pruritis

Classes of banned drugs (*cont*)

Human chorionic gonadotropin (hCG)

Administration of hCG to males induces an increased rate of production of natural androgenic steroids. It is equivalent to administration of exogenous testosterone.

Adrenocorticotropin (ACTH)

Like endogenous ACTH, exogenous ACTH stimulates production of corticosteroids and results in the feeling of euphoria. It is equivalent to administration of exogenous corticosteroids.

Growth hormone (hGH)

Is produced naturally in the human pituitary gland and controls our growth from infancy. The synthetic version is identical to the natural version and hence undetectable. hGH has an overall anabolic effect similar to anabolic steroids, but without many of the side-effects. It stimulates muscle protein and nucleic acid synthesis, increases lipolysis (decreases body fat), and improves musculoskeletal repair. The *adverse effects* include diabetes, gigantism in prepubescents, and acromegaly in adults.

Insulin-like growth factor-1 (IGF-1)

Is another natural hormone which promotes growth of all cells. It can increase natural strength by 5–15% and as such is far more potent than growth hormone. It is extremely expensive but of considerable attraction to the power athletes. *Side-effects* are similarly more potent than for growth hormone and include swelling of the brain, hypertrophic cardiomyopathy, sudden death, and diabetic coma. Administration of the hormone releasing factors for the above hormones is similarly banned.

Diuretics

Common examples: frusemide, acetazolamide, hydrochlorothiazide, spironolactone, mannitol, ethacrynic acid, bumetanide. Diuretics are IOC-banned because of the possibility of weight category sportspeople abusing their acute weight-losing effects to satisfy a weight limit. For this reason, competitors may be asked to provide urine samples at the time of weigh in. Diuretics also tend to dilute urine, making detection of other substances more difficult.

Others

It is important to be aware of the possibility of banned substances being included in natural remedies, herbal mixtures, and over-the-counter (OTC) preparations. Athletes have tested positive after using Chinese herbs and OTC cough preparations for minor complaints.

Table 15.7 Effects of peptide and glycopeptide hormones

Potential benefits	Potential side-effects
EPO Increases blood oxygen-carrying capacity Improves endurance	**EPO** Sudden death Increased blood viscosity Hypertension Congestive heart failure Stroke
hCG Testosterone-like effects Testicular atrophy prevention	**hCG** Headache Mood swings Depression Edema
ACTH Equivalent to systemic corticosteroid therapy Anti-inflammatory effects	**ACTH** Mood changes Hypertension Osteoporosis Glucose intolerance Many systemic long-term side-effects of regular corticosteroid use
hGH Muscle growth Lipolysis Improved musculoskeletal repair	**hGH** Hypertension Cardiomyopathy Acromegaly (adults) Gigantism (prepubescents) Diabetes Creutzfeld–Jacob disease (from contaminated sources)
IGF-1 Muscle growth Increased strength Lipolysis Improved repair	**IGF-1** Swelling of the brain Hypertrophic cardiomyopathy Sudden death Diabetic coma

Classes of restricted drugs

Alcohol

For various reasons, including the image given to a sport by participants, testing may be conducted for ethanol. Positive results may lead to sanctions from, as always, the sport's governing body.

Marijuana

As for alcohol, testing for cannabinoids (marijuana and hashish) may be carried out in agreement with the International Sports Federations. The cannabinoids have an unpredictable detection window period ranging from 1 week for infrequent users to around 10 weeks for longer-term users. This is because the cannabinoids have an affinity for fatty tissue in the body. Here, they may or may not remain dormant or only slowly leach out, remaining detectable in the urine for long periods. Urinalysis detects the active ingredient of marijuana and hashish, THC (delta-9-tetrahydrocannabinol), or its metabolites. (Table 15.8.)

Caffeine

Is an ingredient in coffee, tea, chocolate, cola drinks, and many common medications. At the lower doses very common in society, the stimulant properties of caffeine are not generally considered to be significantly performance enhancing, although conflicting research data exist. Caffeine tolerance may explain some of the individual variability. At levels higher than 400mg, increased physical endurance and performance does occur. In recognition of potential abuse by athletes, the IOC has banned caffeine urine levels measured above 12 *micrograms* per liter. This level will be reached if around 400 milligrams of caffeine is ingested over a fairly short time period (30–60min). (Table 15.9.)

Beta-Blockers

Common examples: sotalol, atenolol, metoprolol, propanolol, oxprenolol, labetolol. These are IOC-banned substances because they decrease tremor and improve steadiness, giving possible benefit to archers, shooters, and biathletes. They are likely to impede performance in endurance sports which require prolonged periods of high cardiac output, so these sports are very unlikely to request testing. (Table 15.10.)

Corticosteroids

Common examples: prednisolone, hydrocortisone, dexamethasone. Corticosteroids have natural antiinflammatory properties and are used to treat asthma, pain and inflammation. They can influence the body's own production of corticosteroids when given systemically, producing some desirable non-specific systemic energizing effects. These include a feeling of well-being or euphoria which may translate into sporting improvement in a way similar to the stimulatory effect of amphetamines, but with more of a psychological component. (Table 15.11.)

In the past, corticosteroids were being taken in many sports by the oral, rectal, intramuscular, and intravenous routes, obviously in excess of their therapeutic value. The IOC thus invoked restrictions requiring a doctor's declaration of use, to try to keep use to genuine

Table 15.8 Detection of marijuana

Drug	Detection window	Detection limit
Marijuana (THC)	1–10 weeks	10ng/ml

Table 15.9 Estimated caffeine content of some common foods

Item	Caffeine content	Quantity required to exceed limit (12μg/L)
Coffee (instant)	50–100mg/cup	4–8 cups
Coffee (fresh)	80–200mg/cup*	2–5 cups
Brewed tea	40–80mg/cup	5–10 cups
Cola	30–50mg/can	8–12 cans
Cocoa/drinking chocolate	40–80mg/cup	5–10 cups
Chocolate	150mg/family block (240g)	2–4 family blocks

*Up to 350mg/cup in extremely strong brews.

Table 15.10 Olympic sports tested for beta-blockers

Summer	Winter
Archery	Biathlon
Diving	Bobsled
Equestrian	Figure skating
Fencing	Luge
Gymnastics	Ski jumping
Sailing	
Shooting (incl. modern pentathlon)	
Synchronized swimming	

Table 15.11 Effects of corticosteroids

Potential benefits	Potential side-effects
Mood elevation	Withdrawal effects (depression,
Generalized feeling of well-being	malaise, tiredness)
Enhanced energy levels	Long-term effects (skeletal muscle
Delayed tiredness	wasting, weakness)

therapeutic cases. Unfortunately, many athletes began abusing the use of inhaled corticosteroids during competition, so stronger restrictions became necessary. Corticosteroids are now banned except under the following conditions:

- topical use on skin, eye, or ear (rectal use is banned)
- inhalants are permitted (pulmicort, becotide, becloforte), but reporting is mandatory
- intraarticular or local injection only is permitted

> **Oral, intramuscular, and intravenous use of corticosteroids is banned. Any team doctor wishing to administer corticosteroids intraarticularly or locally to a competitor must give written notification to the IOC medical commission'.**

Non-steroidal antiinflammatory drugs (NSAIDs) are recommended by the IOC for treatment of sports-related injuries.

Local anesthetics

Injectable local anesthetics are banned except under the following conditions:

- that procaine, lignocaine, mepivacaine, etc. are used **but not cocaine**. Adrenaline and other vasoconstrictor agents are permitted in conjunction with local anesthetics
- intraarticular or local injection only is permitted
- medical justification must be submitted immediately in writing to the relevant medical authority. This includes details of the diagnosis, procedure and the site, dosage and route of administration

Doping methods

Blood doping

A higher level of red blood cells in the circulation increases the oxygen-carrying capacity of the blood and enhances an athlete's endurance. These methods are favored by cyclists, cross country skiers, orienteers, triathletes, and marathoners. Improvements in endurance capacity, VO_{2max}, and race times are undeniable but the exact relationship to the increased hemoglobin level is uncertain.

Blood doping entails reinfusion of 275–550ml of an athlete's own previously stored, or type-matched, packed red cells with saline 1–7 days before competition. Up to 12% increases in hemoglobin levels have been detected after reinfusion. Levels remain high for 4–6 weeks, tapering back to normal levels in 3–4 months. Some risks associated with non-medical transfusion include allergic skin rash, acute hemolytic reaction of mismatched donor blood, transmission of viral hepatitis, or AIDS. (Table 15.12.)

Masking agents (chemical manipulation)

Probenicid and related masking agents alter the integrity and validity of urine samples. They are IOC-banned since they are used by some athletes in conjunction with anabolic steroids to reduce urine steroid concentration.

Epitestosterone is sometimes administered along with drugs designed to increase the testosterone concentration. The testosterone: epitestosterone ratio must remain under 6:1 or suspicion of exogenous testosterone administration is aroused. To counter this practise, testing of the absolute levels of these two hormones are now performed.

Catheterization and urine substitution (physical manipulation)

Some athletes anticipating drug testing carry clean urine samples with them and attempt to somehow provide that as their sample. The athlete may use a catheter, providing the clean urine from a storage bladder inside. Samples may also be stored within clothing or inside the rectum or vagina (uncomfortable for competition). For this reason, the provision of samples is directly observed—the official (of the same sex) directly watches the urine pass from the competitor's urethra into the sample container.

Table 15.12 Effects of blood doping

Potential benefits	Potential side-effects
Improved oxygen-carrying capacity	Allergic reactions
Improved endurance	Acute hemolytic reaction
Faster race times	Kidney damage
	Viral hepatitis
	AIDS

Miscellaneous performance-enhancing techniques

Bicarbonate loading works by neutralizing lactic acid build-up in muscles. It is used by middle-distance runners, who take 300mg/kg common baking soda 30min before their event. Small decreases in running times have been noted. *Phosphate loading* works by elevating the level of 2,3-DPG, which shifts the oxygen dissociation curve to the right and allows increased oxygen unloading at the tissues. Benefits are unclear.

No testing is performed for these two doping methods.

Carnitine and other amino acids, proteins, vitamins, and minerals are variously used by athletes in attempts to improve performance. In general, athletes eating good balanced diets will not benefit, and megadoses of some vitamins (e.g. A, D, E and K) can sometimes be toxic. If specific deficiencies exist then improvements in performance could theoretically occur with use of appropriate supplements. In practise, it appears that diet-obtained vitamins and minerals allow the body to utilize them optimally, better than artificial intake regimes.

533

Drug testing methods and protocol

A positive drug test can wreck an athlete's career and life, so the evidence must be incontrovertible. To protect athletes against any possibility of false accusation, the IOC has strict rules governing sample handling, analysis, and confirmation of a positive result before it is reported to the authorities. Routinely, urine is the specimen sampled, meaning that the use of blood doping or erythropoietin cannot be detected. In certain competitions, provision can be made for sampling of blood from competitors for this purpose, but the invasive nature makes it a highly unpopular method of testing. Urine is preferred by laboratories as a 'cleaner' sample than blood, with better detection limits. Urine will continue to be sampled at the Olympic Games for the foreseeable future, but laboratories are equipped to detect all substances in blood plasma, including erythropoietin and blood doping, if required.

Who gets tested?

In Olympic competitions, all medal winners and a random number of other competitors are required to be tested. In World Championships, Grand Prix series events, national, minor and regional championships, and other competitions, competitors may be chosen for a drug test entirely randomly or based on some formula unknown to the competitors beforehand (e.g. 1st, 3rd, and 5th in every 3rd event). All the banned substances are tested for, as well as those restricted substances relevant to that particular sport.

Out-of-competition testing now operates in several countries, where athletes in training are randomly required to submit samples. Any élite athletes, including those not yet selected for representative competition, may be required to give urine samples within 24h of notification. Normally only anabolic-androgenic steroids, diuretics, and masking agents are tested for in these samples. Up to 50% of tests in some countries may be conducted in this way.

Random testing procedures depend on an athlete being present for testing either at home or at the competition or training venue. There have been cases of competitors quietly disappearing from a venue as soon as rumours are heard that drug testing is taking place, carefully avoiding any official-looking person. If an official cannot contact the athlete, no test can be performed, and no positive result recorded.

Sample collection protocol[1,2]

Very strict regulations govern the collection, transport and handling of samples. After being informed that he/she is required to provide a urine sample for the purpose of drug testing, an athlete is bound to provide that sample. Failure to co-operate in the drug test will be considered a positive result. If extremely good reasons for not complying with the test are provided promptly in writing, an athlete may be excused. Normally, however, the sport's governing body will impose sanctions similar to that for a positive test. An athlete can postpone the drug test for a few reasons including: media commitments, victory ceremony, competing in further events, completing a training session, warm-down, medical attention, or to find a representative to accompany him/her at the drug control facility. The

1 L Badewitz-Dodd (ed.) 1992 *Drugs and sport*. IMS, Sydney 2 Australian Sports Drug Agency (ASDA) internet site: http://www.ausport.gov.au/ asdamain.html

534

athlete does, however, eventually have to provide an 80ml sample of urine. Waiting is often necessary, especially in relatively dehydrated athletes. To hasten the process, drinks from sealed containers can be consumed. Drinks containing caffeine are not recommended. If less than 80mls is produced, the athlete must wait until a further sample can be provided. Then, the two samples are mixed together. Athletes are under constant chaperone observation while providing their urine sample(s) (see Fig. 15.1).

Before being accepted, the specific gravity of the urine is checked to ensure the sample is suitable for all the laboratory tests. If not, a further sample must be provided. The urine sample is divided into two (the A and B samples) which are both sealed, and then labelled with a code to preserve the athlete's anonymity at the laboratory. The samples are then transported, under secure conditions, to the laboratory.

Laboratory accreditation

The B sample is stored at the laboratory and used only if a positive test requires confirmation. Where this is required, testing would be carried out by a different chemist and within a set time limit, usually in the presence of the athlete and/or a representative of the sport's governing authority. All positive tests are checked first using a different analytical technique before being declared positive.

Because a positive test has to be confirmed and may well be subject to legal challenge, there must be no doubt about both the test results and the identification of the sample. Accredited laboratories are continually monitored to ensure that for each test carried out, there is a documented record of the analytical parameters and conditions as well as the results, and a foolproof sample-tracking procedure so there can be no doubt as to the accurate identification of the sample. Daily evidence of faultless machine operation must also be available in the event of a legal challenge to any results.

Analytical techniques

The majority of tests are qualitative rather than quantitative. Any use of banned drugs, in any quantities, contravenes the rules, so detection of any trace of such compounds or their metabolites will give a positive result. For most of the restricted substances, where a positive test result is registered only if a certain physiological cut-off level is exceeded, quantitation is required. Examples include testosterone, caffeine, and certain other substances where the abuse, rather than the use, is prohibited.

Drug testing laboratories (use gas chromatography combined with mass spectrometry (GC/MS) as the 'gold standard' analytical technique. Most operating procedures use capillary gas chromatography with a mass selective detector (MSD) to detect the presence or otherwise of anabolic steroids, stimulants, diuretics, analgesics, narcotics, and beta-blockers. Another procedure uses GC/MS for quantification of such substances as testosterone, caffeine and ephedrine. The epitestosterone:testosterone ratio can be determined automatically using these techniques.

The corticoids are detected using high performance liquid chromatography (HPLC) in conjunction with a mass spectrometer and particle beam interface. HPLC is also used as part of the testing procedure for diuretics. Immunological assays are also used in screening for some banned substances. With the advent of high resolution mass spectrometry (HRMS), detection possibilities have been enhanced even further and will continue to do so as research analysts refine their art. Still, there is pressure to achieve ever-smaller detection limits for the established drugs. Of course, athletes will continue to abuse newer synthetic drugs and doping methods. The IOC banned list is regularly supplemented, and the analysts in turn must develop methods to detect not only the compounds themselves, but also their metabolites, which may provide the only evidence of abuse. (Table 15.13 shows the relative frequencies of detected substances.)

Laboratory accreditation

Stringent initial accreditation of IOC-approved laboratories ensures that they are of the highest standard, and always capable of carrying out IOC-approved drug testing. Throughout these initial tests, a representative of the IOC Medical Commission ensures not only the correctness of the results, but also that the procedures for carrying out tests on the complete range of banned substances were flawless.

To ensure that the quality of the lab's work continues to meet the IOC's requirements, re-accreditation process takes place annually. Proficiency tests occur every 4 months and random checks in between involve control samples sent to the lab as part of the normal routine workload. The IOC demands 100% accuracy in these annual re-accreditation tests. A single false positive result is sufficient for the lab to lose its accredited status, while a false negative will mean suspension of accreditation until the reasons for the mistaken result have been clarified and rectified.

The IOC's rules for accreditation now insist that laboratories take precautions against sports doctors or athletes aiming to discover, by trial and error, the minimum drug levels that the accredited lab is able to detect. Laboratories now, for example, undertake not to carry out testing for medical doctors working with athletes.

There are currently 24 laboratories in the world fully accredited by the IOC for dope testing, mostly in Europe and North America (one in Australia).

Table 15.13 Relative frequencies of detected substances

Substance	1986 tests [a] (18 labs)	1991 tests [b] (21 labs)
Stimulants	177 (26.3%)	221 (23.9%)
Narcotics	23 (3.4%)	72 (7.8%)
Anabolic steroids	439 (65.3%)	552 (59.6%)
Beta blockers	31 (4.6%)	10 (1.1%)
Diuretics	2 (0.3%)	47 (5.1%)
Masking agents	1 (0.1%)	1 (0.1%)
Peptide hormones		1 (0.1%)
Ethanol		7 (0.8%)
THC (cannabis metabolite)		14 (1.5%)
Phenobarbital		1 (0.1%)
Total number of samples with at least 1 substance detected	623 (1.9% of all samples)	805 (0.96% of all samples)

[a] Based on a 1986 sample of 32,982 urine analyses from 18 IOC-accredited laboratories[5]. [b] Based on a 1991 sample of 84,283 urine analyses from 21 IOC-accredited laboratories.[7]

Treatment considerations

Recognizing the athlete using drugs

A potential drug abuser may be very difficult to identify, but a physician having a good rapport with the athlete, together with the knowledgeable coach, may detect subtle but suggestive changes. An athlete displaying formerly uncharacteristic aggression, trouble with relationships and authority, lateness for training, lying, or a heavy reliance on medications for small injuries, should arouse suspicion of drug abuse. Similarly, changes in physical appearance, concentration, training capability, or indeed performance are also suspicious.

Ethical considerations

A physician treating an athlete known to be abusing performance-enhancing drugs has to be aware of the potential implications for the health of his/her patient and of a positive test for the athlete, his/her team, and future. Understandable personal concerns for the physician may include issues regarding legality of the drug, negligence, potential personal malpractice claims, duty to practice management, and patient confidentiality. For the team physician, there are naturally responsibilities to the entire team which may require breach of doctor–patient confidentiality, especially where the consequences of a positive drug test could mean disqualification of the athlete, future bans on his/her team, and shame to the team and perhaps the entire nation.

Declarations of usage to sports governing bodies

Written notice must be given to the relevant sporting bodies if a physician prescribes to an athlete medications from the banned or restricted categories that the IOC has determined to be permitted for legitimate medical reasons. Asthmatics, for example may use the β-2 agonists, salbutamol and terbutaline, by inhalation only. The relevant sporting authority should be able to advise whether continued treatments also require further notification. Where possible, the IOC has minimized the need for these notifications by allowing certain drugs from these categories as treatment for common medical conditions in which other drugs are less effective. For example, codeine is now permitted as an analgesic, adrenaline is permitted when administered with local anesthetic agents, and imidazole preparations are permitted for topical use.

Non-steroidal antiinflammatory drugs (NSAIDs)

Common examples: indomethacin, phenylbutazone, ibuprofen, diclofenac, piroxicam. This class of drug is not banned by the IOC and is, in fact, recommended treatment for athletes with soft-tissue injuries. NSAIDs have antiinflammatory, analgesic and antipyretic properties. They are capable of relieving pain and stiffness, reducing swelling and hastening recovery of function of inflamed joints. When used as an adjunct to the RICE policy (rest, ice, compression, elevation) for treatment, NSAIDs may allow earlier return to competition because of the reduced swelling and pain relief afforded. NSAIDs are also commonly used to relieve menstrual cramp pain. (Table 15.14.)

Interestingly, with the use of NSAIDs, performance can be improved because movement is less impeded by pain and swelling.[1] In a sense, they can be thought of as being ergogenic, but nevertheless have the blessing of the IOC. Since serious side-effects are unusual, NSAIDs are considered valuable drugs for the injured athlete.

1 GI Wadler, B Hainline 1989 *Drugs and the athlete* p162–4. FA Davis, Philadelphia

Table 15.14 Effects of NSAIDs

Potential benefits	Potential side-effects
Analgesia	Gastric irritability
Antiinflammatory effects	Gastrointestinal bleeding
Antipyretic effects	Bleeding in injured joint
Hastened injury recovery	Rash
Menstrual cramp relief	Tinnitus
	Bronchospasm
	Edema
	Hypertension
	Congestive heart failure
	Blood dyscrasias (meclofenamate)

Suggested treatments for selected medical conditions

Table 15.15 Permitted treatments for selected medical conditions

Medical condition	Suggested permitted medications
Asthma	Sodium cromoglycate (high dose, e.g. 6 × 5mg dose puffs), nedocrimil sodium, salmeterol, bitolterol, orciprenaline, rimiterol, salbutamol, terbutaline (all aerosol or inhalant form only)
Soft tissue injuries	NSAIDs (rapid action versions in acute cases, e.g. diclofenac potassium, naproxen sodium), keto-profen, sulindac
Cough	Nedocromil sodium, sodium cromoglycate
Vomiting	Fluids, metoclopromide
Hayfever	Livostin topical & spray for acute attacks, loratadine, astemizole, terfenadine as preventers
Diarrhea	Loperamide
Headache	Paracetamol, fluids

Note: medical assessment should in all cases include differential diagnoses for the athlete's complaint and exclude more sinister pathology).

Gender verification

Determination of gender has been an intriguing aspect of international sport this century. It has had a turbulent and secretive history, with its place in sports testing seemingly permanently insecure. Rumour abounded in the 1960s, especially at the Rome Olympics, that males were possibly masquerading as females. Any female competitor with masculine bodily attributes was regarded with suspicion. These suspicions were not entirely unfounded. At least six cases of individuals with testes, successfully competing in international events as females from 1932 to 1966, have been well documented.[1]

One example concerned the winner of the women's world downhill ski title in 1966. A medical examination in 1967 revealed undescended testes, which were then surgically corrected. The skier married and became a father.

Nude parades

Early attempts to quell the suspicion included gender verification by nude parade in front of gynecologists. This method apparently worked to exclude five world record holders who declined to compete at the 1966 Budapest European Athletics Championships for no apparent reason, presumably because they felt they would fail the inspection. The 'femininity' control in the 1966 Kingston Commonwealth Games took the form of a manual examination of the external genitalia by a gynecologist. The indignation felt among the athletes to these insensitive early measures have created enduring resistance to any form of clinical examination for the purpose of gender verification.

The sex chromatin test

Involves sampling oral epithelial cells (a buccal smear) and examining stained cells for the presence or absence of the Barr body. This genetically inactive X-chromosome becomes condensed and recognizable in female cells. Male cells have only active X-chromosomes and do not normally show up Barr bodies. Although the test itself is non-invasive and reasonably reliable, there have been continuing problems with interpretation of results. It does distinguish XY males from XX females and would detect a male masquerading as a female. The problems arise in certain cases of genetic, metabolic, and endocrine disorders. For example, women with sex chromosomal abnormalities such as Turner's syndrome (a 45, XO karyotype) would fail the chromatin test. A metabolic defect is the cause of congenital adrenal hyperplasia, which involves overproduction of adrenal androgens. Females may have increased muscle mass, hirsutism, and even a well-developed penis. Males with the condition may benefit from increased androgens. Both, however, would pass the chromatin test. Women with androgen insensitivity syndrome (XY females) have male karyotype but since their androgen receptors fail to respond to androgens, they remain with largely female sexual characteristics. Milder forms of impaired androgen sensitivity further complicate the issue. The IOC has determined that these females are entitled to compete, but must submit to further chromosome testing, hormone tests, and gynecological examination. It is here that many retire early or are unjustly disqualified because they are too distressed, embarrassed,

1 MA Ferguson-Smith MA 1994 In M Harries *et al* (eds) *Oxford textbook of sports medicine* p329–37. OUP

and misunderstood to proceed. In many cases, failure in the sex chromatin test is a personal shock and highly distressing. It is felt by many that a person's anatomical sex, even if disagreeing with the sex chromatin test, better determines gender. Perhaps more importantly, it more regularly succeeds in determining the appropriate athletic potential of the person.

The 1968 Grenoble Winter Olympic Games apparently successfully utilized the sex chromatin test on randomly chosen female athletes. No official figures are given for results from Grenoble or from the 1000 or so tests performed at the 1968 Mexico Olympics, or subsequent events. The IOC maintains strict secrecy on gender verification findings, presumably to avoid the rumor which was rife in the early 1960s. In this respect, the IOC claimed femininity control by sex chromatin testing had worked, quelling rumor and deterring males from cheating by trying to compete as females, all with a non-invasive and non-degrading test. It remained a fact, however, that many mistakes and personal tragedies have resulted from failure in the sex chromatin test.

Alternative approaches

A 1990 convention of the International Athletic Foundation (IAF) recommended a 'health check' for all participants, male and female, in international competition. Apart from a general brief medical examination to ensure fitness to compete, the check involved a simple inspection of the external genitalia. A 'health and gender' certificate issued then was required for entry in events.

The convention also finally determined rules for eligibility in women's events. Individuals with any form of masculinization due to any non-drug cause should not be barred from competing in womens events. In particular, this includes 21-hydroxylase deficiency, 5α-reductase deficiency, androgen insensitivity, and all forms of sex chromosome mosaicism, provided that the individual has been reared as a female.

Unfortunately, some athletes felt this health check was a return to the bad old days of genital examinations by nude parades, and the procedures were still not universally accepted. The IOC approved the idea of the health check for National Olympic Committees, but remained convinced that a chromosomal sex test was still required at the Olympic Games. Other sporting bodies believe chromosome testing unnecessarily subjects many women to emotional and social injury and have abandoned them in favor of anatomical observation. The IAF agreed in May 1992 that the arrangements already in place for doping control, which includes direct observation of the provision of a urine sample, obviated the need for separate femininity certification. They resolved that there was no longer a need for gender verification to exclude males masquerading as females.

The IOC, however, remains unconvinced and established a new polymerase chain reaction amplification of the SRY (sex determining region of the Y-chromosome) test at the Albertville 1992 Winter Olympics. All female competitors were tested there (via a buccal smear sample), and it seems this will remain the IOC-favored method for gender verification.

The Olympics and drug tests

In the 1950s, drug abuse became evident among European competition cyclists. In the first ever dope testing program at a 1955 French cycle race, over 20% of the competitors tested positive. In the succeeding decade, a number of athletes died as a result of drug abuse. To combat the perceived rise in Olympic athletes abusing drugs, the IOC developed the first plans to implement formal drug testing in major competition, and other sporting bodies quickly followed. Olympic drug testing began at the 1968 Grenoble Winter Olympics, where no positive tests were returned. This followed an IOC Medical Commission publication in 1967 of a small list of proscribed substances. Since then, the list has grown to include over 150 banned substances, including the introduction of anabolic steroid testing at the 1976 Montreal Summer Games.[1] Testing for all these substances is now achieved on typically around 2000 athletes at the summer games and 600 at the winter games. (Table 15.16.)

Most international sports authorities followed the IOC in establishing drug testing in their sports. Consequently, most major sporting events around the world now operate significant drug screening programs. The Royal Australasian College of Physicians have put out a position paper on the subject.[3]

1 DA Cowan 1994 In M Harries, *et al* (ed) *Oxford textbook of sports medicine* p314–29. OUP 2 International Olympic Commitee Medical Commission internet site: http://www.olympic.org/medical/efdop.html 3 MC Kennedy *et al* 1997 Drugs in sport. A position paper. *Fellowship Affairs* July

Table 15.16 Olympic drug testing[2]

Olympics	Year	Athletes tested	Positive results
Grenoble	1968 winter	86	0
Mexico City	1968 summer	667	1
Sapporo	1972 winter	211	1
Munich	1972 summer	2079	7
Innsbruck	1976 winter	390	2
Montreal	1976 summer	786	11
Lake Placid, NY	1980 winter	440	0
Moscow	1980 summer	645	0
Sarajevo	1984 winter	424	1
Los Angeles	1984 summer	1507	12
Calgary	1988 winter	492	1
Seoul	1988 summer	1598	10
Albertville	1992 winter	522	0
Barcelona	1992 summer	1848	5
Lillehammer	1994 winter	529	0

Appendix: Expanded list of banned substances

Caution this is not an exhaustive list of banned substances. It is provided only to give the reader a more comprehensive list of banned substances. Many substances that do not appear on this expanded list are considered banned under the term 'and related substances'.

Stimulants

Amfepramone
Amineptine
Amfetamine
Caffeine
Cathine
Cocaine
Cropropamide
Crotetamide
Ephedrine
Etamivan
Etilamfetamine
Etilefrine
Fencamfamin
Fenetylline
Fenfluramine
Heptaminol
Mefenorex
Mephentermine
Mesocarb

Metamfetamine
Methoxyphenamine
Methylendioxyamfetamine
Methylephedrine
Methylphenidate
Nikethamide
Norphenfluramine
Parahydroxyamfetamine
Pemoline
Phendimetrazine
Phentermine
Phenylpropanolamine
Pholedrine
Prolintane
Propylhexedrine
Pseudoephedrine
Salbutamol
Strychnine

Narcotics

Buprenorphine
Dextropropoxyphene
Diamorphine (heroin)
Ethylmorphine
Hydrocodone
Hydromorphone
Levorphanol

Methadone
Morphine
Pentazocine
Oxycodone
Pethidine
Propoxyphene
Triameperidine

Anabolic agents (including anabolic-androgenic steroids and β-2 agonists)

Bolasterone
Boldenone
Clenbuterol
Clostebol
Danazol
Dehydrochlormethyltestosterone
Dihydrotestosterone
Drostanolone
Fluoxymesterone
Formebolone stanozolol
Mesterolone testosterone

Metandienone trenbolone
Metenolone
Methandriol
Methyltestosterone
Mibolerone
Nandrolone
Norethandrolone
Oxandrolone
Oxymesterone
Oxymetholone

Beta blockers

Acebutolol
Alprenolol
Atenolol
Betaxolol

Metoprolol
Nadolol
Oxprenolol
Pindolol

Bisoprolol
Bunolol
Labetalol

Propranolol
Sotalol
Timolol

Diuretics
Acetazolamide
Amiloride
Bendroflurmethiazide
Benzthiazide
Bumetanide
Canrenone
Chlormerodrine
Chlorthalidone

Diclofenamide
Ethacrynic acid
Furosemide
Hhydrochlorothiazide
Hindapamide
Hmersalyl
Spironolactone
Triamterene

Masking agents
Epitestosterone

Probenecid

Peptide hormones
hCG
Erythropoietin

HhGH
HACTH

16 Nutrition

LOUISE BURKE

Introduction[1–5]

Why is sports nutrition important and who is it important for? It is easy to understand the search for a competitive edge in the élite world of sport. In many events, the margin between winning and losing is measured in millimeters and hundredths of seconds, and the stakes include international fame and considerable amounts of money. A number of prominent sports scientists have suggested that at this level, where genetics, training, equipment, and motivation are all equalized, nutrition might provide the vital ingredient in success.

However, it is clear that recreational athletes are also interested in sports nutrition, as shown by the recent boom in the market for specialized sports drinks and sports bars. Although some people consider that special sports nutrition strategies are relevant only to the élite athlete (or that these specialized sports foods are a waste of money for the non-elite sportsperson), it is important to realize that the fundamentals of exercise physiology apply to sporting activities, regardless of the talent of the athlete involved. For example, sweat losses and carbohydrate needs are created by muscular activity, whether it be undertaken by Michael Jordan or Joe Public. While for recreational athletes, the rewards of sports nutrition strategies are likely to be the satisfaction of improving 'personal bests' or achieving personal goals, the spin-off of better safety and enjoyment of exercise activities may be an important factor in encouraging population participation in exercise. Finally, since many of the principles of sports nutrition concur with population dietary guidelines, the interest in sports nutrition may independently help to improve the general health and nutritional status of the population.

Sports nutrition is underpinned by the sciences of exercise physiology and biochemistry, and aims to supply the body with the nutrients needed to adapt to a training program, to perform optimally during competition, and to recover quickly after exercise. However, sports nutrition also involves the art of translating nutrient needs into foods and eating practices that are compatible with the busy schedule and commitments of an athlete's lifestyle. This chapter will summarize the current guidelines for achieving both the science and practice of 'eating to win'.

1 KD Brownell *et al* (ed) 1992 *Eating, body weight and performance in athletes: disorders of modern society.* Lea & Febiger, Philadelphia **2** LM Burke, V Deakin (ed) 1994 *Clinical sports nutrition.* McGraw-Hill, Sydney **3** LM Burke 1995 *The complete guide to food for sports performance* 2nd edn Allen & Unwin, Sydney **4** C Williams, JT Devlin (ed) 1992 *Foods, nutrition and sports performance.* E & FN Spon, London **5** I Wolinsky, JF Hickson (ed) 1992 *Nutrition in exercise and sport* 2nd edn CRC, Boca Raton

Goals of training nutrition

The purpose of training is to prepare the athlete to perform at his/her best during key competitions, and in most situations the time and demands of this preparation far outweigh those of competition. Therefore, it is the everyday or training diet of the athlete that has the greatest impact on sports performance. The athlete shares the population nutritional goals of meeting nutrient requirements for immediate health, as well as adopting dietary strategies to reduce the risk of developing Western disease patterns in later life. Additionally, he/she should be able to participate in the enjoyment and social interaction that is provided by food. However, the athlete must also meet special goals of sports nutrition during the training phase including:

- to achieve a body size and composition that is ideal for performance in the athlete's sport
- to meet additional demands for energy and nutrients that arise from the training program
- to undertake dietary strategies that optimize performance during training sessions and enhance recovery after the session
- to practice any competition nutrition strategies in advance so that these can be fine-tuned for success.

The importance and the details of these goals will vary from sport to sport.

What is 'ideal' body shape and composition?

The size, shape, and composition of the body are important determinants of performance in many sports. In some sports, weight divisions or limits are set to encourage fair competition between opponents of equal size and strength. These sports include weight lifting, boxing, judo, light weight rowing, and horse racing. In other sports, a low weight and/or low bodyweight level is a factor in successful performance. This may be to increase the athlete's 'power to weight' ratio, or to reduce 'dead weight' that must be transported over long distances (e.g. in distance running, road cycling, or triathlons) or moved against gravity (e.g. jumping events, hill cycling). In some sports, the esthetic appeal of a lean body provides favorable characteristics for judging (e.g. in body building, gymnastics, figure skating), although this is usually combined with the biomechanical advantages of being small and light (e.g. in gymnastics).

In many situations, the athlete achieves a suitable body size and shape for their sport as a result of the combination of the genetics which have 'selected' them to excel in that sport in the first place, and their training program. However, in other situations the athlete may desire to alter their physique—typically to lose body fat or to gain muscle mass.

Reducing weight and body fat

Sometimes, the need to lose body fat is desirable and achievable. Some athletes become overfat due to poor dietary intake (e.g. as a result of poor nutrition knowledge or erratic eating patterns because of travel) or due to a period of a low energy expenditure (e.g. during the off-season, or while injured). These athletes can be assisted by changes to nutrition, training and lifestyle to regain their 'optimal' body fat level. In general, body fat losses are achieved by a sustained program of moderate energy restriction and appropriate training/increased energy expenditure.

However, there is much concern about athletes who seek to achieve bodyweight and fat goals that are extreme and unnatural. There is considerable pressure on athletes in many sports to achieve very low body fat levels in the belief that 'less is better', or to achieve body fat and weight standards that are arbitrarily set by coaches or other authorities. These practices do not allow for individual variability in physique, nor do they encourage safe and healthy methods to achieve loss of weight and body fat. This situation is particularly true for female endurance athletes, whose desired body fat levels often seem below the 'natural' level for the individual, despite their heavy training program. The problem is compounded in the case of females in 'esthetic' sports (e.g. gymnasts and figure skaters), where training is skill-based and energy balance must be changed primarily through energy restriction. Problems also occur in weight division sports where the tradition is to compete in a weight class which is considerably below 'normal' training weight, and to 'make weight' by 'dieting' to reduce body fat levels, superimposed by acute dehydration during the day(s) prior to the event. Performance in 'weight making' sports is likely to be impaired owing to the effects of fuel depletion and dehydration. However, in the wider view there appears to be an increased risk of disordered eating and eating disorders among athletes in sports in which low body fat levels are emphasized.

It is a challenge of sports nutrition to assist athletes to set and achieve bodyweight and body fat goals that are truly 'ideal'. This should include the notion of individuality, allowing the goals to be set according to the athlete's history and realistic potential. Studies of élite sports show that, although there is a 'typical' physique that seems favorable for performance, there is considerable variation in the physique of well-performing athletes. Athletes should be aware of the disadvantages of fad diets and of extreme fat/weight loss techniques. They should also recognize that there may be penalties for achieving very low body fat levels. These include hormonal, physiological, and psychological disturbances and may result from the low body fat level itself, as well as from the methods involved in achieving it (i.e. restricted eating, overtraining, stress). An 'ideal' weight and body fat level for any athlete should guarantee consistently good performances over a long-term period, promote good health, and allow the athlete to consume a diet of sufficient energy and nutrients that allows all goals of training to be achieved. The need for individualized and expert advice on management of bodyweight and fat is the most common reason for an athlete to seek the services of a sports dietitian.

Increasing muscle mass

The other physique change desired by athletes is an increase in muscle size and strength. This is principally achieved by a suitable resistance training program and genetic potential; however, an adequate energy intake and usually, a positive energy balance is required. Although the protein needs for optimal muscle gain remain an emotive area for many athletes (and scientists), the primary dietary requirement for gain in muscle mass is energy. For some athletes, dietary counseling is required to provide strategies for increasing energy intake in an already high energy diet or in a busy timetable.

Energy requirements

Vary markedly and are influenced by the size of the athlete, the need to lose or gain weight, growth, and the training load (frequency, duration, and intensity). Dietary surveys of athletes find that male athletes generally report energy intakes varying from **10 to 25 MJ/day (2500–6000 cal/day)** over prolonged periods.

However, while the energy requirements of female athletes might reasonably be 20–30% lower than their male counterparts, principally to take smaller size into account, some surveys of female athletes often report an 'energy imbalance' whereby reported intakes of 4–8 MJ/day (1000–2000cal/day) are lower than expected and sometimes do not seem to cover the costs of the training program itself. There appears to be no physiological explanation for this. Rather, systematic under-reporting of food intake or 'restricted' eating during the period of the food diary due to concerns about body fat levels are suspected.

Protein needs

Are increased by training. This results from the small contribution of protein oxidation to the fuel requirements of exercise as well as the protein needed to support muscle gain and repair of damaged body tissues. While athletes undertaking recreational or light training activities will meet their protein needs within population protein recommended dietary intakes (RDIs), a guideline for increased protein intake for heavily training athletes, both endurance and strength training, has been set at **1.2–1.6g/kgBM(body mass)/day**. These targets are easily met within the increased energy requirement enjoyed by athletes who undertake such training. Indeed, most dietary surveys show that athletes who eat a typical mixed diet report protein intakes within or above these goals. Despite this evidence, many body builders and weight lifters eat unnecessarily large amounts of protein-rich foods or buy expensive protein supplements.

Vitamins and minerals

A moderate to high energy intake and a varied diet based on nutritious foods are the key factors that ensure an adequate intake of protein and micronutrients. Dietary surveys of athletes show that when these factors are in place, the reported intakes of vitamins and minerals are well in excess of RDIs and likely to meet any increases in micronutrient demand imposed by exercise. Thus, the generalized need for micronutrient supplementation is not justified. Furthermore, studies do not support an increase in performance with such supplementation except in the case where a pre-existing deficiency was corrected. However, not all athletes eat varied diets of adequate energy intake. It has already been discussed that some athletes are 'restricted eaters', who eat low energy intakes for prolonged or intermittent periods in an attempt to control body fat and weight levels. Restriction of dietary variety is also found among, but not limited to such athletes. While fad diets and disordered eating are typical causes of reduced food range, other underlying problems include poor practical nutrition skills, inadequate finances, and the limited access to food, and erratic meal schedules that may be typical of an overcommitted lifestyle. Nutrition education to increase dietary quality and quantity is the preferred management route. However, low dose, broad range multivitamin/mineral supplementation may be of benefit where dietary restrictions are resistant to change, or where the athlete is traveling to places with an uncertain food supply and eating schedule.

Iron

Is involved in sports performance through its role in oxygen transport in the blood (hemoglobin) and muscles (myoglobin), as well as its action as a cofactor for many of the enzymes involved in fuel oxidation. A low iron status can reduce performance, although it is still uncertain how to distinguish true iron deficiency from some of the alterations in iron status measures that are caused by exercise. For example, endurance training causes a drop in hemoglobin levels due to an increase in blood volume. This hemodilution, often termed 'sports anemia', does not impair exercise performance, but has probably caused an overdiagnosis of the true prevalence of iron deficiency in athletes.

Nevertheless, some athletes are at true risk of becoming iron deficient when increased iron needs (e.g. due to growth, or small but consistent iron losses from gastrointestinal bleeding, or 'foot-strike' damage to red blood cells) are compounded by a poor intake of bioavailable iron. Low iron consumers include 'restricted' eaters, vegetarians, and other athletes eating high carbohydrate (CHO), low meat diets. The heme form of iron found in red meat, liver products, and shellfish is much better absorbed than non-heme iron found in plant foods such as wholegrain cereal foods, legumes, and green leafy vegetables. Low iron status, such as that indicated by serum ferritin levels lower than 20ng/ml, should be considered for treatment. Present evidence does not support that iron deficiency without anemia reduces exercise performance. However, many athletes with such low iron status, or a sudden drop in iron status, frequently complain of fatigue and inability to recover after heavy training. Many of these athletes respond following an improved iron status. At the very least, treatment may prevent the situation from progressing to clinical anemia.

Evaluation and management of iron status is best done on an individual basis by a sports medicine expert. Prevention and treatment of iron deficiency may include iron supplementation. However this should be considered as a part of the management plan along with dietary counseling to increase the intake of bioavailable iron, and appropriate strategies to reduce iron loss. Mass supplementation of athletes with iron, or self-diagnosis of low iron deficiency, are to be avoided since they exclude the opportunity for a more holistic plan. Dietary guidelines for increasing iron intake should be integrated with the other nutritional goals of the athlete, so that goals of high CHO intakes or reduced energy intake to reduce body fat can be met simultaneously. This is where the expertise of a sports dietitian is most useful.

567

Calcium

Since exercise is considered to be one of the best protectors of bone density, the recent discovery of low bone density in some female athletes seems contradictory. It appears that some female athletes are either losing bone density, or failing to optimize the gaining of peak bone mass that should occur during the 10–15 years after the onset of puberty. One confounding factor appears to be menstrual disturbances found in greater prevalence among some groups of female athletes, particularly those undertaking sports in which there is an emphasis on low body fat levels. Although the situation is complicated and multifactorial, it is likely that reduced estrogen levels and other hormonal abnormalities associated with menstrual disturbances are involved. 'The female triad' has been used to describe the concurrence of stress fractures/low bone density, menstrual dysfunction, and disordered eating among some female athletes. While this highlights attention to the serious problems involved, it also tends to simplify complex issues an independent problems into a single syndrome. Clearly, each of these problems, whether they appear together or independently, requires expert diagnosis and management. Often a team, including a sports physician, dietitian, psychologist, coach, and parents may be involved.

Optimal nutrition is important to correct factors that underpin the menstrual disturbances, as well as those that contribute to suboptimal bone density. Adequate energy intake and reversal of disordered eating or inadequate nutrient intake may be important. Calcium requirements must be met, and may include an increased goal of 1200mg/day in those athletes with impaired menstrual function. Strategies to meet calcium needs must be integrated into the total nutrition goals of the athlete. Where adequate calcium intake cannot be met through dietary means, usually through use of low fat dairy foods, a calcium supplement may be considered.

Supplements

It is considered that more than one in every two athletes is a consumer of the supplements that fill health food outlets, sports magazines, and specialized sports shops. Such supplements can be divided into two categories: sports supplements and nutritional ergogenic aids. Sports supplements have been described as products that allow an athlete to achieve known nutritional goals, and in addition to micronutrient supplements that are part of a prescribed dietary plan, this category includes products such as sports drinks, sports bars, and liquid meal supplements. These latter products have been specially manufactured to help an athlete meet known specific needs for fluid and CHO, or generalized energy and nutrients, in situations where normal foods are not practical. This is particularly relevant to intake immediately before, during, or after exercise.

These supplements can be shown to improve performance directly or indirectly by allowing the athlete to achieve his/her sports nutrition goals. However, since it is the use of the product rather than the product itself achieves this effect, there is an important role for nutrition education of the athlete. The cost of these products is greater than that of normal food and must be balanced against the convenience that they provide.

Meanwhile it is nutritional ergogenic aids, products that promote a direct and 'supercharge' benefit to sports performance, which best capture the imagination of many athletes. These products continually change in fashion, and include micronutrients in megadoses, free-form amino acids, ginseng, bee pollen, inosine, and carnitine. In general, these supplements have been poorly tested, or have failed to live up to their claims when rigorous testing has been undertaken. Exceptions to this are creatine, caffeine, and bicarbonate, each of which may enhance sports performance in certain athletes under specific conditions. However, the athlete should seek expert advice about these supplements to ensure that such conditions apply to their own situation, and that these ergogenic aids are used correctly. Meanwhile, the remainder of these products are considered to offer only a placebo effect to athletes, which should be balanced against their considerable expense. In many cases the athlete would be better rewarded by directing their money and endeavor to a more credible area of sports performance, such as better equipment, improved training techniques, or advice about nutrition or psychological preparation.

Optimizing training and recovery

An important dietary energy need is for adequate CHO to meet the fuel requirements of the training program. The energy requirements for exercise are met largely by oxidation of fat and CHO. Whereas body fat stores are adequate to supply the energy cost of exercise for may days, CHO stores are vulnerable. With prolonged training each day the body may turn over in excess of its total body CHO stores. Furthermore, there is an obligatory need for CHO oxidation when the intensity of exercise is high (e.g. >70% VO_{2max}). Therefore, daily replacement and supplementation of CHO intake may be needed to provide the fuel needs for a strenuous training program, particularly to maintain the intensity of training sessions. Inadequate CHO intake will gradually lead to a depletion of muscle glycogen stores and may reduce the ability of the athlete to complete their desired training load.

The guidelines for healthy eating in most countries recommended an increase in CHO intake, particularly from nutrient-dense CHO-rich foods, such as cereal and grain foods, fruit, starchy vegetables, and legumes. It is generally recommended that CHO intake should provide at least 50–55% of total energy intake. Although the exact CHO needs of athletes vary according to their muscle mass and training load, this general guideline is likely to meet the fuel requirements of most athletes.

For some athletes, it is important to maximize daily glycogen storage. This may be to support the fuel needs of a prolonged and high intensity training program, or to 'fuel-up' in anticipation of a prolonged competition bout. In such a case, an intake of approximately **7–10g of CHO/BM/24h** is needed. This may represent 50–70% of total energy intake of the athlete, and requires both planning and good knowledge of nutrition to achieve. Practical challenges which limit the intake of CHO include the bulkiness of many high fibre CHO-rich foods, and the reduced opportunities for eating in a busy day. A pattern of 'grazing' (frequent meals and snacks), together with reliance on portable and compact CHO-rich choices is recommended (see Table 16.1). Eating a CHO-rich snack or meal providing at least *1g* **CHO/kgBM** straight after a training session is considered good practice for enhanced recovery. It appears that the depleted muscle is most responsive to CHO supplied immediately after exercise. More importantly, it allows the athlete to optimize the refueling time before the next training session; a factor which may be important for athletes who undertake more than one training sessions each day.

Fluid needs are also an important consideration in the performance of, and recovery after, training sessions. This issue will be discussed in detail in the competition nutrition session and is summarized in Table 16.2.

Table 16.1 Strategies for high levels of carbohydrate intake

1 The athletes should be prepared to be different—a Western diet is not a high CHO diet. CHO foods and drinks should make up at least half of all meals and snacks:

2 Nutritious CHO foods should be the focus of meals and snacks,
   • wholegrain breads and breakfast cereals
   • rice, pasta, noodles, and other grain foods
   • fruits
   • starchy vegetables (e.g. potatoes, corn)
   • legumes (lentils, beans, soy-based products)
   • sweetened dairy products (e.g. fruit-flavored yogurt, fruit smoothies)

3 Many foods commonly believed by athletes to be CHO-rich are actually high fat foods (e.g. cakes, takeaway foods, chocolates, and pastries). The athlete should be aware of low fat eating strategies.

4 Sugar and sugar-rich foods are useful for the athlete, especially when added to a nutritious CHO food meal, or when needed during and after exercise. Not only do they taste appealing, but they provide a more compact form of CHO.

5 When CHO and energy needs are high, the athlete should increase the number of meals and snacks that they eat, rather than the size of meals. This requires organization to have snacks on hand in a busy day.

6 Lower fiber choices of CHO-rich foods may be useful when energy needs are high, or when the athlete needs to eat just before exercise. These choices are more compact and less likely to cause gastrointestinal discomfort during exercise.

7 CHO drinks (e.g. fruit juices, soft drinks, fruit/milk smoothies) are also a compact source for special situations or high CHO diets. This category includes many of the supplements made specially for athletes (e.g. sports drinks, liquid meal supplements).

8 The athlete who needs to optimize muscle glycogen storage, either to recover between prolonged training sessions, to 'fuel-up' for a competition, should aim to eat 7–10g CHO/kgBM/day. It may require expert advise to design an eating program to achieve these levels.

9 The athlete should eat a high CHO meal 1–4h prior to competition. The type and amount of foods, and timing of this meal will vary with the individual and their event. All strategies should be practiced in training. *Suitable meal choices are suggested in Table 16.3.*

10 Post exercise recovery of muscle fuel stores is enhanced by eating a high CHO meal or snack within 15–30min of exercise. An intake of at least 1g CHO/kgBM is recommended (see Table 4). Nutritious CHO-rich foods and drinks can provide protein and other nutrients that may also be useful in recovery.

11 CHO should be consumed during lengthy training and competition sessions when additional fuel is needed. A guideline of 30–60g CHO/h is suggested, and both CHO foods and drinks can be used by athletes to achieve this. However, sports drinks offer the advantage of looking after fluid and CHO needs simultaneously, and being specially designed for sports situations.

Practising nutritional strategies during training

It is worth noting that many athletes do not appear to optimize fluid and CHO intake strategies during training sessions as well as they do in the competition setting. Sometimes this is simply due to practical limitations: during competitions, access to fluid and CHO is improved due to the provision of aid stations, or to the scheduled breaks which allow intake. However, there is some evidence that athletes may not rate attention to these needs as highly during training. In some cases, the erroneous (and dangerous) belief that an athlete may become 'tougher' by exposing themselves to dehydration during training still persists. It is important that the athlete optimizes his/her performance during training by attending to fluid and CHO needs as well as possible. Furthermore, the training situation provides an opportunity to perfect competition intake strategies. This might include assessing the extent of fluid losses during exercise and learning to tolerate fluid intake while exercising, or assessing the optimal amount to CHO that may be needed during a prolonged exercise event.

Table 16.2 Fluid intake strategies for athletes

1 Monitoring weight changes over an exercise session may provide the athlete with a guide to the extent of sweat losses and their success in replacing these during the session (1kgBM = 1 litre of fluid). This may allow the athlete to devise a fluid intake plan for future sessions as well as to estimate the current fluid deficit that needs to be replaced.

2 The athlete is reminded that they cannot 'toughen' up or adapt to dehydration. Instead they may sacrifice their performance in these sessions.

3 The athlete should begin all exercise sessions well hydrated. This means replacing fluid losses since the last session (including dehydration used to 'make weight'). In some situations aggressive rehydration strategies may be needed.

4 The athlete should drink during the pre-event meal, and again in the hour prior to exercise. This is particularly important in hot conditions. It may also be useful to 'prime' the stomach with a large bolus of fluid immediately prior to exercise (e.g. 200–400ml). Since gastric volume is a factor in promoting gastric emptying, in situations where the athlete requires to drink large volumes during exercise, this technique may optimize the rate of fluid delivery from the stomach. This strategy needs to be practiced to learn individual tolerance.

5 The athlete should drink during all training and competition sessions. The ideal situation is to replace at least 80% of sweat losses (predicted by point 1). However, in many sports, practical issues such as the opportunity to drink and GI comfort may limit the athlete's intake to 400–800ml/h, which may be considerably below this. In any case, the athlete should form a fluid intake plan that optimizes opportunities to drink and minimizes dehydration. The athlete should not rely on thirst or good luck to dictate their fluid intake.

6 The athlete should explore the opportunities for fluid intake to their sport. Access to fluid may be provided by aid stations, by individual handlers, or may require the athlete to carry their own supplies. In many sports there is opportunity to drink during formal breaks in play (e.g. half-time) as well as informal breaks (e.g. stoppage in play due to rule infringement or player substitution). Athletes who drink while they exercise (e.g. runners, triathletes, cyclists) should practice this to learn techniques of grabbing and consuming drinks on the run, as well as to tolerate the fluid.

7 Drinking early in the event is important, with the goal of preventing large fluid deficits rather than reversing them. Drinking the largest tolerable amount at frequent intervals will help to keep the stomach at optimal (comfortable) volume, thus facilitating gastric emptying.

8 A cool, flavored beverage is most palatable to athletes and will enhance voluntary fluid intake.

9 Sports drinks (containing 5–7% CHO and 10–25mmol/L sodium) provide a palatable choice that should match fluid and carbohydrate needs of athletes inmost exercise situations.

10 After exercise, fluid deficits should be replaced quickly, especially if another training or competition session is scheduled within 2–12h. Where fluid deficits are greater than 1–2L, the retention of ingested fluids is important, and will be enhanced by replacing sodium losses simultaneously. Sodium may be replaced by drinking sports drinks or oral rehydration Solutions, or by eating salty foods. In general, salt losses are well replaced by daily eating patterns, but aggressive rehydration techniques may require acute salt intake strategies. However, this will only minimize rather than prevent urine losses during the recovery period. In general, a volume that is 150% of the fluid deficit must be consumed to allow full replacement of fluid losses during the 4–8h after exercise.

Goals of the competition diet

Eating for competition is a challenging area of practice for the sports dietitian or team physician. There is considerable pressure on the athlete (and the sports medicine professional) to succeed, and the outcome may be definite, public, and carry significant financial implications. The nutritional goals of a sports competition may be unique to the specific event, and include:

- In weight-classed sports, to achieve the weight-in target without sacrificing fuel stores and body fluid levels.
- To 'fuel-up' or store adequate CHO stores prior to the event.
- To minimize dehydration by appropriate fluid intake strategies before, during, and after the event.
- During prolonged events or other events where body CHO stores become depleted, to supply additional CHO during the event.
- To avoid gastrointestinal (GI) discomfort during the event.
- To promote recovery after competition, particularly in sports played as a series of heats and finals, or as a tournament.

Preparing adequate fuel stores

Preparation for competition should aim to match the body's CHO stores of liver and muscle glycogen to the anticipated fuel needs of the event. Normalized glycogen stores can be achieved by a high CHO intake, in conjunction with a reduction in exercise volume and intensity for the 24–36h pre-event. This is considered sufficient for most sports events, particularly events lasting less than 60min. Athletes who compete in events longer than this (particularly events longer than 90min) may try to maximize their muscle glycogen stores by undertaking a exercise–diet program known as glycogen (or CHO) loading.

The original CHO loading protocol, as described by Scandinavian researchers in the late 1960s, used extremes of diet and exercise to first deplete the supercompensate glycogen stores. Recent work has demonstrated that trained athletes do not need to undertake the severe depletion phase to subsequently achieve an increase in glycogen stores. Instead, they need only to taper their training and ensure **a high (8–10g/kg BM/day) CHO intake over the 72h prior to an event** to achieve similar increases in muscle glycogen to those reported by the more extreme regimens. Some studies have reported that athletes do not have sufficient practical nutrition knowledge to achieve such CHO intakes and may require dietary counseling.

The pre-event meal

Offers a last chance to fine-tune fluid and fuel levels prior to the event, as well as to ensure GI comfort. An athlete who is well-tapered and has been consuming high CHO meals over the last 2–3 days may already have optimized muscle CHO stores. In this case, the major concern is to top-up liver glycogen stores after an overnight fast should the event be early in the day. Conversely, if preparation for the event has been less than optimal due to inadequate recovery from the last exercise session, food eaten in the pre-event meal (1–4h pre-event) may significantly contribute to muscle fuel availability.

In summary, the optimal pre-event meal obviously varies between individual athletes, and is influenced by factors such as the time of day of competition and the degree to which the athlete has prepared or recovered fluid and fuel status since the last exercise session. The menu recommended for pre-event eating should include high CHO, low fat foods, with reduced fiber and protein content being an additional recommendation for those who experience GI discomfort. Fluid intake is also important, especially in preparation for events carried out in hot conditions. While some athletes may be able to comfortably consume a larger meal or snack 3–4h prior to competition, those involved in early morning events may prefer to consume a smaller snack 1–2h before. Liquid meals, such as commercially available supplements or fruit smoothies, provide a practical alternative for athletes who find it difficult to consume solid foods prior to exercise. The athlete is advised to experiment with various pre-event routines during training to define the optimal strategy. Some suitable pre-event meal choices are summarized in Table 16.3.

Table 16.3 Suitable pre-event meal choices: high CHO, low fat

- Breakfast cereal + low fat milk + fresh/canned fruit
- Muffins or crumpets + jam/honey
- Pancakes + syrup
- Toast + baked beans (note this is a high fiber choice)
- Creamed rice (made with low fat milk)
- Rolls or sandwiches with banana filling
- Fruit salad + low fat fruit yogurt
- Spaghetti with tomato or low fat sauce
- Baked potatoes with low fat filling
- Fruit smoothie (low fat milk + fruit + yogurt/icecream)
- Liquid meal supplement (e.g. Sustagen Sport, Exceed Sports Meal, GatorPro)

Fluid and carbohydrate intake during exercise

Maintenance of body temperature is a major concern for the athlete, particularly during exercise in hot, humid conditions. Evaporation of sweat from the skin provides a major mechanism of heat dissipation, with the athlete's sweat rate being determined by exercise intensity, the state of heat acclimation, and the prevailing environmental conditions. Sweat rates as high as 2–3L/h have been reported in some athletes exercising at high power outputs in hot and humid conditions. However, during more prolonged, moderate intensity exercise such as running and cycling, sweat rates in most athletes are closer to 1.0–1.2L/h. Unless this fluid is replaced, the athlete will eventually become dehydrated.

Dehydration of as little as 2% of an athlete's body mass has been shown to significantly reduce high intensity exercise capacity. Furthermore, the effects on exercise response appear to be directly related to the degree of dehydration, and the athlete cannot acquire a tolerance to dehydration as is popularly believed in some sports. It appears that the effects of dehydration on exercise performance are related to the type of event or sport being undertaken. While aerobic exercise, particularly in the heat, is impaired at such low levels of dehydration, events requiring strength and power do not seem to be affected by such small fluid losses. However, minimal dehydration may negatively impact on mental function and should therefore have a greater impact on team and racquet sports which involve skill and decision-making processes, than endurance sports such as running and cycling. Dehydration has also been shown to reduce the rate of gastric emptying which may further compromise exercise performance. For these reasons, the athlete should aim to minimize net fluid losses during all types of exercise.

In terms of optimal fluid balance, the athlete might be advised to consume fluids to keep pace with sweat losses; or at least 80% of sweat loss rate. However, in most competition and training situations, athletes are limited to drinking what is practical rather than optimal. This appears to be **400–800ml of fluid per h under most sports conditions.** Whether this is done at aid stations, at formal breaks between quarters or halves of a game, or from drink bottles carried by the athlete will vary according to the sport. However, athletes should be encouraged to establish a drinking routine that takes into account their sweat losses and their opportunities to drink fluid (see Table 16.2). This may not be optimal when sweat losses greatly exceed the general rate of gastric emptying (about 1L/h), but the athlete should aim to minimize dehydration. The athlete should drink early and frequently **e.g. 150–250 ml every 15–20min)** to prevent rather than try to reverse dehydration. Special consideration should be given to athletes who need to consume fluids during events, literally 'on the run' (e.g. marathon runners, cyclists, cross country skiers, triathletes). These athletes may need to balance their intake against the possibility of GI discomfort or upset, as well as the time lost while eating/drinking (i.e. slowing down to approach an aid station or to handle fluids/food). Fluids that are palatable are likely to be consumed in larger quantities; for this reason, cool and sweet-tasting drinks are promoted.

CHO depletion is a common cause of fatigue during prolonged intense, caused by muscle glycogen depletion and/or hypoglycemia.

Many endurance and ultra-endurance events challenge the athlete's carbohydrate reserves despite pre-exercise strategies to maximize fuel stores. Carbohydrate intake during such exercise may benefit performance, both by preventing hypoglycemia in those individuals susceptible to small changes in blood glucose concentration, and by supplying additional fuel for muscle glucose oxidation. Numerous studies have reported benefits to endurance capacity and/or performance in prolonged exercise events when CHO is consumed.

Both solid foods and CHO drinks have been used successfully to supply CHO during exercise. CHO drinks are particularly useful because of the decreased risk of GI side-effects, and the simultaneous supply of fluid. Although early studies reported that gastric emptying was reduced following the intake of CHO drinks greater than 2.5% in concentration compared to plain water, there are now many studies that report that CHO drinks of 5–7% concentration are emptied rapidly and do not compromise fluid replacement. Today, commercial sports drinks are manufactured using a combination of carbohydrate types (glucose, sucrose, glucose polymers, etc.) to achieve a palatable beverage with a carbohydrate content of 5–7% and a moderate sodium level 10–25mmol/L). These sports drinks provide a practical way to achieve CHO and fluid needs during exercise and post-exercise recovery. The athlete should experiment with carbohydrate intake strategies during training to perfect a competition (see Table 16.3).

Recovery after exercise

In some sports, competition is conducted as a series of events or stages. Examples include track and field and swimming events where athletes may compete in a number of brief events, or heats and finals, all in the one day. In tennis tournaments and cycle tours, competition may extend for 1–3 weeks with competitors being required to undertake one or more lengthy bouts each day. The value of rapid recovery between events is clear; and recovery strategies must consider the extent and type of nutritional stresses involved as well as the time interval between competition bouts. Even where athletes compete in a weekly fixture, optimal recover is desired to allow the athlete to undertake training between matches or races.

Immediate intake of carbohydrate food has already been identified as a key strategy in enhancing glycogen refueling (see Table 16.4). Despite the intake of fluid during exercise most athletes finish the session at least mildly dehydrated. From a practical standpoint, the success of post-exercise rehydration is dependent on how much the athlete drinks, and then how much of this is retained and re-equilibrated within body fluid compartments. Flavored drinks may encourage greater intake than plain water, in addition to the benefits of CHO content on muscle fuel needs. Urine losses appear to be minimized by the replacement of lost electrolytes, particularly sodium, simultaneously with fluid replacement. The inclusion of sodium in the drink (particularly in levels as high as in oral rehydration solutions used in the treatment of diarrhea), or the concurrent consumption of salty foods, may be an important strategy in the rapid recovery of moderate–high fluid deficits. Since caffeine and alcohol promote diuresis, consumption of large amounts of alcohol and caffeine-containing drinks may also impair rapid fluid restoration. The current practices of some athletes, particularly in team sports, to consume excessive amounts of alcohol after competition requires re-education. Disadvantages include impairment of rehydration and thermoregulation, exacerbation of soft tissue damage, as well as behavior that provides a high risk of accidents.

While eating for optimal competition recovery may simply represent an extension of everyday nutrition patterns, it is important to remember the practical implications of the competition situation. Some consideration may need to be given to ensuring the availability of suitable foods at the competition venue, particularly where athletes are often competing interstate or overseas. The post-event phase is often a time of conflicting priorities, with the athlete being distracted by requests for drug testing, equipment checks, travel, media interviews, and team activities. **It is vital that the athlete is aware of the importance of recovery nutrition**, and that creative and practical ways of achieving this can be organized. Nutrient-dense supplements in liquid (e.g. liquid meals) or solid form (e.g. sports bars) may provide a practical alternative to food in some situations.

Table 16.4 Suitable post-exercise recovery snacks

These serves provide 50g of CHO–the athlete may need 1–2 serves depending on their bodyweight. Many other CHO snacks or meals may be eaten according to the athlete's appetite or availability of these foods.

- 800–1000ml sports drink
- 500ml fruit juice or soft drink
- 250ml high CHO supplement (e.g. Exceed High Carbohydrate Source, Gatorlode)
- 250–350ml fruit smoothie
- 250–350ml liquid meal supplement (e.g. Sustagen Sport, Exceed Sports Meal, GatorPro)
- 50g jelly beans or lollies
- 70–80g chocolate bar
- 1 round jam or honey sandwich (thick-sliced bread + lot of jam or honey)
- 3 muesli bars
- 3 medium–large pieces of fruit (e.g. apple, orange, banana)
- 2 cups breakfast cereal + skim milk
- 2 × 200g carton low fat fruit yoghurt
- Cup of thick vegetable soup + large bread roll
- 2 cups fruit salad + $\frac{1}{2}$ carton of low fat fruit yogurt
- 1 large bread roll + banana filling
- 1–2 pieces of thick crust pizza

Summary

Sports nutrition combines science and practice to assist athletes to be healthy, train effectively, and compete at their best. The special nutritional needs of athletes must be met within a busy schedule and with creative strategies that combine a number of nutritional goals simultaneously. Special fluid and food intake strategies before, during, and after exercise can improve athletic performance and enhance subsequent recovery.

17 Dermatology

DIANA RUBEL

Introduction

The skin plays an important role in protecting the body from noxious external stimuli such as mechanical forces, temperature changes, and harmful chemicals. It is no surprise, therefore, that cutaneous disorders are an important factor in every athletic specialty. Sports dermatology is concerned with skin disorders related to athletic activity, manifesting either as a primary disorder or as an exacerbation of a pre-existing dermatological dermatosis. Sports dermatology is an expanding field and this chapter summarizes some of the more commonly encountered problems.

Skin infections

Fungal infections

Dermatophytic fungi live in the stratum corneum (most superficial epidermal layer) and can cause superficial infections. *Tinea pedis* or 'athlete's foot' affects the interdigital and lateral areas of the feet and is characterized by pruritis, scaling, and occasional soreness. The classic 'wet form' presents with white macerated scale, fissures, and occasionally with vesicles and bullae. Less commonly a 'dry form' or 'moccasin foot' is seen as a dry, rough, diffuse white scale affecting the sole. The problem is often bilateral and the toenails may also be involved (manifest by discoloration, thickening, crumbling, and subungual scale of one or more toenails). Tinea pedis is a chronic disorder and patients may be afflicted for decades. Infection occurs by person-to-person or by contact with infected fomites such as a towel or floormat. It is undoubtedly influenced by the microenvironment of the clad foot, and factors that exacerbate the condition include a moist, warm environment; a sweaty foot enclosed in a nonabsorbent sock and occlusive shoe such as a 'trainer' is a likely target for tinea pedis. Secondary bacterial infection is sometimes seen and may present as cellulitis, lymphangitis, or inguinal lymphadenopathy. The diagnosis of tinea pedis is confirmed by examining scrapings of keratinous debris in a 10% potassium hydroxide (KOH) preparation and observing the characteristic hyphae. Culture permits identification of the causative fungus (usually *Trichophyton rubrum, T. mentagrophytes,* or *Epidermophyton floccosum*).

The **differential diagnosis** includes pompholyx, pustular psoriasis, pitted keratolysis, and allergic contact dermatitis to shoes; a positive skin scraping, however, does not necessarily exclude these dermatoses, as a superficial dermatophyte infection may be superimposed upon an area of already broken skin. **Treatment**: acutely inflamed 'wet forms' of superficial fungal infections should be treated with a combination of shooting antiseptic soaks or paints (e.g. Castellan's) and topical antifungals. Soaks should be lukewarm and contain potassium permanganate 1 in 10,000, and the feet immersed in the solution for 15min 3 times daily. Effective topical antifungals include the newer imidaoles such as miconazole, econazole or clotrimoxazole in a cream or tincture base; these should be applied twice daily for approximately 2 weeks. Careful attention should be given to avoidance of exacerbating factors such as sweat, heat, and occlusion. Socks should be cotton or wool, and preferably changed once or twice during the day. Footwear such as thongs or clogs should be worn while using communal showers or change rooms. Athletes should alternate pairs of sneakers or shoes if possible to allow airing in between periods of wear. Infection of the nails is an indication for oral antifungal therapy as dermatophyte in the nail are relatively resistant to topical agents. A new allylamine drug, terbinafine, can achieve a mycological cure of toenail onychomycosis in 70–80% of patients following 12 weeks of therapy.[1] Other oral agents used include griseofulvin, ketoconazole, and intermittent itraconazole. Although generally safe agents, **ketoconazole is contraindicated** in patients with hepatic disorders and can interact with other medications (e.g., warfarin). Itraconazole has fewer hepatic side-effects but is considerably more expensive than other oral antifungals. Amorolfine 5% nail

1 A Tosti *et al* 1996 *J Am Acad Dermatol* **34** 595–600

lacquer can be applied to affected nails 1–2 times/per week and has shown to cure approximately 40–55% of patients with toenail onychomycosis.[1]

Other fungal infections include *tinea cruris*, *tinea versicolour*, and *tinea incognita*.

Tinea cruris ('*jock itch*')

Commences in the groin folds and extends out in an annular or circular fashion with a scaly, inflamed border. Hyphae can also be identified on KOH preparation of scale taken from the active advancing border. **Treatment** of tinea cruris is with oral griseofulvin and concomitant topical treatment with one of the newer imidazole creams.

Tinea versicolour

Not actually a dermatophyte infection but is due to the saprophytic yeast *Pityrosporum orbicular* which develops into is parasitic fungal form *Malasezia furfur*. This transformation may be provoked by humidity, ambient heat, as a result of exercise, secondary to diabetes mellitus, or iatrogenic immunosuppression (e.g. systemic corticosteroid treatment or immunosuppressives for solid organ transplants).

Tinea versicolour infection produces hyper- or hypopigmented macules on the torso and proximal limbs with fine bran-like scale. Infection can be chronic and recurrent with exacerbations following climatic changes in humidity. Organisms can be detected in a KOH preparation of skin scrapings. Treatment of pityriasis versicolour has traditionally been with selenium sulphide (Selsun® shampoo) applied as a cream to the affected areas twice daily or more recently with imidazole creams or foaming washes. **Treatment** needs to be applied to skin beyond the disappearance of the eruption, however, relapses are common with topical therapies. A course of oral ketoconazole or itraconazole for 7 days is effective in eliminating the reservoir of *Pityriasis* organisms and helps prevent further relapses.

Tinea incognita

Refers to the specific clinical picture seen when a potent topical corticosteroid preparation is mistakenly applied to a tinea infection. Inflammatory features such as erythema may be absent; typically a mild, pink, scaly annular macule with central clearing is seen. Skin scrapings stained with KOH show abundant hyphae and permit the correct diagnosis.

Bacterial infections

Impetigo

A superficial bacterial infection characterized by honey-colored crusts or vesicles on a moist erythematous base. Impetigo is highly infectious and is spread by direct contact or fomites and can infect intact skin. The organism(s) responsible are usually *Streptococcus* or *Staphylococcus aureus*. High ambient temperatures, humidity, low altitude, and poor hygiene may favor development and transmission of impetigo. Streptococcal impetigo has spread among footballers

1 M Haria, HM Bryson 1995 *Drugs* **49** 103–20

and those playing American football.[1] **Treatment** consists of topical or systemic antibiotics directed against both streptococcus and staphylococcus. Removal of crusts by gentle soaking with warm compresses of potassium permanganate (1 in 10,000) dilution followed by a topical antibiotic such as mupirocin or fusidic acid, for approximately 7–10 days is effective. The entire skin, scalp included, should be washed with an antiseptic soap daily for 10 days. Alternatively, a 10-day course of broad-spectrum oral antibiotics active against β-lactamase-producing staphylococci is also efficacious.

The patient should be isolated until clearance of crusts and not allowed to compete in contact sports. In particular, sportsmen such as wrestlers should be free of new lesions for at least 48h prior to competition and should have no moist, exudative or draining lesions prior to tournament participation.

Pitted keratolysis

A bacterial infection of the palmar surface of the feet due to superficial infection with *Corynebacterium* species. It characteristically appears as shallow white pits or dents in the stratum corneum. Increased sweating (hyperhidrosis) is thought to play an etiological role in the condition and thus may be seen with increased frequency in athletes. Maceration and malodor may be associated findings. **Treatment** consists of general preventative measures to control hyperhidrosis (absorbent socks, leather shoes, 'shoe-free' intervals), topical application of antiperspirants containing 20% aluminium chloride, an topical antibiotics such as 1–2% erythromycin or clindamycin solution.

Viral infections

Herpes simplex virus (HSV)

HSV is a double-stranded DNA virus which typically causes recurrent infections of the mucous an periorifical membranes. However, it can infect any skin surface and remain latent in the ganglia of peripheral nerves.

Herpes gladiatorum

Herpes gladiatorum has been described in participants in close contact sports such as wrestling and rugby (also known in the latter as 'scrumpox') and in a recent study of American college wrestlers 7.6% were reported to have had a herpes skin infection in the preceding 12 months.[2] Herpes gladiatorum is transmitted primarily by direct skin-to-skin contact, and abrasions in the skin may allow a pathway of infection. The majority of lesions occur on the head or face, followed by the trunk and/or extremities. A prodromal itching or burning sensation is followed by clustered vesicular lesions on an erythematous base which heal with crusts over about 1–3 weeks. Less commonly headache, malaise, sore throat, and fever may accompany the primary infection. Recurrent episodes may occur following the initial infection and may precipitated by sunburn, illness, and emotional stress. HSV antibodies, acquired from previous cold sores, may be protective from acquiring herpes gladiatoraum eruptions. Because

1 P Bartlett *et al* 1982 *Am J Sports Med* 10 371–4 **2** TM Becker 1992 *Cutis* **50** 150–2

of its unexpected location on the cutaneous surface, herpes gladiatorum any be confused with impetigo, varicella, staphylococcal furunculosis, or allergic or irritant contact dermatitis. Adequate treatment, counseling, and public health strategies depend on making an accurate diagnosis, hence viral immunofluorescence and cultures should be obtained by gently breaking an intact vesicle and firmly rubbing the swab tip across the base of the erosion. **Treatment** of herpes gladiatorum is ideally with oral acyclovir (200mg 5 times a day for the 5 days) and is most effective if commenced at the first symptoms of an outbreak. Topical acyclovir is available but is probably less effective. Concomitant secondary impetiginization should also be treated. HSV can survive for hours to days outside the host if environmental conditions are appropriate[1] hence all contaminated surfaces should be cleaned with antiseptic solution. In the vesicular phase and until the crusts have separated, patients should avoid sports which could involve physical contact.

Molluscum contagiosum

A highly infectious pox virus which can also be spread by human contact. The organism appears to be easily spread in an aqueous medium (e.g. in communal baths, spas, and pools). Athletes, swimmers, and cross country runners have the highest incidence of mollusca. Their incidence may be increased in patients with underlying active atopic dermatitis. They typically appear as solitary or multiple flesh-colored dome-shaped papules with a central umbilication. The differential diagnosis includes multiple basal cell carcinomata, cryptococcosis, and appendageal tumors such as trichoepitheliomas. They can be treated by gently breaking the surface of the lesion and extracting the central *keratinous plug*. Other treatments employed are cryosurgery with liquid nitrogen, electrodessication and topical trichloroacetic acid, or tretinoin. Athletes may resume contact sports 48–72h after the lesions have cleared.

Common warts

Are epidermal growths caused by infection by the human papillomavirus group (HPV). Infection can occur if infected debris from warts comes in contact with abraded skin and can result in either autoinoculation or transmission to susceptible individuals. However, it is not generally thought to be highly infective and thus not limit participation in contact sports. Plantar warts can cause pain with ambulation, thereby limiting performance in sporting activities. Warts may also be more common in callouses which develop in sport.[2] Paring of plantar warts with a no. 15 blade reveals small black spots corresponding to thrombosed capillaries within papillae, thus distinguishing the lesions from callouses or corns, which lack these dots and have a central hyaline core. **Treatment** of plantar warts is challenging and may cause as much inconvenience to the athlete as the presence of the wart itself. Daily application of salicylic and lactic acid preparations under occlusion with concomitant paring with an emery board may be effective, as may repeated cryosurgery and

1 LS Nerurkar *et al* 1983 *J Am Med Assoc* **250** 3081–3   **2** G Kantor, W Bergfeld 1988 *Exercise Sports Sci Rev* **16** 215–53

paring at 2–3-week intervals. For resistant warts, intralesional bleo-mycin injections or carbon dioxide ablation can be used. Oral high dose cimetidine therapy (30–40mg/kg/day) has reportedly been suc-cessful in childhood warts; however, other studies have shown no advantage in cimetidine over placebo in adults.[1]

1 E Yilmaz E *et al* 1996 *J Am Acad Dermatol* **34** 1005–7

597

Sports-related allergic and irritant dermatitis

Urticaria (hives)

Is relatively common disorder and its incidence is highest in young adults. It can be defined as a transient red and/or edematous swelling of the dermis or subcutaneous tissues. Some factors that can provoke urticaria include medications such as analgesics and non-steroidal antiinflammatory drugs (NSAIDs), which may be ingested by athletes from time to time. Of particular interest are the physical urticarias. These are triggered by a variety of physical causes such as pressure, cold, heat, water (aquagenic), and solar irradiation. Most patients suffer from idiopathic urticaria as well (i.e. physical factors may not always contribute to urticarial lesions). Athletes may develop pressure urticaria from tight fitting belts, clothing, or on the soles of feet following running. Cold induced urticaria can be precipitated by food, drinks, and changes in the ambient temperature. If the whole body is cooled suddenly, as when diving into a swimming pool, an episode of urticaria could lead to circulatory collapse. It is thus very important to recognize this uncommon condition and instruct patients to avoid such triggers. Exposure to the sun or artificial light sources may rarely be followed by itching, erythema, and wheals. Cholinergic urticaria is a type of eruption associated with sweating. The weals are characteristically small and surrounded by large red halos, and last less than an hour following the trigger. Flushing, faintness, asthma, nausea, vomiting, and diarrhea may occasionally occur as a result of systemic histamine released by mast cells. Water-induced urticaria presents in a similar fashion. **Treatment** of the physical urticarias is first to eliminate the triggers as far as is possible. An episode of cholinergic urticaria may be followed by a refractory period of up to 24h; athletes may therefore wish to 'warm-up' a few hours prior to a specific event where the unpleasant effects of weals may be undesirable. Non-sedating anti-histamine agents, such as loratadine or cetirizine, are usually effective treatment.

Contact dermatitis

Many natural and synthetic substances can induce dermatitis or inflammation of the skin on physical contact. Sports enthusiasts may be particularly vulnerable to irritant dermatitis from equipment and medicaments. In addition, sweat and local heat and humidity may enhance a substance's allergenic or irritating potential by inter-fering with the normal barrier function of the skin. An irritant reaction will result in dermatitis independently of a specific immu-nological reaction and will tend to produce a similar reaction in all persons exposed to the irritant (e.g. chronic exposure to water and detergents may result in irritant contact hand dermatitis).

An allergic contact dermatitis, however, is a delayed (type IV) immunological reaction involving specifically sensitized T lympho-cytes in a susceptible individual. Some of detective work may be required to identify the offending allergen (e.g. a linear abdominal eruption in a surfer may be attributable to allergic contact dermatitis to nickel contained in the zip fastener of a wet suit). A spectrum of clinical presentations may be seen in both irritant and allergic contact dermatitis. Classically, contact with an allergenic plant (e.g. *Rhus iv, grevillea, primula obconica*) in a sensitized individual results in a bullous, intensely itchy, linear eruption of the forearms. These reactions may be seen in outdoor athletes. Rubber is a known sensitizer and may produce either a delayed type contact dermatitis (usually due to accelerants or antioxidants used in rubber manufacture) or an urticarial type immediate reaction (due to latex allergy). Bathing caps, nose clips, ear plugs, fins and finstraps, swimming goggles, diving suits, and underwater masks and mouthpieces are all capable of producing potentially serious cutaneous reactions in swimmers or divers. *Of particular concern* would be a patient with type I allergy to rubber latex who dived with a rubber mouthpiece and experienced an urticarial reaction while diving. Allergic contact dermatitis to shoes (tanning agents used in leather, rubber, glues, inner soles) may result in a symmetrical bilateral dermatitis affecting the feet, in a distribution reminiscent of actual contact with the allergen (e.g. a rash on the lateral aspect of the soles may correlate with allergy to inner soles). Sports participants may develop allergic contact dermatitis to topically applied medicaments (salicylates, linaments, tea tree oil, antibiotics, antiseptics, and any fragrances or preservatives contained therein) or tapes and plasters (colophony, para-tertiary-butylphenol resin).

PABA—containing sunscreens used by athletes may also result in allergic contact dermatitis, often involving sun exposed skin only. Identification of the offending allergen may be difficult and patients should be referred to specialist dermatology centers for detailed patch testing should allergic contact dermatitis be suspected. **Treatment**: topical corticosteroids with wet dressings, and occasionally oral corticosteroids, along with withdrawal of the offending substance, are used to treat allergic contact dermatitis.

Dermatological manifestations of physical, cold, and electromagnetic injury

Acne mechanica

Is a papulopustular eruption caused by the physical factors of pressure, occlusion, friction, and heat acting on the skin.[1] It is believed that these mechanical stresses, rather than follicular infection by normal skin commensals (as in common acne), play a primary causative role in sports-related acne. Pre-existent acne vulgaris is therefore not necessarily a precursor of acne mechanica, although the mechanical stresses mentioned above certainly aggravate common acne. Acne mechanica is one of the more prevalent dermatoses among athletes. Heavy protective padding, headgear, occlusive synthetic garments such as leotards, and golfers carrying heavy bags can precipitate acne mechanica. It has thus been observed in American football players, hockey players, aerobics participants and golfers. An unusual example of acne mechanica has been described on the neck of a shot putter at the position where the shot is rested against the neck before being thrown.

Acne keloidalis is a specific chronic pilosebaceous disorder affecting the posterior occipital scalp of predominantly black skinned individuals; it has reportedly developed in helmet-wearing football players with no prior history of the disorder.[2] **Prevention** of the condition is important in management and wearing a clean, absorbent cotton T-shirt under uniforms and equipment may be useful. Early removal of clothing and showering after sport will also alleviate aggravating factors. **Treatment**: thorough cleansing followed by keratolytics such as salicylic acid in ethanol, or tretinoin cream. Topical antibiotics such as clindamycin or erythromycin in an astringent base are helpful in visibly infected cases. Systemic antibiotics, used with success in common acne, seem to be of less benefit in acne mechanica. The eruption invariably settles down during seasonal breaks from participation in sports activities.

Foot blisters may result from heat and humidity combined with unaccustomed localized friction. Improperly fitting shoes and sporadic training may contribute to their development. **Treatment**: they are best treated by sterile aspiration, leaving the overlying skin intact to form a natural dressing. The area can then be treated with an antibiotic ointment or antiseptic and covered with a simple dressing. Newer hydrophilic dressings are comfortable and absorbent and may allow the athlete to resume participation. **Prevention** is the key to successful treatment; shoes should be properly fitting and worn with two pairs of cotton socks. Foot powders may help to absorb moisture and thus reduce skin shearing forces. Anecdotal evidence suggests that application of Friar's balsam may 'toughen' skin and reduce the incidence of blisters.

Black heel or *talon noir* are petechiae occurring over the posterior aspect of the heel. They are common in sports such as basketball, squash, or football, where frequent changes in direction occur, resulting in a shearing effect on the skin. The color of the eruption may alarm the athlete and cause them to present. **No treatment** is required apart from reassurance. *Jogger's nipple* is a painful and often fissured dermatitis eruption over the nipples produced by friction from unyielding vests or T-shirts and may also occur in women who

1 RSW Basler 1992 *Cutis* **50** 125–8   2 H Harris 1992 *Cutis* **50** 154–6

do not wear undergarments while jogging. **Treatment** is with an emollient such as emulsifying ointment or white soft paraffin, or a mild topical corticosteroid, and elimination of the underlying trigger. 'Tennis toe', actually observed in a variety of activities including cricket, jogging, and skiing , is due to hemorrhage under the nail plate of the great toe caused by impact between the distal end of the nail plate and the shoe. This may result in an acutely painful subungual hematoma which may require drainage. The injury **may be prevented** in some cases by excising away a small portion of the toe of the shoe, thus reducing the impact effect on the toe.

Repeated low grade trauma or pressure to the skin surface will result in a protective hyperkeratotic response to prevent injury to underlying structures; eventually a callus will form. The type of sport will determine the location and shape of the callus (e.g. the hands of a rower or weight lifter, or the soles of a jogger). *Corns (clavi)* are callosities over bony prominences. Athletes with long second or third toes (*Morton's toe*) may develop buckling of the second toe which forces the second metatarsal head into the ground and results in clavus formation in this position. Clavi are exquisitely tender to lateral pressure or squeezing. Treatment of callosities and clavi begins with correction of the abnormal mechanical stresses and consultation with a podiatrist may help to identify these. **Treatment**: the lesions can be pared with a scalpel blade and keratolytics applied to help remove excess keratin. Cryotherapy of clavi requires relatively long freezing times (approximately 90s); the resultant crust is shaved in t3 or 4 weeks, and often one treatment can abolish the clavus.[1]

Athlete's nodules

Are connective tissue naevi (collagenomas) at sites of recurrent trauma and friction. They may appear in knuckles, pretibial areas or dorsal aspects of the feet, in an area directly related to the particular sport. '*Nike nodules*' appear on the dorsal foot from repetitive trauma associated with jogging[2] *Surfer's nodules* develop on the dorsal foot from trauma associated with surfboards. *Piezogenic papules* are small, painful herniations of fat through areas of damaged dermis, often appearing on the mediolateral aspects of the feet. They may only be apparent when the foot is in a weight bearing position. Support stockings may afford some symptomatic relief.

1 C Sheard 1992 *Cutis* **50** 138 **2** RSW Basler RSW, Jacobs Senior Lecturer Orthopaedic Surgery Reply (letter) 1991 *J Am Acad Dermatol* **20** 318

Heat- and cold-related skin disease

Intertrigo

An inflammatory dermatosis affecting the body folds, in particular the submammary and genitocrural areas. Obesity, sweat and friction predispose to its development, and the clinical appearances can range from mild erythema to frank dermatitis with secondary bacterial or candidal infection. In refractory cases, diabetes mellitus should be excluded. **Prevention**: avoidance of tight clothing, carefully applied wet dressings in the acute phase, and the application of one of the imidazole preparations alone, or with a topical corticosteroid, may help control the condition. *It is important to remember that flexural psoriasis occasionally presents a similar clinical picture* and may lack the characteristic silvery scale in the moist flexural region. Flexural psoriasis is generally more erythematous with a well defined border, and there is often evidence of psoriasis elsewhere on the body such as the scalp, elbows, or knees.

Miliaria ('prickly heat')

Occurs in a hot and humid environment when sweat becomes trapped within ducts before it reaches the epidermal surface. It mainly affects the torso. Three types of miliaria are seen depending on the level of obstruction with the skin. *Miliaria crystalline* occurs when obstruction is very superficial in the epidermis, resulting in fragile vesicles. *Miliaria rubra* is the most common type and is due to obstruction in the intraepidermal sweat duct, and presents as erythematous papules associated with pruritus and stinging. *Miliaria profunda* is rarely seen outside of the tropics and is due to obstruction of deeper dermal sweat ducts. **Treatment** of miliaria consists of reducing environmental heat and humidity, use of mildly astringent lotions to help relieve ductal obstruction, and mild topical corticosteroids to reduce inflammation. Miliaria may be followed by a period of hypohidrosis or defective sweating, and may put athletes at risk for overheating injury for several weeks.

Erythema ab igne

Is a characteristic cutaneous eruption consisting of a well demarcated area of livedoid erythema and pigmentation, most commonly seen on the lower legs of older women who sit too close to a heater in winter. Vascular injury secondary to heat damage is thought to play a role. Similar eruptions may be seen in athletes who apply heat packs to the skin for musculoskeletal injuries. Cold compressions are also used for such injuries and cryogenic damage to skin following their correct usage has been reported.[1] The eruption consisted of bullae and erythema 24 hours following a 25 minute exposure time to the cold compress. The degree of hypothermia delivered by such cold compresses may be potentiated by applying an elastic bandage and/or actually sitting on the cold compress thus firmly immobilizing it against the skin. This method of application should therefore be avoided.

1 V Cipollaro 1992 *Cutis* **50** 111–12.

603

Ultraviolet-related skin disease

Sunburn

Is a preventable skin injury which has acute and chronic effects on the skin. Acute effects include erythema, edema, and desquamation. Chronic effects comprise increased incidence of cutaneous tumors (including malignant melanoma, squamous and basal cell carcinomata, keratoacanthoma), photoageing, and atrophy. Malignant melanoma is of particular concern because of its aggressive behavior and strong correlations between frequency of sunburn in youth and the development of melanoma. **Prevention** of sunburn and excessive photoexposure in sports participants is an area of preventative medicine which should be endorsed by all sports enthusiasts—spectator, athlete, and official alike. Sporting activities should ideally be timed for early morning or mid to late afternoon in order to avoid the harsher midday ultraviolet (UV) rays. Broad-spectrum sunscreen agents (which block out UVB, UVA, and infrared rays) with a sun protection factor (SPF) of at least 15 times normal should be applied and reapplied frequently during outdoor exposure. Use of hats and protective clothing, preferably also with good UV blocking abilities, should also be endorsed.

UV light exposure may also result in phototoxic reactions to substances either orally ingested (e.g. NSAIDs, or applied topically, i.e. perfumes and essential oils). Even brief exposure to UV light may cause intense reactions in persons who have used photosensitizing agents, and this can persist long after cessation of the offending agent.

Exacerbation of pre-existing skin disease

A variety of dermatological conditions may become exacerbated by sport activity. Although acne may arise *de novo* following trauma from sport, it is also a common condition of young people and may worsen with activity. It is important to remember that treatments for acne, such as isotretinoin (oral synthetic vitamin A derivative), may give rise to side-effects, such as photosensitivity, skin fragility, and myalgias, which can interfere with sporting performance. Minomycin, a commonly used oral antibiotic for acne, can also result in photo-sensitivity.

Psoriasis is a common skin disorder with quite varied clinical manifestations. Psoriasis is often exacerbated by trauma (the Koebner or isomorphic response) and palmoplantar psoriasis may also be influenced by chronic mechanical pressure. Retinoids and tar pre-parations may result in photosensitivity.

Many patients with atopic dermatitis find that sweating aggravates their condition. Seasonal exacerbations in spring and autumn are also frequent. Chlorinated, as opposed to saltwater, pools can be very drying for atopic individuals, and frequent showering may also exacerbate eczema. Exposure of the skin to irritant chemicals or physical trauma should thus be avoided as far as possible.

Dermatological effects of anabolic-androgenic steroids

The use of self-administered anabolic-androgenic steroids by athletes and body builders may be widespread and under-recognized. Anabolic steroids are synthetic derivatives of testosterone. High doses may stimulate the production of sebum by sebaceous glands and increase the numbers of normal follicular bacteria. Acne, oily hair and skin, sebaceous cysts, hirsutism, and rogenetic alopecia, striae (stretch marks), seborrheic dermatitis, and secondary bacterial infections occur with increased frequency in this group of athletes. Cutaneous-side effects are often the initial clinical manifestations of anabolic steroid usage.[1]

1 MJ Scott, AM Scott 1992 *Cutis* **50** 113–17

Introduction

Sport psychology is practised by psychologists specializing in the domain of sport psychology and by sport scientists specializing in psychological aspects of sport and the athlete. It concerns itself with the maximization of sporting performance by developing the mental strength and addressing the general psychological well-being of athletes. Sports psychologists from both backgrounds, have most often worked with athletes on mental or psychological skills training, which deals with topics such as motivation, confidence, arousal control, concentration, mental rehearsal, and life skills; usually addressed through an educational approach. Additionally, psychologists have become involved in a range of clinical issues with athletes and interpersonal issues between members of a team or between coaches and athletes. Contemporary sport psychologists endeavor to follow a scientist–practitioner model, where applied intervention is grounded in theory and research. However, intuition and clinical experience are also drawn upon, especially when there is no documented theory of significant research findings to guide intervention.

From a psychological perspective, athletes are best considered first as the same as non-athletes. Athletes have the same amount of psychological problems as non-athletes, although they do tend to have certain problems (e.g. eating disorders) a little more than the general population, while a slightly lower rate of chronic mental health problems (e.g. schizophrenia). This chapter is written with adult athletes in mind. However, it must be recognized that young athletes have a number of differing and special needs. Coverage of issues in relation to child and adolescent athletes are addressed in a number of specialist texts in the area.[1]

Sports physicians need to know about a number of psychological factors, including those related to peak athletic performance, and those that effect injury recovery or contribute to injury. They also need to be aware of common psychological problems that an athlete may experience, and be able to recognize the signs and symptoms of an actual mental disorder. It is useful for physicians consulting with athletes to know basic treatment processes for psychological problems in order to undertake initial intervention with athletes, and for physicians to have some understanding of the type of intervention strategies applied by psychologists. Whenever referring to a sport psychologist, it is important to check their qualifications and enquire as to their background and experience. Aim to match the psychologist's training and area of expertise with the athlete's needs. There are a number of difficulties with the psychologist seeing the athlete separate from their sporting environment. The ideal mode of operation for a sport psychologists is for them to work as part of the sports' science team, interacting with physicians, coaches, trainers and other support staff.

1 T Morris, J Summers 1995 *Sports psychology; theory, applications and issues.* Wiley, Australia

Psychological principles of peak performance

Athletes endeavor to perform consistently to their maximum. Psychological factors are important determinants of peak sporting performance. A state indicative of peak performance has been coined 'being in the flow'. Features of the 'flow' state include:

- Being composed, but alert and energized (not too relaxed but not over aroused). Thriving on pressure, wanting to be involved in the action and being proactive.
- Feeling of 'knowing what have to do', and belief that it can be done. Being 'focused' on the tasks at hand (not affected by distractions, a loss of self-consciousness), and having extraordinary awareness (clarity and certainty).
- Displaying spontaneous and automatic activity (merging of action and awareness). Having timing, space, and rhythm.
- Well-prepared physically and mentally, with both aspects peaking in harmony.

Through attention to these mostly mental aspects, athletes can move toward the achievement of peak performance. Five psychological principles evident in the description of the flow state are activation, concentration, motivation, confidence, and preparation.

Activation

The optimal level of activation is the most fundamental prerequisite for peak performance, and excessive anxiety the most common pre-competition worry for athletes. The relationship between arousal (the physiological component of anxiety) and performance is best understood diagrammatically (Fig. 18.1). Although other models (e.g. reversal theory) have become more popular, the 'inverted-U hypothesis' portrayed in Fig. 18.1 remains the most applied model of arousal control. The model indicates, that as arousal improves performance to a certain point—performance declines if arousal continues to climb. A curvilinear relationship exists between arousal and performance. Too much or too little arousal impairs performance. The desirable state (optimal arousal level) is at the point before the curve arches downwards or where the line levels off. This point (Fig. 18.1) varies according to sporting task and across individuals. A variation on this model, the 'catastrophe theory', indicates that the arousal–performance relationship is not symmetrical. Instead, once anxiety exceeds appropriate levels, performance deteriorates rapidly rather than gradually.

Treatment: if an athlete is experiencing too much anxiety, intervention at both somatic and cognitive levels should be conducted. Arousal can be lowered through relaxation exercises (e.g. deep diaphragmatic breathing, progressive muscle relaxation, biofeedback). Psychologists train athlete's in mental strategies to help control dysfunctional thoughts (which are essentially perceptions of environmental demands), effectively plan for sporting tasks, and build self-confidence. Behavioral interventions such as systematic desensitization (where through gradual exposure athletes come to tolerate situations that created anxiety or discomfort for them, see Anxiety disorders, p624) and performance simulation are also applied if appropriate. Additionally, coaches can be educated on how to lower the pressures on their athletes. In extreme cases, athletes may be experiencing symptoms of an anxiety disorder which require clinical

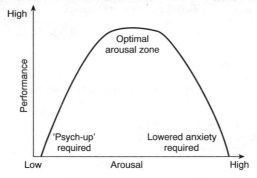

Fig. 18.1 The 'inverted-U hypothesis': relationship between arousal and performance

attention (see later). *It must not be neglected that athletes can also be underaroused*, a state often associated with apathy and a lack of focus or wandering thoughts. As with over arousal, multimodial intervention needs to be conducted to 'psych-up' lethargic or unassertive athletes.

Concentration

Concentration, attention, or focus are also significant elements of successful sporting performance. Athletes (as with humans generally) have limitations in what they can attend to at any one time. Athletes need to display *selective attention* or be 'focused on the right thing at the right time'. Athletes need to:

- Concentrate on task-salient cues (events or things in the environment) while simultaneously ignoring extraneous or irrelevant information. This includes focusing on the present and putting aside previous errors.
- Display flexibility or shiftability in their concentration (i.e. alter width and direction of attention). This includes switching to relaxing cues after or in between intense mental efforts in order to regulate mental energy.
- Sustain alertness (sensitivity to environment) throughout sporting events, and respond quickly to events.

A widely applied model of attentional focus (Nideffer) is presented in Fig. 18.2. The dimension of direction refers to the source of things attended to; either in the sporting environment (external) or within the individual (internal). The dimension of width refers to the number of cues that receive attention at one time; ranging from broad (many cues) to narrow (a few cues only). Skilled athletes switch between cues that are optimally task-relevant (including refocusing after distraction). For example, they move attention from play in general (broad focus) to the particular motor skill they are performing (narrow focus). If athletes do not maintain the *appropriate attentional style* (i.e. broad–internal, narrow–internal, broad–internal, narrow–external) for the various tasks they perform (examples shown in Fig. 18.2) they will have problems. Athletes can also be negatively affected by overloads of internal (e.g. to many instructions or game plans to apply) or external (e.g. lots of other competitors to watch) stimuli.

Treatment: for some athletes, a clear and practical description of the Nideffer model (Fig. 18.2) is sufficient for the self-development of positive attentional strategies. Other athletes, may require more intensive training in concentration. Generic and sport-related interventions include: exercises for clearing the mind (letting thoughts go), the maintenance of focus on a particular object/s, the performance of mental tasks while confronted with distractions, and cognitive structuring (e.g. parking thoughts); controlled breathing; goal setting/performance planning; positive self-talk; mental rehearsal; the development of cue words or checklists (events, things, or thoughts for an athlete to associate with specific concentration points, e.g. 'head down' when shooting for goal); performance simulation; and the use of biofeedback and video feedback equipment. Regular practice of skills is essential if athletes are to improve. An individualized training program can be developed according to the assessment of attentional deficits (the TAIS questionnaire, based on the Nideffer

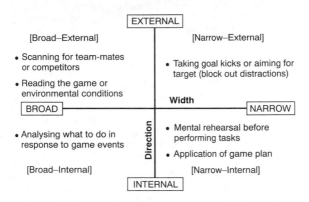

Fig. 18.2 The Nideffer model of attentional focus

model, can be used). Long-term or consistent deficits in an athlete's concentration may be due to, or symptomatic of, some psychopathological problem requiring clinical attention.

Motivation

It is essential for athletes to be motivated and confident. Motivation involves the energization and direction of behavior. Individuals vary in the degree they are influenced by intrinsic/internal (e.g. fun, personal mastery) or extrinsic/external (e.g. approval from significant others, material rewards, winning) sources of motivation. Similarly, achievement orientation (an ego or task goal approach to performance, and desire for success or fear of failure) differs among athletes. Furthermore, as an athlete experiences transitions in his/ her life, sources of motivation are likely to change in a corresponding manner.

Treatment: an understanding of what is important to each particular athlete, is a prerequisite for intervention to increase motivation. Also, any reasons for a loss in motivation should be assessed. Research has found that internal sources of motivation (because these involve factors which athletes have control over) and a positive task orientation (which leads to greater intensity and persistence) are most related to successful performance. These factors, in conjunction with each individual athlete's identified sources of motivation, should be addressed in an enthusiastic manner with the athlete. It is useful to bring in a person who is held in high regard by the athlete and has good communication skills to discuss such issues with the athlete. As a protocol, *it is important*: to never assume what motivates each athlete, to not overestimate the importance of personality factors (traits) relative to environmental influences, and to have athletes focus on achieving positives rather than avoiding negatives. The setting of specific, challenging, but realistic goals is the most commonly used strategy to aid motivation.

Confidence

618

An athlete's self-confidence encompasses their general state of being and their confidence in undertaking specific sporting tasks of relevance. Self-confidence has a large cognitive element, whereby a person forms subjective judgments about their ability to perform successfully certain tasks or meet certain environmental demands. The point that perceptions and attitudes are involved forms the basis for interventions aimed at improving an athlete's self-confidence.

Treatment: strategies that can be used (in conjunction with coaches) to raise an athlete's confidence in relation to sporting tasks include: imagery of successful performance accomplishments, actual successful performance accomplishments (through favorable game simulations and drills at training), utilization of genuine and credible verbal reinforcement from coaches and peers, frequent self-affirmations, self-talk and thought control during performance, and the setting and subsequent achievement of appropriate attainable goals. Since athletes perceptions of their actual performance can override gains from most confidence-building techniques (performance accomplishments provide the most potent information for judgments related to self-confidence), mental skills trainers should aim to use previous successful performance as the primary catalyst for efficacy of future performance.

If an athlete is experiencing a general loss of confidence in their life, a psychologist can employ global strategies or undertake personal development focusing on the 'whole' person. As a first step in this therapeutic process, athletes explore their self-image and personal belief systems, identify aspects which provide barriers for them or which they require healing on, and emphasis the productive attitudes they hold. Changing confidence at this level takes time. Unconstructive thought patterns (e.g. constant attributions in external or 'uncontrollables' terms) are usually entrenched.

Preparation

Surprisingly, the obvious prerequisite for success, preparation or organization, is frequently given insufficient attention by athletes. Athletes often need reminding about the importance of looking after themselves physically, following appropriate pre-competition routines, and having game plans, etc.

Stress management

Because of the amount of exercise athletes undertake, they are often regarded as not being stressed. However, athletes engage in exercise to achieve a high performance level, which places immense pressure on them, and means that they do not always achieve the health benefits that come with non-competitive physical activity. Both sport-related rigors and non-sporting pressures (relationships, shortage of time, developing a career outside of sport, financial concerns) lead to specific performance problems (e.g. excessive self-focus, 'choking') and a general proneness to stress. Furthermore, with numerous physical and psychological demands due to intense training and competition over the course of their careers, athletes are susceptible to injury, overtraining and burn-out. In cases of *burn-out* (characterized by exhaustion, negative responses to others, depressed mood, and being overwhelmed by stressors), time away from sport for reassessment of goals and the undertaking of stress management is a necessity. Interventions in regard to injuries and overtraining are discussed in detail in later sections of this chapter.

Stress management intervention involves techniques employed in anxiety control for somatic and cognitive aspects (see p626), training in planning and organizational skills, and coping strategies for dealing with pressure. A role of the sports psychologist is to facilitate the personal development of athletes; to assist them to develop, and effectively use, a range of coping strategies and problem-solving processes. This includes removing maladaptive strategies an athlete has applied (e.g. excessive avoidance behavior or withdrawal, substance use—see p630), and devising interventions that improve the ways he/she copes with sports-specific and life stressors. Assessment of the athlete's current coping strategies is an important part of the process of determining the most useful intervention mix. An athlete's coping style can be monitored through questionnaires such as the Ways of Coping With Sport (WOCS), and Mental Attributes of Performance (MAPS). Response patterns can be considered in relation to sports-specific research on the most effective or adaptive coping styles. A model for training coping skills involves instruction in the control of emotions, organizing and filtering feedback information, planning responses, and executing responses. It should be particularly noted, that in team sports, each individual athlete has additional resources to draw upon (team-mates), but also additional stressors.

Individual differences

It is of interest to know, that the existence of intuitively appealing relationships between sport and personality can be accorded only mythological status. Research has failed to show either that success in sport depends on the possession of certain personal characteristics, or that certain individuals are best suited to certain sports or positions. Although personality traits offer little discrimination between athletes, or between athletes and non-athletes, there are some individual differences (IDs) in sport to consider:

1 There are IDs on the dimensions of anxiety, concentration, and mood. These vary according to sporting tasks and /or whether athletes are skilled or novice performers. Psychometric tests such as the SCAT (Sport Competition Anxiety Test, and the later version,

CSAI-2), the TAIS (Test of Attentional and Interpersonal Style), and the POMS (Profile of Mood States) measure athletes' level of anxiety, style of attention, and mental strength, respectively. Athletes with inappropriate scores on these factors can benefit from the interventions outlined in the previous sections of this chapter.

2 There are IDs in the prevalence of certain mental disorders across sports. Suggestions that a higher prevalence of personality disorders exists among martial arts participants has anecdotal support, while there is epidemiological data to validate the assumed higher prevalence of eating disorders among gymnasts.

Clinical problems: psychological disorders

Athletes will generally display positive, goal-driven behavior and behave in such a way to facilitate improvement or maximal performance. They typically do not concern themselves with being psychologically 'sick' or 'ill'. Nevertheless, athletes can develop mental illness, often in reaction to certain environmental events. Because of the athletic environment they are in, athletes can be reluctant to acknowledge they have a mental disorder, but in most cases an early diagnosis improves prognosis considerably. Treating an athlete's underlying disorder will help improve both their sporting performance and life in general. Three notable categories of disorder most relevant to athletes, depressive, anxiety, and eating disorders (all classified in the *Diagnostic and statistical manual of mental disorders*, version IV: DSM IV; American Psychiatric Association 1994), are considered in this section. Descriptions of symptoms (diagnostic criteria are taken directly from the DSMIV), prevalence rates, features specific to an athlete population, and treatment models are provided for each disorder.

The DSMIV is a widely used classification system which meets the need for a coherent diagnosis of disordered behavior. The DSMIV is somewhat linked to the ICD9 and ICD10. Often, athletes do not display all the symptoms required for a classification of a specific mental disorder, but commit behavior that can be regarded as maladaptive and inappropriate for the team or sporting environment they are a part of, and thus still require alleviation of symptoms.

Treatment of psychological disorders typically involves either psychotherapy or pharmacotherapy. Both treatment approaches typically take a few weeks to show improvement of symptoms. Psychologists cannot legally administer drugs to athletes, so drug treatment is best undertaken by psychiatrists. Because of drug use standards and restrictions in sports, the physician conducting pharmacological treatment with an athlete must be extremely sensitive and knowledgeable in the area. The Australian Drug Agency (ADA), responsible for the drug testing of athletes in that country, can provide information on drugs permissible to be used in competitive sport. Also, the fact that side-effects from drugs can affect both an athlete's training and competition performance needs to be foremost in the mind of those undertaking pharmacotherapy. Additionally, issues of 'duration', 'gradual discontinuation', and 'relapse' are implicated in any drug-based program. Psychologists will use clinical judgment and additional information to determine the nature of an athlete's problems and formulate a specific treatment plan. However, if an athlete is experiencing a severe disorder rendering them fully dysfunctional the only option may be to admit them as an inpatient to a psychiatric institution.

Akin to medical diagnosis, a cautious approach needs to be taken in categorizing athletes' mental problems, as labels can be damaging. Besides being stigmatizing and long lasting, classification may lead an athlete to perceive themselves as intrinsically sick and to not take responsibility for their problems. The focus of diagnosis should be the presenting behavior or disorder, not the athlete *per se*. Also, the severity and course of symptoms should always be considered. An athlete may have more than on disorder, which may (e.g. major depressive disorder and panic disorder) or may not be related. The multiaxial assessment approach recommended by the DSMIV system enables for principal and secondary diagnosis. Additionally, it considers any relevant 'general medical conditions', 'psychosocial and environmental' stressors, and an individual's 'global assessment of functioning'.

Depression

Major depressive disorder (MDD), dysthymic disorder (DD), and bipolar disorder (BD), with both manic and depressive episodes are the most notable metal illnesses which have a disturbance in mood as the predominant feature. Of these, athletes experience major depression, in particular, most often bought on by a stressful event such as a serious injury. Lifetime risk can be as high as 15% (25% for females).

To meet the diagnostic criteria for MD Disorder one (single episode) or more (recurrent) MD episodes need to have occurred, and a manic episode not have occurred. An MD episode constitutes at least 2 weeks of continual depressed mood or loss of interest/pleasure compared to normal functioning, and at least 4 weeks of: changes in weight/appetite, sleep, or psychomotor activity; decreased energy; feelings of worthlessness or guilt-delusional negative self-evaluations; difficulty thinking, concentrating, or making decisions; suicidal ideation, plans or attempts. Symptoms must not be better accounted for by recent bereavement or another source of grief, and need to cause significant distress, or impairment in the athlete's functioning. DD is characterized by at least 2 years of depressed mood for more days than not, accompanied by additional depressive symptoms that do not met the criteria for a MDE: self-esteem; poor concentration; and feelings of hopelessness. DD can be distinguished from MDD by its more chronic and persistent (but less severe) depressive symptoms. Individuals with DD often have superimposed MDD.

Prevalence: about 5% and 3% of the general population are affected by MDD and DD, respectively, in any given year. Females twice as much as males.

Athletes: increased likelihood after serious injury or overtraining. Athletes suffering from depression lack motivation to compete in their sport, but participation can alleviate some of the symptoms of depression. Substances use may exacerbate depression and worsen prognosis.

Treatment: a combination of psychotherapy and antidepressants is best in most circumstances. Clinical assessment is the first part of the treatment process. Drug treatment is required for severe cases, as sufferers are usually not in a satisfactory state for talk-based therapy. Medication can stabilize behavior enabling counseling to occur. In mild or moderate cases, or when depression is related to a particular event or stressor, psychotherapy should be the primary option.

Consideration of the five Ss provides a guide for drug use: if there is high Severity and Stupor, a need for Speed of treatment, Somatic symptoms, and an absence of Suicidal ideation (low overdose risk) then drug treatment can be the preferred option. However, the athlete must be supportive of the use of drugs (and vice versa with therapy) or compliance will be low. Neurotransmitters implicated in the pathophysiology of depressive disorders include norepinephrine, epinephrine, serotonin, acetylcholine, and dopamine. Tricyclic antidepressants (e.g. imipramine), MAOIs (e.g. phenelzine), and newer reuptake inhibitors are all able to be enacted depending on the athlete's situation. For tricyclics, dosages of around 150mg/day are recommended. Prozac (fluoxetine), 20–60mg/day, a selective serotonin uptake inhibitor, is increasingly favored for the treatment of depression, mainly because it can be given less frequently than once a day. All classes of drug have advantages and disadvantages. The choice of antidepressant should take into account the athlete's previous responses to medication and their preferred drug/s, his/her particular symptoms (e.g. if insomnia is present a more sedative drug is required), the speed of therapeutic effect required, the impact of side-effects on sporting tasks, overdose potential, and the clinician's personal preference and previous experience. A combination of drugs is usually applied for resistant depression. Although often maligned, electroconvulsive therapy (ECT) is also an effective option with resistant or life threatening depression. Bilateral ECT is generally more effective than unilateral, but can cause some memory disturbances.

Depending on the nature of the individual athlete (i.e. their education, verbosity, emotional expressiveness) rationale emotive therapy (Albert Ellis) or client center counselling (Carl Rogers) are typically the most useful psychotherapy methods to overcome depression. However, most psychologists take an eclectic approach to the treatment of depression.

Suicide

Up to 15% of individuals with severe MDD commit suicide. Other athletes not diagnosable with a depression disorder also kill themselves. It is important to detect some of the signs of suicide. **Warning signs include**:

- A move from general or transient thoughts of committing suicide, to frequent, specific, and feasible plans (practical and with high lethality) of how to commit suicide.
- Increasingly strong (sincerely held) beliefs that 'others would be better off' if they were dead.
- History of previous attempts themselves, or of friends or family members who committed suicide.
- Apparent sudden change in mood to happiness and calmness after continuous depressed mood.
- Saying goodbye to people, putting personal affairs in order (e.g. selling belongings).
- Statements such as 'I won't be at training next week', 'I will miss our appointment next week'.
- Alcohol or drug use, while an absence of social support in living arrangements, etc.
- Unusual interest in how others are feeling.
- Preoccupation with death and violence themes.

Anxiety disorders[1]

As with those for depression, the consequences of untreated anxiety disorders are poor physical and emotional health, substance abuse,

1 W Coryell, G Winokur 1991 *The clinical management of anxiety disorders.* OUP

and long term impairments in social functioning. Phobias, which involve clinically significant anxiety in relation to objects, places or situations are the most significant (*social phobia is the most common type among athletes*), but are typically the least severe. The DSMIV describes a number of more intense anxiety disorders, including the two addressed in this section, and other such as obsessive-compulsive disorder (OCD) and acute stress disorder. The DSMIV also differentiates disorder 'due to a general medical condition' and that which is 'substance-induced'.

Panic attacks are a part of several anxiety disorders. A panic attack is a discrete period in which there is a sudden onset of intense apprehension, fearfulness, or terror, often associated with feelings of impending doom. Symptoms present during these attacks are the following (at least 4 for diagnosis): pounding heart, sweating, trembling, shortness of breath, choking sensation, chest discomfort, nausea, dizziness, depersonalization (being detached from oneself), feeling of loss of control, fear of death, paresthesia, and chills or hot flushes. Symptoms develop abruptly and reach a peak within 10min. The onset of panic attacks can either be associated with (expected), or not associated with (unexpected), situational triggers (e.g. seeing a certain competitor or performing in front of a large crowd).

Panic disorder is characterized by recurrent unexpected (absence of a consistent situational trigger) panic attacks about which there is persistent concern. To meet the diagnostic criteria, at least one of the attacks needs to be followed by at least 1 month of persistent concern about having another panic attack, worry about the possible implications or consequences of the panic attacks (e.g. 'going crazy'), or a significant behavioral change related to the attacks. Panic attacks better accounted for by phobias or OCD do not constitute panic disorder.

Generalized anxiety disorder (GAD) is characterized by at least 6 months of persistent and excessive anxiety and worry which the individual finds difficult to control. The anxiety or worry causes distress or impairment in social, occupational and sporting areas of functioning. To meet the diagnostic criteria, 3 of the following symptoms need to accompany the anxiety and worry: restlessness, being easily fatigued, difficulty concentrating, irritability, muscle tension, and disturbed sleep. Additionally, the focus of the anxiety can not be confined to features of another specific disorder (e.g. social phobia, OCD). For both disorders, disturbance must not be due to the physiological effects of substance use (e.g. caffeine intoxication) or a general medical condition (e.g. hyperthyroidism).

Prevalence: between 3% and 5% of the population suffer from an anxiety disorder at any one time. For panic disorder, 1-year prevalence rates are between 1% and 2%. Twice as likely with females than males. For GAD, 1-year prevalence rates are around 3%. Two-thirds of cases are female, one-third male.

Athletes: panic attack symptoms may constitute difficulties with sporting performance. With GAD, apprehensive expectation can be about a number of events or activities but typically centers around sporting performance, the focus of which may shift from one aspect to another. Athletes may worry about being humiliated or excessively scrutinized, with anxiety increasing as performance approaches. The intensity, duration, or frequency of the anxiety is far out of proportion to the actual likelihood or impact of the event of concern. In some cases, criteria for GAD may not be met, but symptoms for *social phobia* (see DSMIV criteria) may be present. Adolescent athletes in particular have concern over quality of performance even when their performance is not being evaluated by others. Young athletes (under 18) away from home, may also be experiencing *separation anxiety disorder* which is characterized by anxiety related to separation from parental or personal figures (see DSMIV or diagnostic criteria).

Treatment: referral to a psychologist for clinical assessment enables consideration of the type of cognitive-behavioral and/or drug-based intervention to be undertaken. The athlete's preference should also be taken into account. Two classes of antidepressants (tricyclics and MAOIs) and certain high potency benzodiazepines (e.g. alprazolam, clonazepam) are used to reduce or eliminate the panic attacks associated with panic disorder. Benzodiazepines are most often the medication of choice. In particular, Xanax (alprazolam) approved by the US FDA for the treatment of panic disorder has often been used but is not recommended. However, anxiolytics are not suitable for those athletes who have a predisposition for, or history of, substance use problems. The tricyclic antidepressants have the disadvantages of not being tolerated by a significant proportion (30%) of individuals and taking longer to achieve effect. MAOIs require diet restrictions. Also, all drugs have notable side-effects (e.g. drowsiness, amnesia, constipation, psychomotor impairment) which need to be considered in relation to the athlete's sporting and non-sporting tasks. If after 8 weeks no benefit is seen from a medication, an antipanic drug from another class is usually used. For treatment of GAD, sufferers typically take minor antidepressants or tranquilizers as an adjunct to psychotherapy. SSRIs (fluoxamine, paroxietine, prozac) are more effective and less dependent.

Psychotherapy for panic disorder usually follows a cognitive-behavioral approach. Advanced exposure therapy (beginning with situations that bring the least fear and moving towards those most difficult to tolerate), hyperventilation control (breathing) exercises are the most common interventions employed by psychologists. Therapy is similar for GAD, however, because of the generalized anxiety responses associated with this disorder, there is less emphasis on stimulus control measures and more on anxiety management in general (e.g. allocation of worry time, sophisticated relaxation techniques).

Preliminary research suggests that combinations of cognitive-behavioural therapy and pharmacological treatment have the potential to show the highest clinical effectiveness for panic disorder and GAD.

'Eating disorders'[1,2]

Athletes are a population prone to eating disorders. This is particularly the case for those involved in sports where a thin figure or controlled weight are desirable or necessary (e.g. gymnasts, synchronized swimmers, runners, boxers, figure skaters, wrestlers, jockeys,

1 KD Brownell *et al* 1992 *Eating, body weight, and performance in athletes.* Lea & Febiger, Philadelphia 2 YR Thompson, R Sherman 1993 *Helping athletes with eating disorders.* Human Kinetics, Champaign, IL. USA

divers). Furthermore, weight management is necessary part of most athletes' training. However, it can go awry. Eating disorders are characterized by disturbances in eating behavior and in the perception of body shape and weight.

Anorexia nervosa is diagnosed when: an athlete refuses to maintain bodyweight at or above a minimally normal weight for age and height, has an intense fear of gaining weight or becoming fat (even though underweight), and exhibits a signification disturbance in the perception of the shape or size of his/her body. In addition, postmenarcheal females with this disorder are amenorrheic. Actual loss in appetite does not necessary occur, but individuals suffering from anorexia are often preoccupied with thoughts of food (e.g. collect recipes, hoard food). Usually, weight loss is a result of excessive dieting. However, a subtype of anorexia involves purging, with or without binge eating.

Bulimia nervosa is differentiated from anorexia nervosa primarily by the maintenance of bodyweight at or above a minimally normal level (though fear of gaining weight is strong). Bulimia has the essential features of recurrent episodes of binge eating (eating an abnormal amount of food in a discrete period and have a sense of lack of control over its consumption) with inappropriate compensatory methods (e.g. vomiting, use of laxatives, fasting, excessive exercise) to prevent weight gain. In addition, self-evaluation is unduly influenced by body shape and weight. To meet the diagnosis, the binge eating and compensatory behaviors must occur (on average) at least twice a week for 3 months. Individuals with bulimia usually attempt to conceal their symptoms and binge eat and purge in secrecy. They also tend to restrict calorie consumption between binges.

Prevalence: currently around 1% and 2%, for anorexia nervosa and bulimia nervosa, respectively; incidences of eating disorders among young females in the general population appear to be increasing. More than 90% of individuals with either disorder are female, but with athletes this disparity is less. Prevalence rates for athletes are higher than for the general population. Research has reported incidences as high as 20% (40% female) of bulimia among athletes. Gymnastics has been found to have the most incidence for females, while for males, eating disorders are most common among wrestlers and jockeys.

Athletes: the most common method employed by athletes to lose weight is calorie restriction, but self-induced vomiting is not uncommon. The semistarvation characteristic of anorexia and the purging behavior of bulimia significantly impair and athletes' physical capacity. Additionally, mental functioning is typically disturbed. In the case of bulimia, athlete's use of exercise as a means to purge food consumed during binge eating can interfere with training schedules.

By recognizing the signs and symptoms that typically proceed the establishment of the full diagnostic criteria for an eating disorder an athlete can be helped earlier. Behaviors such as eating alone, weight loss (or in the case of bulimia, weight fluctuations), and mood changes are of note. Other indications of a developing eating disorder may be apparent through a medical examination. Medical symptoms include anemia, leukopenia, osteopenia, renal and liver problems, peripheral edema, dental problems (from vomiting), and gastrointestinal problems. **Treatment:** raising the issue of treatment with an athlete is not easy due to the secretive nature of the disorders and (as with all major psychological problems) the athlete's fear of being dropped from a team or program. In mild cases, or in the early stages of the disorder, inform athletes about safe and effective methods of weight management. Give them written and video material (which is increasingly available) on eating disorders in sport. In most cases, referral to individual therapy (which focuses on affective expression, cognitive-behavioral work, and a psychological-educational approach), group therapy (involving other supportive athletes, and used as an adjunct to individual therapy), or family therapy (including the coach) is advisable. The assistance of a dietitian or nutritionist is also recommended. Medications that may be useful in conjunction with psychotherapy are benzodiazepines for anorexics and tricyclic anti-depressants for bulimics. The use of thyroid hormones, insulin, diuretics, and laxatives should be avoided. In life-threatening cases, hospitalization is required to restore weight and to address fluid and electrolyte imbalances.

Since the culture of many sports fosters are unhealthy focus on weight concerns (i.e. through weight restrictions, judging criteria, misunderstanding of body–type performance relationship, pressure from coaches and media), any treatment an athlete undertakes can be undone by continual exposure to damaging aspects of their sports culture. A truly effective solution for the problem of eating disorders needs to involve coach and peer education and a changing of the prevailing culture of certain sports.

Other clinical problems

There are other notable clinical problems athletes experience which are either not classified by the DSMIV or are best not considered as actual mental disorders. Three important problems of this class, substance use, injury rehabilitation, and overtraining/exercise addiction are addressed in this section.

629

Substance use problems[1,2]

At various times in his/her career, an athlete may take alcohol, *performance-enhancing drugs*, *recreational/illicit drugs*, or *prescribed* and *over the counter (OTC) medications*. Research shows that athletes use substances more often for recreational or medical purposes than for performance enhancement. Alcohol in particular, is used reasonably frequently by athletes, often in response to stress or injury. While any use of performance aiding drugs is forbidden in sport and thus is of clinical concern, use *per se* of the other three substance types does not constitute illness behavior. More contentious, is whether *abuse* of and *dependence* on these substances can be conceptualized as constituting a mental disorder. Alcohol, amphetamine, cannabis, cocaine, hallucinogen, inhalant, opioid, and phencyclidine categories of dependence and abuse are of interest; along with sedative, hypnotic, or anxiolytic dependence and abuse: all appear as disorders on the DSMIV diagnostic criteria for 'substance abuse' and 'substance dependence'. Substance use problems are best considered from an a theoretical perspective.

Athletes who experience *substance dependence* typically display symptoms of tolerance and withdrawal. *Withdrawal* symptoms vary from drug to drug, but are typically observable and measurable negative physical and psychological experiences whereby the substance needs to be taken to relieve the suffering. However, withdrawal is not evident with all drugs. Likewise, the case with tolerance symptoms (where more and more drug is required to achieve the same feeling). Cannabis, cocaine, and hallucinogens are all usually without physiological dependence (do not have both withdrawal and tolerance symptoms). A contentious point is whether drug dependence can still occur without this physiological dependence. Other symptoms for drug dependence are: compulsive drug taking behavior (including a craving or drive to use the substance) where much time and energy is based around activities related to substance use; a desire, and actual efforts, to cut down use, but excessive use continues; and continual use of substance despite experiencing significant problems related to its use. *Drug abuse* refers primarily to the latter symptoms. Athletes abusing a drug (or drugs) repeatedly use a substance while experiencing recurrent significant adverse consequences related to that substance use (e.g. they fail to met obligations, their performance declines, they have troubled interpersonal relations).

Repeated episodes of *substance intoxication* can lead to drug abuse and dependence. Symptoms of intoxication vary from drug to drug, but usually consist of behavioral and personality changes and observable effects on psychomotor and cognitive performance. Urine and blood tests are the most efficient means for determining intoxication after recent ingestion of drugs. However, depending on the drug, intoxication effects can last for a number of days. A great majority of athletes have experienced drug (usually alcohol) intoxication at some stage in their lives. Frequent substance intoxication does not necessary lead to abuse or dependence (addiction), however, in most cases overly frequent use of drugs (including medications and steroids) is not of benefit to the athlete. For most athletes, minimal drug use is appropriate. Nevertheless, despite perceptions of athletes of athletes as fitness and health fanatics, athletes levels of drug use are in line with those of the general population. Athletes in team sports or those regularly involved in social events or celebrations are particularly subject to peer pressure and sensation seeking which influences drug use. Alcohol is the substance most used by athletes, followed by cannabis. Also regularly used by a small percentage of athletes are, amphetamines, cocaine, anabolic steroids, and anxiolytics. Some individuals use more than one substance, and as with the general population, some individuals use more than one substance. As with the general population, some individuals are more predisposed to excessive or dysfunctional usage of substances than others. Further, male athletes are more at risk for alcohol abuse problems, being at least twice as likely as females to become heavy drinkers, and drinking to intoxication twice as often. Gender differences for other drugs (except anxiolytics) are similar.

Signs and symptoms of substance abuse among athletes include:

- Self-reports of some drinking or drug use, simultaneous with reports of current sporting or life stressors.
- Given the rules that regulate drug use in the athletic environment, denial and secrecy usually surrounds drug use. If an athlete is overt enough to come to practice or competition under the influence of a substance (even if minor), it is very likely symptomatic of more severe abuse or dependence issues in the rest of their life.
- Also of concern is if an athlete frequently misses training.
- Major changes in sporting performance (decline–recreational drugs, improvement–performance enhancers), and increased disturbances in mood, are also indicators. As is, marked changes in personality and behavior, and memory loss.
- Physiological indicators include abnormal blood and urine samples, changes in blood pressure or respiratory rate, vitamin B deficiencies, needle marks (intravenous administration), and erosion of nasal septum (due to snorting, i.e. cocaine and amphetamines).
- Alcohol-dependent individuals can have high levels of substance in blood but few visible intoxication effects. (Although there are few withdrawal symptoms, tolerance is high for alcohol.
- With amphetamine (particularly 'diet pills') and cocaine abuse, significant weight loss, or weight cycling may be apparent.

Treatment: there is a 25% spontaneous remission rate for individuals diagnosed with substance abuse or dependence. Recovery usually follows a severe life threat, such as the pending termination of sporting career. However, all individuals recovering from substance use problems remain vulnerable for relapse. Thus, judgments of remission should be considered provisional, with follow-up work required. Nevertheless, an individual will overcome substance use problems much easier if no withdrawal symptoms were originally present.

Education programs conducted should focus on skills rather than knowledge. For *alcohol and illicit drugs*, education on the health problems associated with abuse (e.g. liver damage (cirrhosis), heart problems, impotence, and loss of brain cells), is of limited value; especially with drug-dependent individuals, who are usually aware of the problems substance use brings them and wish to stop drug use but cannot. It is hard for athletes to accept any negative effects of *performance-enhancing substances* (e.g. irritability, depression, mania, impotence, liver problems, impairment of psychomotor skills), and with physiological dependence unlikely, the threat of getting caught and banned is the main factor controlling usage patterns of these type of drugs. However, promoting alternative methods to get the edge (e.g. hyperbaric chambers, mental skills training) does help to overcome the problem. The biggest barrier to overcoming the abuse of *prescribed and OTC medications* is the easy availability of these drugs to athletes. To be effective, education programs need to be multidimensional (cognitive-behavioral–affective), both information-providing and experiential, and consider the issue of substance abuse in its broadest sense.

All treatment protocols for substance use should involve individual therapy by a drug and alcohol specialist and aim to include group therapy involving family, team-mates, and coach. The focus of individual psychotherapy should be on the acknowledgment of the problem; willingness to change; strategies to moderate or replace behavior; and empowering and skilling the athlete to bring about the necessary change. If receiving outpatient treatment, athletes can still maintain occupational, family, and even sporting pursuits. In severe cases (where major detoxification is required), inpatient chemical dependency programs may need to be accessed. Controlled drinking or drug programs, with a variety of support group sources, are increasingly recommended over AA (or NA, narcotics, CA, cocaine, etc.) as a treatment option for most substances. Recovery and compliance rates for AA are low. Nevertheless, all athletes with substance use problems should initially aim to abstain from their substance of abuse (whether or not they chose to access AA, and irrespective of their long-term wish for controlled use). If an athlete does wish to attend AA, additional counseling is essential.

1 JR May, MJ Asken 1987 *Sport psychology the psychological health of the athlete.* PMA, USA **2** J Orford 1985 *Excessive appetites. A psychological view of addictions.* Wiley, New York

633

Psychological aspects of injury rehabilitation[1,2]

To an athlete, injury can represent a loss of ability, identity, esteem, and social support. In addition to physical pain, athletes often feel frustrated at not being able to participate in a significant part of their life, experience trouble undertaking other daily life activities, are fearful of losing their place in the team and/or feel bad about letting the team down, are uncertain about the future, and may experience a loss of income (lifestyle) and a break-up in their social system. Psychological problems impact strongly on recovery from injury and can also be antecedents to future injuries. This section considers the rehabilitation and prevention of non career-ending injuries. (The issue of career transition due to injury provides a separate topic not discussed here.)

Although a grieving process occurs after an injury, it is debatable whether it is akin to that which follows the loss of close friend or relative, or similar to that experienced by terminally ill patients (5 stages of: denial, anger, bargaining, depression, acceptance). In the medium term, responses to injuries range from coping positively, to extremely maladaptive responses. Mood disturbance and lowered self-confidence are two negative correlates on injury. In some cases, sporting injury can lead to major depression or to substance dependency. Furthermore, poor adjustment to injury often leads to exacerbated injuries or delayed recovery.

Signs and symptoms: there are warning signs of poor adjustment to injury:

- Extended social withdrawal (but nomal in the short term)
- Prolonged depression
- Suffering of high levels of stress
- Evidence of persistent anger, confusion, apathy, or feelings of helplessness
- Notable changes in mood or personality
- Repetitive (obsessive-like) focus on 'When will I be able to play again', etc
- Excessive impatience
- A history of problematic injury rehabilitation
- Injury appears to be taking control of athlete's life (i.e. they make comments such as 'I have to see how pain is before I do anything')
- Additionally, there are situational factors which make recovery more difficult:
  - evidence that athlete bought injury upon him/herself to save face (e.g. to leave team they did not want to be in, to avoid being dropped) or that secondary gain occurred from injury (e.g. get out of training)
  - athlete has high ego involvement in the sport (i.e. it is the most important thing in his/her life)
  - Athlete's support network (family, coach) react negatively to injury circumstances surrounding it's onset
  - Recovery progress is slow and the athlete is negatively affected by this.

1 A Petitpas, Danish 1995 *Sports psychology. Interventions.* In S. Murphy (ed) Human Kinetics, IL **2** D Yukelson, S Murphy 1992 In P. Renstron (ed) *Sports injuries. Basic principles of prevention and care.* Blackwell Scientific, USA

Treatment should focus on attending to the person and not just the injury. It is important to understand what injury means to each individual athlete. Assessment of the specific intrapsychic, interpersonal and situational factors impacting on the athlete provides a useful starting point. Treatment should aim to alleviate the distress caused by injury (primarily psychotherapy, PST, methods). Psychologists are a useful part of the rehabilitation team. The athlete's support systems (family, coach, and team-mates) should also be bought into the healing process.

A protocol for those involved in an athlete's rehabilitation to follow is:

1 If necessary, grief issues should be worked through.

2 Encourage the athlete to adhere to the physiotherapist's rehabilitation program; to follow guidelines, resist playing and to undertake prescribed exercises. Adherence is moderated by motivation, social support, and life stress, but the athlete also needs to believe in the treatment program (check if they do).

3 Efforts should be made to keep the athlete involved in some capacity with the sport (provided they do not dwell on what competition they are missing, and do not get diminished attention). Coaches need to be educated not to neglect athletes who are injured, which often happens when they are not partaking in training or playing. This is especially important as injured athletes typically require more sensitivity and attentiveness than on injured athletes. It is also important to get assurances that the athlete will not necessary be dropped from the team if they take the necessary time to recovery.

4 Generate alternative activities for the athlete to do in the extra time they now have. These may include other sporting activities.

5 Be conscious of not rushing the athlete's psychological progress. Changes in an athlete's stress level can be monitored through the use of questionnaires (see section on injury prevention below). Anxious and concerned athletes are more likely to take short cuts in their rehabilitation programs, and end up prolonging the recovery process.

6 Strategies to deal with set-backs in progress should be planned. PST work can be done in the areas of:

- *Increasing coping resources* (stress management).
- *Imagery* is a practice where the athlete creates certain mental images of the self, a particular idea or situation, or a desired or experience emotional response. Both technical and kinesthetic images utilizing all the senses can be produced. For an injured athlete, imagery can be used as a substitute for physical practice (mental rehearsal), and to facilitate the healing process (visualization of fibers mending and tissue being restored).
- *Goal setting*
- *Positive self-talk* to overcome negativity associated with injury.

Due to a loss in confidence and a more cautious approach, athletes returning to competition after injury may not push themselves as much as before their injury. Coaches need to be considerate of this. However, if such behavior persists beyond the short term it is likely to lead to negative performance outcomes and negative psychological states. Attention to this issue may be required in follow-up rehabilitation sessions.

Injury prevention

The likelihood of both injury recurrence and fresh injuries can be reduced by appropriate preventive intervention. Stress seems to increase the likelihood of injury. Education on the value of thorough sporting preparation (i.e. arriving at training or competition in time so not rushed and not tense), on lowering arousal during games (so concentration is broad enough to see potential dangers), and on how to reduce or cope with life stress, are all useful.

An athlete's level of stress can be assessed through scales such as Daily Hassles, Occupational Stress Inventory, Athletic Life Experiences Survey (ALES), and the Social and Athletic Re-adjustment Scale (SARS). Overly stressed athletes should consider treatment before further participation, just as they would if they had a physical condition requiring attention.

Overtraining/exercise addiction[1,2]

Some athletes seem to cope with high training loadings well. However, others overextend themselves physically and psychologically in training, leading to chronic fatigue, injury, illness, and underperformance (also see above section on stress management—burnout). Additionally, for some athletes, exercise behaviors constitute obsessive or addictive behavior (over-reliance on sporting activity for daily well-being and/or personal identity) ultimately leading to depression and other psychological problems. *Excessive training or exercise behavior is most common in running-based training.* **Signs and symptoms:**

Sports signs:
- inappropriate increments in training schedules, or resumption in sporting activities too soon after injury (including neglecting to follow rehabilitation program)
- staleness in performance
- intolerance to training and decreased maximum work output
- nagging injuries
- concentration lapses
- unable to met non-sport commitments, or an absence of life outside of sport

Physiological signs:
- hormonal changes (increased serum cortisol levels, decreased testosterone)
- chronic muscle soreness
- loss of bodyweight and percent body fat
- lowered immune system
- higher resting heart rate

Psychological signs:
- negative mood states (irritability, depression)
- loss of appetite
- sleep disturbance
- excessive concern with amount of training (tolerance effects, feelings of guilt if miss a training session)
- mental fatigue
- increasingly frequent feelings of a motivation, apathy

Unfortunately, it seems that many of these symptoms accompanying overtraining typically become evident only after a fully developed overtraining syndrome exists.

Treatment: clearly, pleasure from the release of endorphin an feelings of a great cardiovascular system are not solely responsible for an athlete's compulsion for excessive training or exercise. An understanding of the differing causes or reasons behind each individual athlete's excessive behavior is a prerequisite for any treatment approach. Following assessment, treatment strategies include:

- Rest (abstinence) from training, if possible, or greatly reduced and controlled training loads (realistic and reasonable), determined in conjunction with coach. Aim to get assurances that an athlete will not necessary be dropped from team if they cut back their training.

1 R Nideffer 1989 *Attention control training for athletes.* Enhanced Performance Services, USA   2 E Etzel et al (ed) 1991. *Counseling college student athletes: issues and intervention.* Fitness Information Technologies, USA

- During break or reduction in training, a psychologist can conduct stress management sessions, increasing an athletes coping resources in relation to training.
- Education of athletes and coaches about risks of overtraining, including emphasizing its negative impact on performance. However, this may fall on deaf ears if an athlete is addicted to their pursuits. For athletes concerned more about the 'buzz' from exercise, than performance outcomes, education can be focused on the fact that their excessive behavior is subject to tolerance effects and will result in increased time periods of dysphoric feelings and diminished pleasurable feelings (withdrawal effects).
- A psychologist looking to the generation of behavioral alternatives to replace some of the training. Or the use of indirect (somewhat manipulative) strategies to get athlete to stop or change behavior.
- The facilitation of improved coach–athlete communication. Athletes may feel that the coach is pushing them to hard. Conversely, coaches may be concerned an athlete is training too much, but are unable to say anything about it.

Interpersonal problems

The best way to react to an athlete reporting interpersonal problems is to listen attentively with empathy and regard. Assessment as to whether the athlete is involved in a specific interpersonal conflict, or whether they have insufficient interpersonal skills in general for success in their sport (and life) roles, provides information to guide intervention. Some athletes find sport too frustrating, and may need to address the issue of whether to give up their sport or make behavioral and attitudinal changes necessary to continue.

Clarification of certain issues (e.g. what the coach requires of the athlete) may need to be sought from other parties. On referral, a psychologist could facilitate conflict resolution (if appropriate and other parties available) and/or undertake communication training with the athlete. Depending on the athlete's needs, communication training (experiential in nature) could include:

- Assertiveness training
- Strategies for getting messages across in a clear and non threatening ways
- Effective/Active listening
- Leadership training
- Application of problem solving methods (individual and group)
- Career counseling
- Performance profiling (use of objective data to provide feedback to athlete)

19 Rehabilitation of sports injuries

PHILIPPA HARVEY-SUTTON,
STEPHEN F WILSON, SAUL GEFFEN

Life is movement, movement is life. Aristotle

Introduction

'Rehabilitation' is a generic term for the comprehensive treatment of injury and/or medical conditions. It has active and passive elements. It focuses on the whole person not just the injury and aims to restore the greatest possible degree of function in the shortest possible time. The factors implicated in the cause of injury should be addressed to prevent injury recurrence. Three concepts help with the understanding of the rehabilitation process: *impairment*, *disability*, and *handicap*.

Injury causes an individual an **impairment**. This is the injury at the tissue level e.g. ruptured medial collateral ligament of the knee. Impairment usually causes a **disability**. This is a loss of function e.g. walking with a limp and unable to run. This in turn may cause a **handicap** this is an individual's inability to perform tasks or engage in activities e.g. the professional footballer is unable to compete for the rest of the season due to the knee injury which causes loss of playing time, reducing his income and prematurely ending his career.

From these examples the need for the physician to consider the medical, physical, psychosocial, vocational and leisure requirements of the injured athlete is apparent. The areas covered in this chapter are:

1 Principles of rehabilitation
2 Key concepts
3 Treatment modalities
4 Complications of inadequate or incorrect rehabilitation
5 Prevention

Principles of rehabilitation

The process of athletic injury rehabilitation aims to minimize tissue damage and allow a safe return to activity. It is based on the science of tissue healing, knowledge of joint biomechanics, physiology of muscular strength and endurance, and the neurophysiological basis of skill retraining. Successful programs are based on an understanding of these constraints, which, when properly applied, permit the progressive activity of joints and muscles. Muscular strength, endurance, and power are redeveloped while flexibility and cardiovascular fitness are maintained. Precipitating factors are identified and addressed to minimize reinjury (1).

To understand, grade, and treat injuries the physician needs to identify the tissues involved. This chapter focuses on muscloskeletal injury and rehabilitation of bone, ligament, muscle, tendon, connective tissue, and neuromuscular structures combining to produce co-ordinated, purposeful movement. The treatment of other injuries is covered in the relevant chapters.

The healing process involves inflammatory, repair, and remodeling phases. There are detrimental effects of immobilization, muscle wasting and weakness, and subsequent joint damage. This leads to further immobilization and reflex inhibition, 'a vicious cycle' (see Fig. 13.15). Early mobilization is usually indicated. Lack of motion of joints results in shortening of capsular and other connective tissue structures supporting the joint, loss of lubrication, and alternating compression between joint surfaces deprives articular cartilage of nutrition (2). There are *detrimental systemic effects of immobilization*, these begin within hours and become clinically important within days. They include cardiovascular deconditioning, nervous system depression, skin sores, gastrointestinal complaints (constipation), thromboembolic genesis, bone resorbtion, and respiratory impairment (3). Thus the expression '**move it or lose it**'.

An understanding of the sport or activity is required, many injuries are sport-specific and communication is enhanced if the physician has some basic knowledge of the sports requirements. 'Profiling' is a concept that matches an individual's physiognomy with the type of athletic activity and in team sports their role.

647

Key concepts

Team approach

Rehabilitation is facilitated by a team approach. The basic team comprises:

- The injured athlete.
- The physical therapist.
- The doctor.
- Others; orthotist, brace maker, strapper, coach, exercise trainers, dietitian, psychologist, dentist, nurse, first aid personnel, peer group, family, and friends.

Diagnosis

History
present injury, past, athletic, social, family and psychological histories where required.

Examination
including measurement of impairment and function, comparison with unaffected limb, and review of biomechanical factors.

Investigations
these may include specific functional tests, pathology, radiology and nuclear medicine investigations where appropriate.

Problem list
particularly if the injury is complex or severe (4).

Acute injury management

Begins immediately and can be performed by the athlete or any other capable person. This phase lasts the first 24–48 hours. It consists of protecting the individual from further harm, resting, and iceing the injury. Compression and elevation are used to minimize oedema and hemorrhage and drugs are used for analgesia, anti-inflammatory properties and muscle spasm relief. Acute injury management is summarized by the acronym **PRICE** (Table 19.1). Occasionally, more extensive treatment or surgery is required.

Drugs

In general the authors feel that drug use should be minimized and the other components of injury management emphasized. Drugs used in rehabilitation of sports injuries are of four main groups:

1 **Analgesics**: paracetamol, codeine, opiates, and local anesthetic agents.
2 **Antiinflammatory** medications are used extensively and have analgesic properties as well as causing moderation of the inflammatory response to injury. A short course of 3–7 days can be useful. Compliance is better with once or twice daily dosing. Topical and parental antiinflammatory medications are now available. Gastric ulceration, hypertension, and renal impairment are among the side-effects of NSAIDs.
3 **Antispasmodics** and sedatives are utilized to reduce muscle spasm and consequent pain, stiffness, and immobility in the first 48h. They also induce drowsiness and can aid sleep. Benzodiazepines are used with caution as they affect balance, co-ordination, and judgment (5).

Table 19.1 Acute injury management: **PRICE**

Protection	is to prevent further injury and may involve the use of tape, padding, or external supports
Rest	is relative; the injured body part is 'rested' while the unaffected parts are exercised. Rest should not mean inactivity
Ice	up to 20min every 2–4h while the patient is awake for first 48–72h
Compress	Bandage, tape, or brace for majority of acute period
Elevate	affected limb for 1–2h periods during the day, a pillow under an injured limb at night

649

4 **Corticosteriods** are usually used in chronic injuries. They have antiinflammatory, immunological, and metabolic effects. They are injected intraarticularly or into connective tissue around tendons (e.g. in subacromial bursitis). Their efficacy has been established (6). There are severe potential complications such as septic arthritis and tendon rupture. These agents should be used by experienced practitioners only. Do not use on the Achilles tendon (7).

Treatment modalities

Passive physical treatments

Use alone or in combination:

- **Ice**
- **Heat**
- **Ultrasound**
- **TENS** (transcutaneous electrical nerve stimulation)
- **Laser**
- **Manual therapy**

Ice has beneficial effects in the acute and intermediate phases (8). Cold decreases spasm and slows nociceptor nerve conduction. Once swelling and pain have diminished sufficiently, ice is combined with active and passive range of motion within pain tolerance. The ice is used both prior to and during the therapeutic exercise session. This is done for 20–30min twice a day. In between the injury site is protected. Induce analgesia with ice for 20min, exercise (static stretch, isometric contract, static stretch), rest 30s and repeat (2–3 times) several times per day. Once the effects of swelling and pain have subsided and the athlete has progressed to more vigorous exercise and functional activity, the ice is used for 20–30min after the therapeutic exercise bout. **Note**: ice can cause burns and superficial nerve palsies (peroneal and ulnar). Use ice pack, plastic bag, crushed ice, and toweling. Caution should be exercised with gel packs which freeze below 0° Celsius. These should be wrapped in toweling.

Heat causes vasodilatation (increased delivery oxygen, nutrients, and immune mediators), increased metabolic rate, altered pain sensation, increased collagen extensibility, and decreased sensitivity to muscle stretch (9). Acute use helps relieve muscle spasm. Most useful for chronic inflammation, joint stiffness, pain syndromes.

Note: may cause increased oedema and local burns and should be supervised by the physical therapist.

Modern use of heat relies on hot packs 40–70 °C applied for 20min in conjunction with range of motion exercises. The widespread use of rubifactents to cause peripheral vasodilatation and local heating is not recommended due to the relative difficulty in controlling timing and dosage.

Ultrasound. High frequency soundwaves (0.8–1.1MHz), produce heating at fascial planes. When pulsed at low frequency ultrasound produces a mechanical effect. Together they produce an analgesic and antiinflammatory effect by increasing local perfusion and metabolism (1). Thrombolysis is aided and there is a role in hematoma treatment (11). There are complications of overzealous or incorrect treatment. Usually employed after the acute phase (**12**).

TENS produces analgesia and is used extensively in chronic pain syndromes (**13**). Works via spinal gate mechanism and direct effects on nociceptors. *Interferential* is a form of TENS in which alternating electrical stimulation is used to produce various levels of muscle contraction. This reduces oedema and helps minimize disuse atrophy. There is some evidence that it has antispasmodic action in spinal injury patients (**14**).

Laser. Cold laser is used for small localized lesions (e.g. long head biceps strain). It is claimed to reduce pain and spasm and to have beneficial effects on local metabolism. Evidence exists for alteration of nerve conduction (**15**) with laser. Clinical effect in controlled *in vivo* studies (**16**) has not been proven.

Manual therapy differs from the above modalities in that it requires 'hands-on' treatment. It encompasses all forms of massage, mobilization, manipulation, traction, and neural stretching. The ultimate manual treatment consists of surgery. The individual techniques and combinations applied vary and are beyond the scope of this chapter. Manual therapy is the most ancient form of medicine, the 'laying on of hands'. Several practitioner groups make claims that are unscientific and misleading. The authors recommend that athletes be guided to therapists who have scientific training, experience in sports injury, and who can work in a team. There are **potential risks with manual therapy**, particularly rotational spinal manipulation which has caused disk prolapse, corda equina lesions, and vertebral artery dissection (**17–20**). There are clear benefits in reduction in muscle spasm and oedema, relaxation, flexibility and increased joint range of motion from manual therapy. There is also a placebo effect in some patients. Psychological benefits are often observed.

Active physical treatments

Are the foundation of the rehabilitation process. When an injury occurs immobile muscle rapidly atrophies, connective tissue contracts, and detrimental joint changes may occur. Active physical treatment requires the interest and compliance of the athlete to minimize injury consequences and return to activity.

Strengthening exercises (Fig. 19.1–19.14).

These aim initially to minimize disuse atrophy, increase circulation and maintain muscle condition. As healing continues gains in strength, control, coordination, and endurance facilitate recovery. There are several types of strengthening exercises and these are combined for maximum effect (**21,22**).

Isometric exercises are conducted without movement across the joint on which the muscle acts. There are two program types prolonged contraction involves a 20–30s contraction performed 10–20 times with a 20s break. These can be performed from the acute phase of injury up to 10 times per day. Basmajian (**21**) recommends brief (5–6s) repeated isometric maximal (added weight) exercises with a 20s delay. This minimizes cardiovascular stress (hypertension) which has been observed with prolonged isometric exercise. Exercise can be performed with the joints in various angles and achieve improved strength of muscle.

Isotonic. In which muscle contraction moves a joint through a range of motion. Thus, if the muscle shortens while contracting (e.g. biceps curl) it is termed a concentric contraction. The act of lowering a weight from height (e.g. lowering a biceps curl back to the start position) is termed *eccentric* as the muscle is lengthening while contracting. Daily progressive resistance exercise (PRE) using weights or other resistant devices is prescribed and begins after the acute phase. Multiple repetitions are used and the number and resistance can be varied (**22**). The tempo or rest periods can also be progressively altered. Careful instruction and supervision is required. Typical examples are provided later. A variety of machines have been designed to improve strengthening throughout the joint range for different muscle lengths. One type is a command system with increased weight at mid range and reducing at full extension and flexion (Nautilis).

Various machines have been developed to perform **isokinetic** exercise. This allows constant velocity with variable resistance as the muscle moves the joint through its range. An example is the isokinetic dynamometer machine which was originally designed for rehabilitation of knee injuries. It can be applied to other joints.

Balance around a joint is essential in any exercise program with a balanced ratio of agonist and antagonist training (23). Co-ordinated patterns of training are covered in the section on Functional training.

Plyometric exercises are also useful in developing muscle power. They use a stretch–shortening cycle to elicit a more forceful concentric contraction. Associated with rapidly changing eccentric to concentric action, it has been suggested that these exercises may develop reciprocal reflex training which may be useful in injury prevention. It is used 2–3 times per week but discontinued if the athlete develops pain, swelling or other signs of overuse. It has also been employed as a strengthening technique in fit athletes.

Flexibility

Exercises have two benefits (1) in allowing and encouraging joint range of motion (ROM) exercises, they are a factor in return of normal joint mechanics; (2) the effect of graduated stretching over time increases the length of contractile units and connective tissue elements within the muscle. As the muscle, tendon, and enthesis are part of the same contractile unit this helps reduce injury. Blood supply to the tendon is predominantely from the muscle with less from the bone attachment/enthesis. There is a critical area in the tendon which is susceptible to injury and ischemia (**24**).

Flexibility exercises have the effect of improving the efficient range of muscle contraction and preventing avulsion at tendon bone junction by reducing the chance of end range 'bow stringing'. After injury stretching after physical therapy such as ice or heat reduces the activity of the fusimotor system, provides analgesia and often allows a greater ROM (**25**).

Stretching regimes range from 30 to 60s, 3 repetitions; twice daily. Ballistic (bouncing) exercises or passive stretches by weights machines or trainer, run the risk of muscle tears. A slow stretch and creep technique is preferred, progressive to the limit of discomfort and **not** beyond. The desired muscle length may require twice daily stretching for 6 weeks with maintenance once daily. Specific stretching exercise programs are available in many forms. A basic lower limb stretching program is provided (Fig. 19.5).

Proprioceptive neuromuscular facilitation (PNF) stretching reduces muscle tone by stimulating the Golgi tendon organs. It relies on synergies using agonist activities to relax antagonists. PNF involves proprioceptive and tactile techniques to cause muscle relaxation and repetitive activities to establish patterns of muscle contraction (**17**).

Various movement and flexibility paradigms are promoted by diverse groups. These include yoga, Bowen and Alexander techniques, and Feldenkrais. The authors believe that each has its merits although blindly following the teachings of self promoting 'gurus' is unscientific.

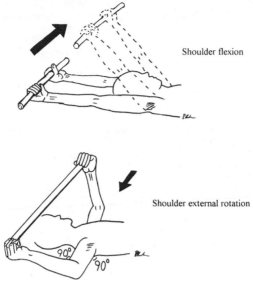

Shoulder flexion

Shoulder external rotation

Fig. 19.1 Shoulder strengthening exercises

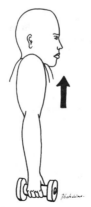

Fig. 19.2 Shoulder strengthening exercises

Endurance

Refers to the ability of a muscle to perform a static (isometric) or dynamic (isotonic) task. It depends on the state of the individual muscle and the cardiovascular status of the individual.

A guide to endurance can be made by using physical work capacity measures, or pulse vs workload. A linear relationship exists between oxygen uptake and pulse rate. Using the Astrand nomogram a predicted VO_{2max} may be determined. (**26**) Other protocols have been used in cardiovascular testing. An example is the step test whereby the number of steps of a given height from the floor, up to a bench, taken in a given period is recorded.

At a minimum, *cardiovascular and endurance training should occur for 20min, 3 times a week*. Most athletes will easily exceed these guidelines. For an indepth description of cardiovascular fitness and aerobic exercise readers are referred to exercise physiology texts. The benefits include cardiovascular training, metabolic stimulation, maintenance of muscle bulk release of endocrine hormones, and immunological modulation. There is evidence that endurance training of unaffected body parts has trophic effects on the injured area. It also may have positive psychological effects in individuals (**27**). Many methods are available to provide aerobic and endurance training for the injured athlete. They include:

- Swimming
- Water exercises (hydrotherapy)
- Brisk walking
- Circuit training
- Calisthenics/Aerobics
- Stationary bicycles
- Machines (stepper, rowing, arm crank, etc.)

Swimming is the preferred exercise in most cases as the activity is non-weight bearing and is less prone to cause reinjury. The particular regime will depend on the site, nature and age of injury, and the individual's circumstances and skills.

Proprioceptive retraining

Ligaments and to some extent tendon injuries are accompanied by an impairment of proprioception which may persist after the inflammatory phase of the injury has resolved (**28**). The three cues to balance are vision, vestibular function, and lower limb position sense—proprioception.

Following an injury, position sense of a body part in relation to space or other objects is often diminished or lost. The goal of proprioceptive exercises is to reduce the time between neural stimuli and muscular response, thus reducing the stress on the injured joint during functional activities. Rehabilitation of injuries to the knee and ankle require proprioceptive retraining. Whiplash injuries cause abnormal neck proprioception and upper limb injuries may also require retraining. The components of lower limb proprioceptive training include:

- Taping or external supports to provide increased sensory input and protection during the early phases.

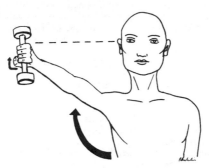

Fig. 19.3 Shoulder exercises: supraspinatus strengthening

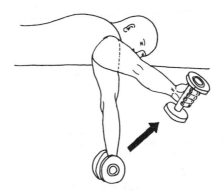

Fig. 19.4 Shoulder exercises: prone horizontal abduction

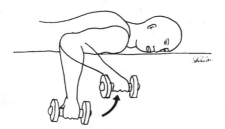

Fig. 19.5 Shoulder exercises: prone external rotation

- Static balance exercises standing on one leg initially then graduating to less firm surfaces (e.g. foam and eventually wobble board).
- Reduction of visual cues using blindfold or distracting activities during balance exercises (e.g. throwing a ball to and from trainer or against a wall and catching).
- Dynamic training such as jogging in soft sand progressing to figure-of-eight or zig-zag patterns. During the later stages of recovery jogging on firm surfaces, then finally on uneven surfaces

Functional training

Training begins when the healing process allows. It is composed of the components already mentioned. Strength, flexibility, propioception, and endurance are required (**11**).

Muscle groups are exercised in tandem allowing co-ordinated purposeful movement. Specific weakness patterns and technique errors can be addressed. This has benefits on strength and endurance allowing further functional training. These exercises may begin with partial squats, leg presses, step-ups, lunges, or closed-chain terminal knee extension. As symptoms subside and function improves devices such as reciprocal (vertical or stair) climbers, lateral slide boards, treadmills are used. A progressive walk-jog-run program can begin as healing proceeds. *For example*, a basketball player with a knee injury could perform a compound exercise such as a set of body weight squats, when pain-free. This could progress with increased weights and gradual introduction of standing jumping exercises. This could be enhanced with a plyometric program of exercises.

Functional training can be general or sports-specific. It can be supervised by trainers, therapists, coaches, or parents. Athletes enjoy it as a part of a graduated return to full activity. It is useful for both acute and chronic injuries and been shown to decrease time off employment and speed return to sport. (**29**)

Psychological factors

The athlete with an injury requires consideration, understanding, and empathy. He or she may be suffering not only an injury but financial and emotional stress. Body image is very important to athletes as well as the endorphin drive they have to exercise. Research suggests that athletes respond to injury with mood disturbance and lowered self-esteem (**30**). Calm explanation of the diagnosis, education, and involvement in the rehabilitation plan are important aspects of the therapeutic relationship (**31**). More time is often required than with other patients but the often excellent results offer the clinician satisfaction. The recruitment of the athlete to taking an active role in their rehabilitation will facilitate the process.

In extreme cases a reactive depression or post-traumatic stress may intervene (**31**). These may be treated by supportive psychotherapy and appropriate medication. Following physical recovery, confidence and athletic performance may be slower to return. Education, explanation, and support are required. A sports psychologist may help.

Biomechanical factors

Understanding the mechanism of the injury will help modify the activity to prevent reinjury. If this is not corrected adaptive protective

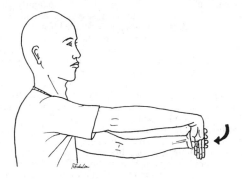

Fig. 19.6 Forearm extensor stretch

Stretching flexors

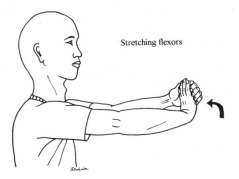

Fig. 19.7 Forearm flexor stretch

behavior may lead to a second and apparently unrelated injury. Biomechanical factors can be assessed by attending the events and being involved as team doctor. A detailed history and examination of the athlete is essential. Some sports have inherent physical demands which cause particular injuries (e.g. female gymnastics forces girls to hyperextend their backs and weight bear on the upper limbs, leading to injury rates approaching 30% per year!) (**32**).

Some injuries are caused by combinations of athletic activity, technique, and individual anatomy. Plantar fasciitis in which biomechanical factors are crucial in the prevention, treatment, and rehabilitation is a good example (**33**).

Subtle abnormalities at a high level of skill may only be diagnosed by video, gait, and force plate analysis. A coach may help in these areas for technique advice. Footwear modifications may be the logical starting point for runners (e.g. iliotibial band friction syndrome may be improved by reducing tibial rotation by insertion of an antipronation shoe or orthoses) (**34**).

Return to sport

When the components of the rehabilitation process have been applied correctly, the synergistic nature of the treatment should enable return to sport. After a subjective assessment from the therapist or trainer that the athlete is able to use the injured extremity well. The athlete's ability to demonstrate enough self-confidence to fully participate in these activities without experiencing pain, swelling, or giving way is assessed. The athlete progresses to sports-specific activities in a noncompetitive environment. Their performance should be critically evaluated by the rehabilitation team. Specific stress testing may be performed. (Table 19.2.)

Table 19.2 Guidelines for return to sport after injury

- Acute signs and symptoms have passed
- Full functional use of all joints, adequate strength, and proprioception to perform tasks
- Normal mechanics of movement
- Successful performance of sport-specific activities at or above pre-injury level should be documented

Gradual isometric contraction of quadriceps

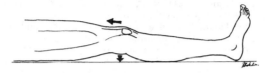

Straight leg raise

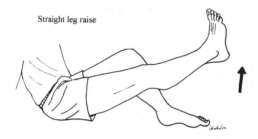

Hip abduction exercise

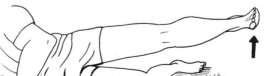

Fig. 19.8 Leg exercises

Rehabilitation of four common injuries

1 Tennis elbow

Is an enthesopathy (see also Fig. 9.3). Inflammation occurs at the common extensor origin of the wrist and finger extensor muscles on the lateral humeral epicondyle. On the first presentation Rest, Ice, Compression, Elevation (RICE) and optional drug analgesia is provided. Within 24h the program starts. Stretching the extensor and opposing flexor groups of muscle is taught. This is followed by graduated weight training for forearm and wrist consisting of sets of 20 repetitions with weights ranging from 100g to 500g for each movement of the wrist, i.e. flexion, extension, pronation, supination, and radioulnar movement. This regime is aimed at improving strength and endurance in the muscles and increasing the range of movement in the joints. The regime is repeated 4 times daily with ice applied over the lateral epicondyle for antiinflammatory and pain relief at the end of each session (35). *Passive treatment* such as ultrasound, interferential, and gentle massage may help. Antiinflammatory drugs are sometimes employed. *Biomechanics* may be altered by a change in wrist action during backhand and increasing the size of the racket grip by wrapping with layers of tape and foam. *Maintaining range of motion* in the shoulder and cardiovascular fitness can be achieved by swimming sessions (crawl or backstroke) 30min 2–3 times weekly. Active participation in running, cycling or other aerobic activities is encouraged. *Psychological issues* can usually be resolved by explanation, education, and providing support. *Rehabilitation* may take 6–8 weeks (35).

2 Sprained ankle

The most common ankle injury is an anterior talofibular ligament strain on the lateral side. More severe injuries cause damage to the calcaneal-fibular ligament with the possibility of medial deltoid ligament injury as the ankle is forced through more extreme inversion. After the immediate period of **PRICE** (Table 19.1X), diagnosis and exclusion of fracture occur. Appropriate antiinflammatory and analgesic measures are taken and a rehabilitation plan implemented. *Initial treatment* days 2–5 focuses on protection with reduced weight bearing, oedema management, and analgesia. *Passive physical treatment* is used together with medication and gentle active range of motion exercises. Simultaneously, cardiovascular and endurance training using the unaffected limbs commences. *Weight bearing proprioceptive retraining* is required commencing 5–7 days post injury. The program involves twice daily sessions of standing on one leg at a time for periods from 1 to 5min. Once standing has been achieved, then distraction of visual cues to balance, such as standing on one leg and throwing a ball against the wall, bouncing and catching drills are used. This can be progressed with the athlete standing on a wobble board. These sessions increase to 20min twice daily. At the same time that static proprioception is being achieved, *dynamic proprioception* will be promoted by jogging in sand. Progressing to figure-of-eight running, jog run, sprint cycles, and rapid changes of direction on a variety of soft, hard, and uneven surfaces (36). The proprioceptive retraining can be facilitated by ankle strapping or bracing which provides increased sensory feedback and some protection from overinversion movements.

Hip flexion exercise

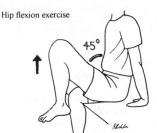

Hamstring curl

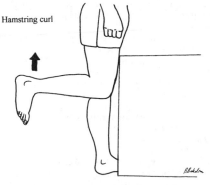

Hamstring stretch

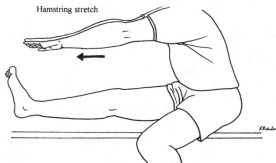

Fig. 19.9 Leg exercises

The total treatment time varies by individual and sport but most injuries take from 2–4 weeks to functional return. Karlson *et al.* report excellent results from early aggressive proprioceptive and functional retraining with mean return to sport in treatment group of less than 10 days (**29**).

3 Hamstring

Muscles run from the pelvis and posterior femur to the tibia and fibular head. They contract concentrically to extend the hip, flex the knee, and contract eccentrically for pelvic stabilization and during the gait cycle. Because of their long length and crossing of two joints (hip and knee) they are susceptible to muscle and connective tissue tears and recurrent injury (**37**, **38**). Strains often occur during periods of acceleration. *Prevention* by prewarming stretches and warm-ups is encouraged. After the initial period of **PRICE** (Table 19.1) and diagnosis a *rehabilitation plan* is formulated. *Local passive treatment*, such as ultrasound and massage, is commenced with the therapist. Antiinflammatories may be prescribed. Isometric exercise can begin within 24h.

A graduated stretching program is begun (**39**). Stretching of hamstrings using stretch and creep technique for 30–60s, 5 repetition times, twice daily with quadriceps and Achilles tendon stretches is essential. Simultaneously, *progressive resistance exercise* (PRE), is prescribed based on a 10-repetition set repeated 2–3 times performed daily. Resistance is progressively increased as pain allows. Iceing is combined with the stretching and exercise program. Balance must be achieved around the knee at a ratio of 3 quadricep/2 hamstrings. Therefore, PRE is used to maintain quadriceps and calf muscle condition. *Isokinetic exercise* if available may speed muscle strength return. *Biomechanical factors* such as pelvic alignment, leg length, and gait patterns may need review. Aerobic exercise to maintain endurance and cardiovascular fitness is integral. Swimming or other injury protecting forms are used.

As recovery proceeds, functional exercises such as squats, jogging, running, and sprinting are reintroduced into the program. Caution is required as hamstring injuries seem prone to recurrence.

4 Stress fractures

Are overuse injuries typically in the lower limb of endurance athletes. They are caused by repetitive cyclical loading of bone which exceeds its repair capability (**40**). They occur most commonly in the tibia, malleoli, and metatarsals (March fractures) but have been reported at other sites.. They cause pain and disability. If training continues stress fractures can progress to complete fractures. There is considerable variation in susceptibility to such overtraining injuries. **Diagnosis** is confirmed by x-ray, bone scan, CT or MRI alone or in combination.

The *principle treatments* are rest, maintenance of cardiovascular fitness and correction of underlying biomechanical factors. Endurance/cardiovascular fitness is maintained by non-weight bearing exercise (e.g. swimming, water exercises, circuit classes, and machines). Rest is required. If compliance is poor, use a plaster of Paris to immobilize the limb. Walking for usual daily tasks is not detrimental. Some fractures (e.g. navicular require strict non-weight-

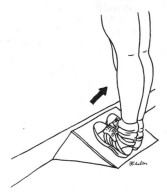

Fig. 19.10 Calf, Achilles tendon stretch

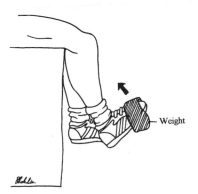

Weight

Fig. 19.11 Foot dorsiflexion exercise

Single leg

Wobble board

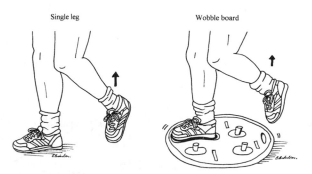

Fig. 19.12 Ankle exercises: proprioceptive retraining

bearing) (**41**).Others (e.g. anterior tibial epiphyseal stress fractures) may require surgery. *Education, counseling, and support* are the keys to treatment of stress fractures. The psychological concerns of these athletes must be addressed. Behaviorally based regimes to reduce uncertainty are recommended (**30**).The athlete must be alerted to tissue limitations from training. Overtraining has detrimental effects on the immune system and endurance, with poorer performance and high injury rates.

Confidence of the athlete and compliance with treatment will be more likely if the sports physician is specific about periods of complete rest and a guaranteed return to training with a rehabilitation training schedule.

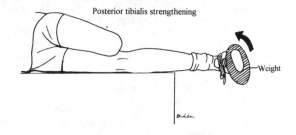

Posterior tibialis strengthening

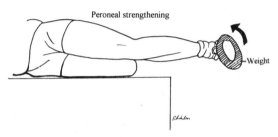

Peroneal strengthening

Fig. 19.13 Ankle exercises

Complications of rehabilitation

The commonest problem is reinjury occurring due to return to sport before injury recovery is complete. This may be due to the athlete, inadequate rehabilitation, or external pressure such as from the coach. Other injuries may occur owing to athletes trying to protect their original injuries and subsequent altered behavior or biomechanics. Injury may occur in another area from trying to protect the primary injury. Overaggressive rehabilitation may be detrimental.

Myositis ossificans occurs in some young athletes following a blow to the thigh and subsequent quadriceps hematoma. Hematomas are common injuries in contact sports. Overzealous stretching, strengthening, and massage can provoke a further hemorrhage which promote fibroblasts to differentiate into osteoblasts, and for formation of bone within the hematoma. This can lead to pain, decreased range of knee motion, and residual disability.

Drug treatment always carries significant risk of side-effects. Passive physical treatment can cause injury if incorrectly applied.

Failure of rehabilitation may precipitate psychological and emotional distress.

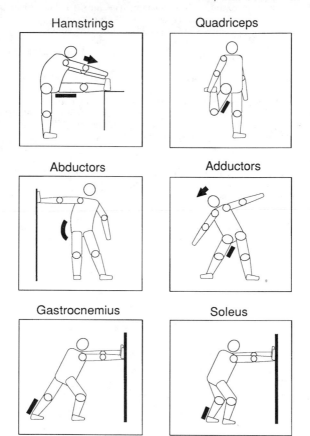

Fig. 19.14 Lower limb stretches

Prevention

The prevention of injury is important. The duty to the patient is greater than the team or sporting event. If injury occurs assess prior to continuing. If health is in danger, discontinue the activity. *General principles*:

- Adequate training and preparation prior to competition (weeks/months).
- Consider body physiognomy, maturity, and experience to compete. 'Profiling' is a concept that matches an individual's physiognomy with the type of sport, and in team sports to their role.
- Sports facility factors, such as state of competition area, equipment maintenance, injury treatment equipment, and air pollution.
- Rules and aims of sporting contest.

Individual factors:
- Treat illness or injury.
- Some athletes should be prevented from high-risk sports (e.g. epileptics should not scuba dive).
- Maintain equipment.
- Adequate warm-up (stretching, cardiovascular, and psychological preparation).
- Protective equipment used.

References

(1) DN Kulund 1988 *The injured athlete*. 2nd edn. Lippincott, Philadelphia
(2) C Hubley-Kozey *et al* 1994 JC Delee *et al* (ed) *Orthopaedic sports medicine* p184–207. Saunders, Philadelphia
(3) *Krusen's Handbook of physical medicine and rehabilitation* 3rd edn 1971. Saunders, Philadelphia
(4) W Stolov 1971 Evaluation of the patient *Krusen's handbook of physical medicine and rehabilitation* 3rd edn. Saunders, Philadelphia
(5) LS Goodman, A Gillman 1990 *The pharmacological basis of therapeutics* 8th edn. Pergamon, Oxford
(6) K Nelson *et al* 1996 *Am Fam Phy* **52** 1811–16
(7) I Shrier *et al* 1996 *Clin J Sport Med* **6** 245–50
(8) SK Hillman, G Delforge 1985 *Clin Sports Med* **4** 431–8
(9) J Lehmann 1984 *Therapeutic heat and cold* 3rd edn. Williams & Wilkins, Baltimore
(10) AM Gam, F Johannsen 1995 *Pain* **63** 85–91
(11) H Luo *et al* 1996 *Circulation* **94** 775–8
(12) J Falconer *et al* 1990 *Arthrit Car Res* **3** 85–91
(13) P Wall, R Melzeck 1989 *Textbook of pain* 2nd edn. Churchill Livingstone, Edinburgh
(14) C Goulet *et al* 1996 *Scand J Rehab Med* **28** 169–76
(15) GD Baxter *et al* 1994 *Exp Physiol* **79** 227–34
(16) B Mokhtar *et al* 1995 *Laser Surg Med* **17** 74–81
(17) MD Ryan 1993 *Med J Aust* **158** 718
(18) WJ Assendelft *et al* 1996 *J Fam Pract* **42** 475–80
(19) G Maitland 1987 *Peripheral manipulation* 2nd edn. Butterworth, Guildford, UK
(20) M Knapp 1982 *Krusen's Handbook of Physical medicine and rehabilitation* 3rd edn. Saunders, Philadelphia
(21) JV Basmajian 1984 *Therapeutic Exercise* 4th edn. Williams & Wilkins, Baltimore
(22) RM Poole 1994 RB Birrer (ed) *Sports medicine for the primary care physician* 2nd edn. p599. CRC, Boca Raton
(23) D Schram 1980 *Resistance exercise, therapeutic exercise*. McMaster University
(24) H Takami *et al J Hand Surg Am* **20** 474–7
(25) WF Ganong 1995 *Review of Medical physiology* 17th edn. Appleton & Lange, East Nowalk, CT
(26) P Astrand, K Rodahl 1986 *Textbook of work physiology. Physiological basis of exercise* 3rd edn McGraw-Hill
(27) A Dickinson, *et al* 1985 *Clin in Sports Med* **4** July
(28) J Leanderson *et al* 1996 *Am J Sports Med* **24** 370–4
(29) J Karlsson *et al* 1996 *Scand J Med Sci Sports* **6** 241–5
(30) AM Smith *et al* 1990 *Sports Med* **9** 352–69
(31) AM Smith *et al* 1990 *Mayo Clin Proc* **65** 38–50
(32) KJ Lindner, Caine 1990 *Can J Sport Sci* **15** 254–61
(33) TJ Chandler, WB Kibler 1993 *Sports Med* **15** 344–52
(34) G Rose 1986 *Orthotics principles and practice*. Heineman, Oxford
(35) S Wilson 1985 *J Occup Health Safety ANZ* **2** 126–9
(36) JL Seto, Brewster 1994 *Clin Sport Med* **13** 695–718
(37) TW Worrell 1994 *Sports Med* **17** 338–45
(38) PA Upton *et al* 1996 *Br J Sports Med* **30** 57–60
(39) BF Taylor *et al* 1995 *J Orthop Sports Phys Ther* **21** 283–6
(40) MT Reeder *et al* 1996 *Sports Med* **22** 198–212
(41) KM Khan *et al* 1994 *Sports Med* **17** 65–76

Part IV
Special groups

20 The athlete with a disability

STEPHEN F WILSON

Philosophy

Ability, not disability

The aspirations of the athlete with a disability are those of any participant in sport. The athlete aims to achieve a level of physical and psychological fitness for their chosen sport and demonstrate that ability in competition. The self-discipline, positive effect on self-esteem and body image, and friendship is an integral part of the sport. The athlete will generally choose a sport based on his or her abilities. This may be in open able-bodied competition or in competition modified for people with similar disabilities. The emphasis is on the ability for a sport, not the disability.

Mind, body, spirit

This is encapsulated in the three tear drops of the Paralympic logo symbolizing mind, body, and spirit participating on land, wheel, and water.

Athletes, not patients

The athlete expects the sports physician to have an intelligent understanding of his/her disability and its implications for participation in sport. Doctors practicing sports medicine often view sport as a part of rehabilitation of a disability in a hospital setting. This doctor–patient relationship should be replaced by the doctor–athlete adviser. This is particularly so when advising in the area of classification (grading), exercise physiology and exercise prescription.

Integration

Sport has been a medium to push social change in society with equal opportunities in work and recreation. Integration within the sporting groups has occurred with the introduction of sports-specific functional classification vs impairment-based grading and classification.

Terminology

Referring to athletes as 'the handicapped' is no longer acceptable. The intention should be to concentrate on the person not the disability. Reference should be made to 'a person with a disability' (e.g. 'An athlete with an intellectual disability').

Mind · Body · Spirit

International Paralympic Committee

677

History

The oldest continuing sports association for athletes with disabilities is the International Committee of Sports for the Deaf, established in 1924. The credit for the formation of the modern sporting movement for people with disabilities goes to the neurosurgeon Ludwig Guttman who founded the Stoke Mandeville Spinal Injuries Unit in England in 1944. He promoted the therapeutic benefit of sport with the benefits for physical social, and psychological rehabilitation following spinal cord injury. He established the first Stoke Mandeville Games which subsequently developed into an international event contributing to the formation of the Paralympic movement. Hans Linstrom contributed to the formation of the Winter Paralympics which was first held in Sweden in 1976.[1] The Special Olympic movement has developed separately as an event for people with more severe intellectual disability. Athletes with intellectual disability will be integrated within Paralympic competition in Sydney in 2000. The World Games for the deaf are conducted every four years (Summer Games 1997, 2001, Winter Games 1999, 2003). Table 20.1 is a summary of some events in the history of sport for people with disabilities.[1]

1 *Paralympic spirit*. Atlanta Paralympic Organizing Committee 1996

Table 20.1 The disabled athlete: some events of note

Year	Significance
1924	International Committee of Sports for the Deaf
1944	Ludwig Guttman established Stoke Mandeville Spinal Unit, Aylesbury, UK
1948	First Stoke Mandeville Games: 16 ex-servicemen and women competed in archery
1952	International Stoke Mandeville Games established
1956	Olympic Committee recognized Stoke Mandeville Games, Melbourne, Australia
1960	First Disabled Olympics, Rome, thereafter Paralympics (Parallel Olympics)
1962	First British Commonwealth Games
1974	Far East South Pacific Games (FESPIC), Osaka, Japan
1976	First Winter Paralympics. Alpine and Nordic skiing, blind and amputee competitors, Sweden
1984	Olympics included wheelchair demonstration sports, Los Angeles, USA
1988	Paralympics. Disability-based, Seoul, Korea
1992	Paralympics. Functional (ability based) classification system swimming, Barcelona, Spain
1996	Paralympics. Demonstration sports, sailing, quad rugby, Atlanta, USA
2000	Paralympics, Functional classification for track and field and swimming, Sydney, Australia

Organized structure of international sport

Athletes' disabilities may be divided into the following 4 categories:[1]

1 Locomotor: *cerebral palsy* (CP). Congenital or acquired brain injury or stroke. This group will include athletes with spastic or flaccid quadriplegia, hemiplegia, or diplegia with or without choreiform or athetoid movements.

Amputee: congenital or acquired limb deficiency.

Wheelchair: congenital or acquired complete or incomplete spinal lesion (e.g., spina bifida). Some amputees and other groups compete as wheelchair athletes.

Les autres others: poliomyelitis with paralysis; muscular dystrophy; rheumatoid arthritis; multiple scleroses; small stature (dwarf).

2 Sensory: hearing impaired (deaf); vision impaired (blind).

3 Intellectual disability (ID) or mental handicap (MH; USA).

4 Transplant: organ transplant (e.g. renal, heart).

The organizations representing these bodies are listed below. Many are associated with the International Paralympic Committee and others are autonomous. Most organizations have links with international sports organizations (ISOs). The following organizations are affiliated with the International Paralympic Committee (IPC):

- International Sports Organizations for the Disabled (ISODs) Les Autres, Amputees
- International Blind Sports Association (IBSA)
- International Stoke Mandeville Wheelchair Sports Federation (ISMWSF)
- Cerebral Palsy International Sports and Recreation Association (CP–ISRA)
- International Sports Federation for People with Mental Handicap (INAS–FMH)
- Disabled Skier Federation (DSF) Snow Skiing
- Riding for the Disabled International (RDI) Equestrian
- International Sailing Federation/International Foundation for Disabled Sailing (ISAF/IFDS)

The following organizations are autonomous:

- International Committee of Sports for the Deaf Comité Internationale des Sports des Sourds (CISS)
- Special Olympics International (SOI) Mental Handicap Intellectual Disability
- World Transplant Games Federation (WTGF)

1 S Goodman 1995 *Coaching athletes with disabilities: General principles* 2nd edn. Australian Sports Commission

681

The athlete

General considerations in treatment of injury:
- *correct lifting* with assistant, avoid tugging limbs to avoid subluxation of hip and shoulder
- *avoid pressure* on insensate areas particularly hip and sacrum to prevent skin ulceration. Use cushioned bench or examine in wheelchair
- *support athlete* to prevent falling from chair or bench (quad, high para)
- *active joint motion* before slow passive range to avoid increase in muscle tone, clonus or spasm
- *position and secure ice packs* and monitor. The athlete may not be able to hold in place due to poor dexterity
- *communicate* with the athlete taking time to comprehend slow or dyarthric speech
- *be aware of drug interactions*. The athlete may be taking multiple prescribed medications
- *Do not assume that physical disability or communication difficulty is associated with intellectual disability*

Cerebral palsy

'Cerebral Palsy is a disorder of movement and posture due to damage to an area or areas of the brain that control and co-ordinate movement' (Little 1862). This disorder may occur *in utero*, intrapartum, or postpartum. **Causes**: (incidence, etiology), 2.5/1000 live births,[1] cerebral hypoxia, hemorrhage, obstetric trauma, meningitis, abruptio placenta. Diplegia, 32%; hemiplegia 29%; quadriplegia 24%; dyskinesia/ataxia, 14% (subtypes CP at age 7).[2] **Physiology**: increased muscle tone leads to risk of muscle strains. There is a higher incidence of epilepsy 30%[3] and intellectual disability 50%, (more likely in quadriplegia). Primitive reflexes (i.e. asymetric tonic neck reflexes, ATNR, may be present). Osteoarthritis in the neck is common with ageing.

Management of injury and associated conditions:

Spasticity: muscle strains treated with RICE. Prevention by regular stretching. Slow prolonged 5–10 min, 4 times daily until desired range, then 1 min twice daily. Maintenance stretching is more effective combined with muscle relaxation, heat, cold, or massage. M*uscle relaxation medications*: dantrolene, monitor liver function (LFTs) regularly (6-weekly). Baclofen, rarely used in cerebral spasticity. Diazepam used rarely, due to effect on alertness, balance, and co-ordination. *Selective muscle paralysis*: botulinum toxin intramuscular injections, 3- to 6-monthly to decrease spasticity and strength, may improve function and ambulation. *Motor nerve or motor point blocks* with phenol or alcohol.

Epileptic seizures: consider low anticonvulsant blood level, timing of medication, travel, dehydration, hyperthermia, intercurrent febrile illness. Beware recent fall, if on anticoagulant exclude extra or subdural hematoma (CT scan). Most fits resolve within 1min, place in coma position, check airway.

1 E Blair, FJ Stanley 1982 *Develop Med Child Neurol* **24** 578–85   2 KB Nelson, JH Ellenberg 1978 In BS Schoenberg (ed.) *Advances in Neurology*, Vol 19, p421–35. Raven Press, New York   3 J Gage 1991 *Clin Develop Med* No. 121. MacKeith Press

If status epilepticus: diazepam, intravenous infusion. Clonazepam. These medications *may be given rectally* if unable to administer IVI.

Neck: new weakness in arms/legs in older athlete with or without bladder, bowel dysfunction. X-ray neck MRI to exclude cervical myelopathy due to spinal cord compression.

Common surgery in CP: Adductor tenotomy for scissoring gait due to adductor spasticity not responding to medication, or obturator block . Achilles lengthening for equino varus foot, with toe walking . These procedures may be used in the future less with the introduction of selective muscle paralysis with botulinum toxin. *Assistive devices*: ankle foot orthosis in polypropylene, resin, or steel (caliper) to control ankle/foot, often used with boot with medial/lateral flare for stable base of support. A lateral or medial T-strap may be attached to the shoe or caliper.

Amputee

Acquired limb deficiency is described in relation to the residual limb Partial foot—transmetatarsal, midfoot (Lisfranc), hind foot (Chopart), through ankle (Symes).

Common amputation sites: below knee (BK), through knee (TK), above knee (AK). Partial hand, through wrist, below elbow (BE). Above elbow (AE), shoulder disarticulation.

Congenital limb deficiency frequently involves partial deficiency or dysplasia of elements of the limb. An international classification system has been established. (ISO: 8548–1: 1989). **Causes (aetiology)**: congential (thalidomide), cancer (osteogenic sarcoma), peripheral vascular disease, diabetes, osteomyelitis, leprosy, traumatic (landmines, occupational, motor vehicle). **Physiology**: traumatic amputees may have phantom sensation, pain, and psychological adaptation to body image. Pain may be related to poor-fitting prosthesis with or without neuroma. Due to decreased surface area thermoregulation may be slower and should be considered in extreme heat and cold. The energy cost of ambulation is greater than able-bodied.[1]

Management of injury and associated conditions

Lower limb stump abrasion: clean, antiseptic non-stick dressing (e.g. silicone gel pad). If the patellar tendon is ulcerated then check prosthetic alignment. Walking and running alignment are different and should be adjusted prior to competition. *Recurrent or chronic amputation stump breakdown*: consider silicon stumpsock, roll on silicon socket (ICEROSS) or polyurethylene socket liner (TEC). *Above knee amputee*: discuss with prosthetist, rotator or vertical shock absorber type pylon.

Stump hyperkeratosis: continual pressure and abrasion makes diagnosis difficult as lesions may not have a typical appearance. Consider the following possibilities:

(1) *Tinea*: fungal scraping, clotrimazole 1% cream topical 3 times daily for 3 weeks

(2) *Contact dematitis*: if new prosthetic liner, exclude contact dermatitis from glue

683

1 JH Bowker, JW Michael 1992 *Atlas of limb prosthetics* 2nd edn. Mosby, St. Louis

(3) *Psoriasis*: check other sites (e.g. scalp, elbows)
(4) *Verrucous hyperplasia*: warty appearance due to poor hygiene, sweating, and poor distal prosthetic contact. Any keratolytic cream (e.g. sulphur 2%, salicylic acid 2%, aqueous cream to 100%)

All athletes should wash prosthetic liner with soap and water and change sockets daily. If all else fails then correct the problems by modifying the prosthetic socket or recasting for a new socket.

Lower limb amputee (lower back pain): adjust height of prosthesis up or down 0.5cm prior to commencing investigation unless signs of nerve root compression.

Prosthesis too tight due to stump edema: for BK amputee, bandage stump with 10cm elastic bandage for 30min then retry. For AK amputee, bandage stump 30min then retry. Try 'wet fit' with aqueous cream to stump prior to donning the suction socket prosthesis.

Pain phantom or stump: exclude referred pain, infection or ischemia. If true phantom pain, self-massage stump 10min 2 to 4 times daily, apply *cetromacrogole* or aqueous cream. *Physical therapy*, transcutaneous electrical stimulation (TENS) applied to popliteal fossa, sciatic nerve 15–30min at night. *Medication*: subtherapeutic doses of anticonvulsants, carbamazepine, at night. *Or* sodium valproate, at night, *or* tricyclic antidepressants, amitriptyline, at night. *Neuroma*: check prosthetic fit. Inject with bupivicaine. Often effective alone. *Or* bupivicaine mixed with methyl prednisolone acetate.

Assistive devices: prostheses consist of the following components: suspension, socket, shank, articulation, terminal device (foot or hand). (Fig.20.1.)

Spinal

Congenital or acquired complete or incomplete damage to the spinal cord or nerve roots within the spinal cord. Athletes competing include those with cervical cord injury (quadriplegia) thoracic, lumbar cord, and cauda equina lesions (paraplegia). **Causes**: traumatic spinal cord injury frequently occurs as a result of motor vehicle and motorcycle trauma, diving, rugby football, and horse riding accident. Spina bifida occurs in 0.7/1000 births. Polygenetic factors and folic acid deficiency in pregnancy. May have associated myelomeningocele with cerebral interventricular shunt inserted. **Physiology**: altered response to exercise occur in the spinal athlete due to a number of factors.

684

Skeletal muscle paralysis: the active muscle mass is limited to the arms and trunk in paraplegics. The inability to utilize lower limb muscle mass will limit the maximal oxygen uptake (VO_{2max}).[1] Increases in aerobic fitness may be achieved,[2] particularly in low spinal with normal cardiorespiratory function, and approach that of a sedentary able-bodied person.[3] *In the quadriplegic* the oxygen demands of the upper limb muscles during exercise are unlikely to exceed cardiac reserve. *Peripheral rather than cardiac factors may be more important.* Adaptive changes in upper limb muscles may occur with the development of a higher percentage of slow twitch fibers in long-term wheelchair users compared to the normal population.[4]

1 GC Gass and EM Camp 1984 *Medicine and Science in Sports and Exercise* **16** 355–9   2 GC Gass and EM Camp 1979 *Medicine and Science in Sports* **11** 256–9   3 S Nilson *et al* 1975 *Scand J Rehab Med* **7** 51–6   4 G Davis *et al* 1981 *Can J Appl Spit Sci* **6** 159–65

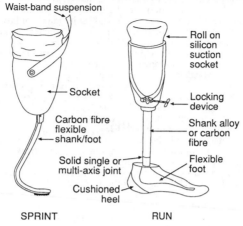

Waist-band suspension

Socket

Carbon fibre flexible shank/foot

SPRINT

Roll on silicon suction socket

Locking device

Shank alloy or carbon fibre

Flexible foot

Solid single or multi-axis joint

Cushioned heel

RUN

Fig. 20.1 Below knee (BK) athletic protheses

Sympathetic autonomic dysfunction spinal cord dysfunction above T4 isolates the sympathetic from the CNS. This results in a loss of sympathetic regulation of heart rate and limits maximal heartrate to 120 or lower. There is a loss of innervation to the arterial and venous smooth muscle, and sweating and thermoregulation is profoundly affected.[1] There is also a phenomenon known as paradoxic hypotension with exercise which improves with training.

Respiratory function: Spinal cord injury impairs respiratory function by paralysis of accessory, intercostal, diaphragm or abdominal muscles depending on the level of lesion. *The quadriplegic is particularly at risk of pneumonia and atelactasis.* Decreased tidal volume with diaphragmatic breathing may be affected by intraabdominal pressure and posture. The reduction of forced vital capacity (FVC) has been implicated as a risk factor for respiratory complications. Exercise training may improve FVC in persons with quadriplegia.[2]

Blood pooling: venous return is impaired due to loss of muscle pump and sympathetic vasoconstriction resulting in orthostatic hypotension.

Spasticity: biomechanical limitations to exercise occur due to spasticity and contracture. Self-implemented daily stretching is recommended. Ballistic stretches or passive stretches by an assistant risk muscle damage. Static sustained stretches are preferred (e.g. 3 repetitions of 60s, 2–3 times daily).[3]

Neurogenic bowel: bowel management is usually daily or second daily with continence achieved between evacuation. Daily management with adequate fiber and intermittent use of peristaltic agents (e.g. senna) to achieve rectal filling and rectal stimulation manually or by enema to achieve evacuation. The defecation reflex is preserved when sacral segments (S2–S4) are intact. Cauda equina lesions result in a patulous anus and regular manual evacuation may be required.

Neurogenic bladder: three types of bladder function occur in spinal injury:

1 *Disinhibited bladder*. In this type of bladder voluntary control is partially retained. Filling of the bladder to a certain point results in reflex emptying and incontinence. The bladder usually fully empties and there is a minimal risk of urinary tract infection. It is managed by regular toileting.

2 *Spinal reflex bladder* (*suprasacral*). The person has no awareness of bladder filling. The bladder fills to a certain limit and then reflexly empties. This is initiated through the S2, S3, S4 sacral reflex arc and emptying may be initiated by tapping the abdomen. A person with this type of bladder may develop a 'balanced bladder' with regular toileting and use of a collecting device (e.g. Uredome and leg bag). The reflex bladder may also be managed by intermittent self catheterization depending on hand function. Anticholinergics (e.g. oxybutinin) are frequently used to block the reflex detrusor contraction if catheterization is the chosen management.

3 *Autonomous bladder*. This occurs in cauda equina lesions (e.g. spina bifida) where and there is insufficient bladder contraction to result in emptying. This type of bladder is usually managed with an indwelling catheter, suprapubic catheter, or intermittent self-catheterization.[4]

Pressure care: Factors that influence the formation of pressure sores in areas insensate to pain temperature, and touch include:

1 SF Figioni 1993 *Medicine and Science in Sports and Exercise* **25** 433–41
2 L Crane *et al* 1994 *International Medical Society of Paraplegia* **32** 435–41
3 SO Kennedy 1988 *Sports N' Spokes* **13**   4 DC Burke and DD Murray 1975 *Handbook of spinal cord medicine* Macmillan, London

- Sustained local pressure
- Friction
- Shearing forces
- Skin maceration
- Infection, burns, and poor nutrition

Sacral and ischial pressure points are most common or any other bony prominence (e.g. heel, toes, trochanter).

Regular lifting of buttocks (self-implemented) by wheelchair athletes at the rate of 3 times per hour and the use of a pressure-relieving cushion (e.g. air floatation) or gel may prevent the problem. Regular inspection of the pressure points by the athlete should be encouraged. Medical examinations should be conducted in the wheelchair or on a cushioned couch. *Thermoregulation*: loss of sweating and vasodilation vasocontriction in the high lesion spinal athlete affects the ability to regulate core temperature. Adequate fluid intake immediately prior to and after competition[16] is essential. Access to ice fans in hot conditions, and blankets and heaters in cold conditions are essential. Increased spasticity may be a symptom associated with low body temperature.

Management of associated conditions

Autonomic hyperreflexia (dysreflexia): this condition occurs in athletes with spinal cord injury above the splanchnic sympathetic outflow (levels higher than T6). Distension of bladder or bowel, initiates excessive reflex activity of the sympathetic nervous system below the level of injury. This causes high blood pressure (BP) which cannot be controlled by centers in the brain. If BP becomes very high, it can cause a cerebral hemorrhage and fitting.

These spinal athletes have an altered cardiovascular response to exercise and in an attempt to increase their performance by up to 10% an illegal technique called 'boosting' has developed.[1] This technique is initiated by placing nociceptive stimuli in the wheelchair (e.g. sharp objects, or tight leg straps). Another method is to increase the bladder volume prior to a race. The intention is to bring on a degree of autonomic hyperreflexia, which is a potentially fatal condition.

Symptoms of autonomic hyperreflexia (dysreflexia):

- Pounding headache which increases in intensity as BP rises
- Bradycardia (slow pulse rate)
- Flushing/blotching of the skin above the level of spinal cord injury
- Profuse sweating particularly above the level of spinal cord injury
- Goose bumps
- Chills without fever
- Nasal stuffiness
- Hypertension. The normal BP for this group of people is commonly 90/60–100/60 lying and lower when sitting. A BP of 130/90 is therefore high for them. If untreated, it can rapidly rise to extreme levels (e.g. 220/140)
- Blurred vision
- Nausea

1 R Burnham *et al.* 1994 *Clin J Sport Med* **4** 1–10

Common causes:
– Bladder irritation (e.g. distended bladder, urological procedure, urine infection)
– Bowel irritation (e.g. distended rectum, chemically irritant suppositories)
– Skin irritation (e.g. pressure sores, infected toe, ingrowing toenail, burns)
– Other (e.g. distended or contracting uterus, fractured bones, ingrown toenail)

Treatment (Two people are required to control the situation unless the condition is easily reversed):
1 Place person in a sitting position with head elevated (BP is lowered by gravity) and ask if cause is known or able to be predicted.
2A For person with an indwelling catheter:
  (a) Empty leg bag and estimate the volume, to determine whether or not the bladder is empty. Ask if volume is reasonable considering fluid intake and output earlier that day.
  (b) Check that catheter or tubing is not kinked or flow is not impaired by clogged inlet to leg bag or perished valve in leg bag.
  (c) If catheter is blocked irrigate *gently* with no more than 30ml sterile water. If this is unsuccessful, recatheterize, using a generous amount of lubricant containing a local anesthetic (e.g. lignocaine jelly).
  (d) If BP declines after the bladder is emptied, the person still requires close observation as the bladder can go into severe contractions causing hypertension to recur.
2B For a person with a balanced bladder (bladder-trained):
  (a) If the bladder is distended and the person is unable to void on gentle abdominal expression or tapping, lubricate the urethra with a generous amount of local anesthetic jelly (e.g. lignocaine jelly), wait 1–2min and then empty the bladder, by passing a catheter.
2C For fecal mass in rectum:
  (a) Gently insert a generous amount of lignocaine jelly into the rectum and gently remove fecal mass—*note*: symptoms may be aggravated initially.
3 If the markedly elevated BP does not start to subside within 1min of above treatment, or the cause is unable to be determined, give nifedipine (Adalat/Anpine) 10mg capsule; the patient should bite the capsule and swallow the liquid like water. The hypotensive response begins within 5min after administration, reaches a peak at 30min, and persists for several hours.
  Glycerol trinitrate (Anginine) can be given instead of nifedipine. It is placed under the tongue or used as an aerosol. If nifedipine or glyceryl trinitrate do not lower BP, IV diazoxide (Hyperstat) 300mg/20ml ampoules can be used. The initial dose is 75–150mg (5–10ml) IV over 30s. Further doses can be given at intervals of 5–15min or a continuous infusion commenced at 15mg/min. (Adapted from Austin Hospital Melbourne, Australia emergency treatment card, personal communication, D. Brown.)
  Peripheral nerve entrapment: upper extremity nerve entrapment in wheelchair athletes is very common with prevalence up to 23%.[1] *The*

1 RS Burnham, RD Steadward 1994 *Arch Phys Med Rehabil* **75**, May 1994 519–523.

commonest injuries are to the median and ulnar nerve at the wrist. The ulnar nerve may be damaged near the elbow and may occur concurrently with median neuropraxia.[1] *Wheeling a chair creates pressure over the carpal tunnel* during the propulsive phase. The use of a glove is not totally protective of the carpal tunnel although designed with padding to reduce trauma to the wrist and palm. Repetitive trauma to the volar aspect of the wrist in extreme forced extension is an important factor.[2] *The ulnar nerve may be damaged* at the distal aspect of the cubital tunnel possibly due to heavy repetitive contraction of the flexor carpi ulnaris and/or pressure from the armrest or the outer rim of the wheel.[3] At the wrist the ulnar nerve and artery enter an osseofibrous canal, *Guyon's canal'*. The nerve travels through a groove between the pisiform and the back of the hamate[4,5] where it is susceptible to damage from repetitive trauma, ischemia, ganglia, or fracture of the hamate.

Treatment: conservative treatment aimed at nerve protection and avoidance of surgery which is unlikely to solve the causative biomechanical factors. *Padding* to gloves and push rims should be checked. *Techniques* to avoid extreme wrist extension and ulnar deviation while pushing and transferring. *Substitute alternative training* (e.g. arm ergometer or swimming), until symptoms subside. *Assess transfers and crutch use* where weight bearing and forced wrist extension occurs with unprotected hands. Prevent arms hitting the outer rims.[6] *Consider night resting splints.*

Shoulder injury: shoulder pain occurs in more than half the number of people with spinal injury using wheelchairs. The shoulder becomes a weight bearing joint for transfers or if using crutches.[7] This results in a high incidence of rotator cuff impingement and subacromial bursitis. Wheelchair propulsion creating overuse injury is also a factor.

Treatment: rest may be difficult to achieve as the problem is often bilateral. Assessment of transfer techniques by a physical, or occupational therapist may assist.

Down's syndrome

People with Down's Syndrome are characterized by an intellectual disability and short stature. Their facies have been described as oriental due to the epicanthal fold of the eye partly covering the medial angle of the palpebral fissure, and poor development of the bridge of the nose. They have an enlarged tongue and their hands are broad with a single palmar crease, hypoplastic middle finger and short little finger.[8] They have a high incidence of cardiac abnormalities (septal defects) and atlantoaxial (C1–C2) instability with the risk of high cervical spinal cord injury. Most compete within the intellectual disability classification and Special Olympics. **Causes**: trisomy of chromosome 21 occurring more frequently to children of mothers with increasing age of parity 1.3/1000 (age 30–34), 1.9/1000 (age 35–39).[9]

1 J Aljure *et al* 1985 *Int Med Soc Paraplegia* **23** 182–6 **2** K Dozono *et al* 1995 *Int Med Soc Paraplegia* **33** 208–11 **3** R Burnham *et al* 1995 *Arch Phys Med Rehabil* **75**, May 513–518 **4** SM Weinstein, SA Herring 1992 *Clin Sports Med* **11**, January 161–188 **5** LE Bloomquist 1986 *Physician Sports Med* **14**, September 97–105 **6** PJR Nichols *et al* 1979 *Scand J Rehab Med* **11** 29–32 **7** JC Bayley *et al.* 1987 *J Bone Joint Surg* **69A**, June 676–678 **8** K Isselbacher *et al Harrison textbook of medicine* 13th edn. *McGraw-Hill, New York* **9** MS Schimmel *et al* 1997 *BMJ* **314** 720–1

The athlete (*cont*)

Management of injury and associated conditions

Intellectual disability may affect the athlete's ability to follow complicated treatment regimes (e.g. application of ice packs). Communication should be brief, simple, and clear. Safety issues and prevention are most important, particularly hydration and application of sunscreens where prompting may be necessary. The doctor should be patient, tolerant, and tactful.

Atlantoaxial (C1-C2) instability[1] occurs in 10–20% of people with Down's syndrome. Since 1983, athletes with Down's syndrome have required a medical examination including flexion and extension x-rays of the head and neck to diagnose the condition. Athletes with atlantoaxial instability, or those who have not received a medical clearance, are prohibited from participation in gymnastics, diving, swimming butterfly stroke, high jump, and pentathlon.[2]

Polio

Paralytic poliomyelitis is due to a loss of anterior horn cells. Muscle paralysis may result in segmental, paraplegic quadriplegic, or bulbar loss. **Causes**: RNA enterovirus with 3 strains spread through feco–oral route. 0.1% of all infections progress to paralysis. Infections are rare in developed countries since the introduction of Salk and Sabin vaccines, 1955–60. **Physiology**: after the initial paralysis a recovery phase occurs with neurological recovery. During this phase 'orphaned' muscle fibers may be reinnervated by terminal axon sprouting from unaffected motor neurones. This results in giant motor units forming with one motor nerve innervating up to five times the original number of muscle fibers.[3] Loss of muscle in the extremities results in blood pooling, intolerance to cold and gait abnormalities. Many athletes require assistive devices such as wheelchair, caliper, and crutches.

Management

Muscle weakness, muscle pain, fatigue, and joint pain are common symptoms as late effects of polio.[4] Strengthening exercises in weakened muscles may result in a decrease in strength. Aerobic fitness programs and biomechanical efficiency and energy conservation is preferred. Compression neuropathics from crutches and wheelchairs are similar to those occurring in spinal athletes. Pressure sores are less common than in spinal athletes due to normal protective sensation.

690

1 TKF Taylor, WL Walter 1996 *MJA* **165** 27 448–450   **2** LE Bloomquist 1986 *Physician Sports Med* **14**   **3** LS Halstead 1988 *Top geriatr rehabi* **3** 9–26 Aspen   **4** JC Agre *et al* 1991 *Arch Physiother Med Rehabil* **72** 923–31

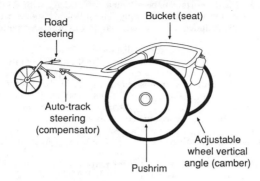

Road
steering

Bucket (seat)

Auto-track
steering
(compensator)

Adjustable
wheel vertical
angle (camber)

Pushrim

Fig. 20.2 Example of a lightweight custom Road racing chair with semi-
automatic steering and small diameter racing pushroms

The sports

General Most sports can be adapted for athletes with disabilities. The rules of the ISOs usually apply. The following sports consist of those sports included in International Paralympic competition or demonstration sports.

Archery Athletes shoot from a distance of 70m at 122cm-diameter targets. Competition scores range from 1000 to 2500 points. Amputees, cerebral palsy, and wheelchair athletes compete in these events.

Athletics All disability groups may compete in these events. Track (10 events): 100m, 200m, 400m, 800m, 1500m, 3000m, 5000m, 10,000m, 4×100 relay, 4×400 relay and marathon. These events may be may be competed in as a running event, or as a wheelchair event depending on the disability. *Field* (9 events): shotput, discus, javelin, club throw (cerebral palsy), long, high, triple jump, pentathlon.

Basketball This is a wheelchair event played in accordance with the regulations of the International Basketball Federation. There are a number of rules of play. The athletes must dribble the ball after two pushes. Touching the ground with the feet or rising from the chair results in a foul.

Boccia (pronounced 'botcha') The athletes throw 6 leather balls as close as possible to the target ball (jack). It is played individually or in teams. Cerebral palsy classes C1, C2, and C1 with assistive devices compete (see p596).

Cycling These events are divided into 3 groups. Cerebral palsy in bicycle and tricycle events. Athletes with visual impairment compete in tandem with a sighted cyclist. Amputees compete with or without a prosthesis.

Equestrian Riders of all disability groups compete in dressage competitions before 3 judges.

Fencing All disability groups compete in wheelchairs fixed to the floor using épée, sabre, and foil. The competitor may duck, lean forward, back, or half turn to avoid touches without rising from the chair.

Football (soccer) This is open to male athletes with cerebral palsy. The game is divided into two 25min halves with up to 7 players on the field from each team of 11 players. Two substitutions per game are permitted.

Goalball Athletes with visual impairments compete in opposing teams of 3 players. The ball contains bells and a goal is scored by throwing or rolling into the opposing team goal which is the width of the court.

Judo Played by athletes with visual impairment. Touch, balance, strength, and agility are highly developed skills in these athletes.

Lawn bowls Disability groups who may compete are amputee, cerebral palsy, visually impaired, and wheelchair. It is played on a lawn bowling court with a target ball (jack). Large wooden balls are rolled towards the jack, and balls lying closest to the jack score more points.

Power Lifting This is a bench press starting with arms extended bringing the bar to the chest. The athlete then presses the bar back to its original position. Male paraplegics, amputees, cerebral palsy, and polio athletes compete. Classification is determined by bodyweight.

Quad rugby This is open to male and female wheelchair athletes. It is played on a basketball court by two opposing teams of 4 players.

The team passes a volleyball while advancing into the opponent's half court with the intention of crossing the goal line in possession of the ball to score. The ball must be dribbled or passed within 10 seconds.

Sailing   All disability groups may compete in the 3-man keel boat division. The selection of a team is based on a total points system based on functions required to compete in sailing. These include stability, hand function, moveability, visibility, and hearing. A single-handed division is developing based on the international 2.4m class. The sailor sits facing the bow and controls sails and steering by sheets and joystick.

Shooting (air and .22 calibre)   Men and women mixed teams compete in SH1 class if no support of the upper limbs is required or SH2 class if arms are unable to support the weight of a rifle, requiring a support stand. Pistol shooting is a standing event and rifle shooting is in prone, kneeling, and standing. Amputees and wheelchair athletes compete.

Swimming   Athletes with locomotor disabilities compete with the 10 functional classes for freestyle, backstroke, breaststroke, and medley. Blind and visually impaired compete in separate competition.

Table tennis   All disability groups compete standing or in a wheelchair. The rules are those of the International Table Tennis Federation with only minor modifications (e.g. player may grip the side of the table).

Tennis   Wheelchair athletes compete on a conventional tennis court. The ball may bounce twice before being returned. There are mens and womens singles and doubles.

Volleyball   Standing volleyball is played with standard configuration. Seated volleyball is played with a smaller court and lower net.

Management of events

Access

Consider that some attendees, athletes, judges and classifiers, and spectators may have disabilities. Access should be available to spectator areas, prize presentation areas, toilets and accommodation and the sporting arena. Wheelchair, ramps of 1:12–1:14 gradient are recommended. Extended ramps 50–100m requires 'pusher' volunteers on standby. Transport by motor vehicle may need ramped access or wheelchair lifts fitted to the vehicles. Amputees, particularly above the knee, develop prosthetic knee instability on ramps therefore steps may be better if a handrail is fitted.

Staff

Small events require a first aid officer with a good referral network. Athletes with severe disabilities often travel with well-informed carers and parents who render first-line treatment. For major events (e.g. state, national, or international, where records may be set), then an organized sports medicine team is required. This should comprise:

1 Medical co-ordinator who may also be the chief medical officer (CMO) for medical emergencies and review of medical certificates
2 Nurse for triage and assistance to CMO in an emergency
3 Physiotherapists for treatment of musculoskeletal injuries
4 Massage therapists for precompetition massage of cerebral palsy and spinal injury athletes with spasticity
5 Sports trainers/first aiders for 'on field' and finish line response to injury. The ratio differs from able-bodied events due to the greater need for precompetition massage:
   doctor (1): nurse (1): physio (3): masseurs (4): sports trainers/first aiders (5): prosthetist/orthotist—optional.

The greatest number of injuries are likely to occur in athletics with fewer injuries in other sports.

Drug/dope testing

The same conditions apply as for able-bodied sport. Prescribed medications taken at the prescribed dose may be acceptable on presentation of a medical certificate to the CMO. Evidence of prescribed medications is generally presented at least 2 days prior to competition, *not* on the day of competition. Prescribed medication should be for an existing medical condition and not prescribed or increased in dose to enhance performance.

Additions to standard doctors bag/kit

Medication: nifedipine capsules, 5—10mg. For sublingual use in dysreflexia, or glyceryl trinitrate aerosol
Diazepam 5mg—for injection
Clonazepam 0.2 mg—for injection
50% dextrose—for injection
Lignocaine jelly lubricant for catheterization
Equipment: Tube gauze for prosthetic 'pull through'
Lubricant cream for 'wet fit' prostheses (aqueous cream)
Stretch stump bandage 10cm × 200cm
Silicon gel pads
Sterile dressing tray, sterile glove, disposable gloves
Neoprene catheters × 4
Screwdriver, pliers, and Allen (hex) key, to assist prosthetist/orthotist with prosthesis and wheelchair repair.

695

Classification

Is a process of grading athletes according to their ability to perform the functional tasks of the sport. The older system of classifying athletes by their medical diagnosis or impairment is being replaced by a *functional integrated classification*. This has enabled many different disability groups to compete in the same events classified as equal to other competitors in terms of their ability to perform the tasks required for the sport. *Athletes are classified prior to an event* and generally retain their classification over many years. Improvements in technique and performance related to training should not change the classification. However, the athlete or the classifier may initiate a new classification if a change of function has occurred through medical or surgical intervention or based on observed performance at events which may be above or below that expected for the class.

Medical and technical classifiers require considerable training and accreditation. The systems of classification consist of three components:

1 *Medical*: assessment by doctor or physiotherapist
2 *Technical*: assessment often by a coach familiar with the tasks and movement potential related to the sports
3 *Review*: classifiers watch training and competition

There are *three basic types of classification*:

1 General
2 Functional
3 Team

1 General

This is the older system based on impairment, diagnosis, and disability. These classifications have little relationship to the sport. Examples are:

- **Visually impaired**

Class B1—No light perception at all in either eye up to light perception but inability to recognize the shape of a hand at any distance or direction.
Class B2—From ability to recognize the shape of a hand up to a visual acuity of 2/60 and/or a visual field of less than 5°.
Class B3—Front visual acuity from 2/60 up to a visual acuity of 6/60 and/or visual field of more than 5° and less than 20°.

- **Cerebral Palsy**

Class 1—Severe involvement in all four limbs. Limited trunk control, unable to grasp a softball. Very poor functional strength in upper extremities, necessitating the use of an electric wheelchair.
Class 2—Severe to moderate involvement in all 4 limbs. Able to slowly propel wheelchair with either feet or arms. Poor functional strength and severe control problems exist.
Class 3—Moderate involvement in 3 or 4 limbs. Fair functional strength and moderate control problems in upper extremities and torso. Uses a wheelchair..
Class 4—Lower limbs have moderate to severe involvement. Good functional strength and minimal control problems in the upper extremities and torso. Uses a wheelchair.
Class 5—Good functional strength and minimal to moderate control problems in upper extremities. May walk with or without aids for ambulatory support.

Class 6—Moderate to severe involvement in all limbs. Ambulates poorly. Severe co-ordination and balance problems which tend to be less noticeable when running, swimming, and throwing.

Class 7—Moderate to minimal involvement in both limbs on the same side of the body. Good functional ability in the non-affected side. Walks and runs with a limp.

Class 8—Minimally affected athlete. May have minimal co-ordination and functional problems affecting only one limb. Able to run and jump freely. Has good balance.

- **Amputee**

AK Above or through knee joint

BK Below knee, but through or above talocrural joint.

AE Above or through elbow joint

BE Below elbow, but through or above wrist joint.

Class A1—Double AK

Class A2—Single AK

Class A3—Double BK

Class A4—Single BK

Class A5—Double AE

Class A6—Single AE

Class A7—Double BE

Class A8—Single BE

Class A9—Combined lower plus upper limb amputation

The classification for winter sports is combined for locomotor disabilities. The prefix in winter sports classification is therefore LW (Locomotor Winter).

- **Wheelchair**[1]

Quadriplegics are classified as T1 or T2 for track and F1, F2, or F3 for field events. The '1' indicates the highest level of disability. Paraplegics are classified as T3 or T4 and F4, F5, F6, F7, or F8. In this system a double leg amputee would be classified as T4 for track events.

2 Functional

These classifications are based on the sport and assessment of the athletes abilities related to the sport. Athletes are classified according to:

A clinical assessment or 'benchtest' by a medical classifier (doctor/physiotherapist) examining the following features as appropriate to the athlete:

1 Muscle strength

2 Dysfunction/coordination

3 Range of motion of joints

4 Limb length in amputees

5 Trunk length in small stature (dwarfs)

B Sports-related test in the pool or on the track by a technical classifier familiar with the tasks required for the sport.

697

---

1 NSW Wheelchair Sports Association (Per comm J McCullough)

Classification (*cont*)

- **Swimming**:
    - Freestyle, Backstroke, Butterfly = S1–S10
    - Breaststroke = SB1–SB10
    - Individual Medley = SM1–SM10

The '1' indicates the most disabled, through to 10 indicating minimal disability. The swimming classification system is 'functional' and caters for various physical disabilities (e.g. in one race there could be competitors with cerebral palsy, paraplegia, polio, and amputations).

- **Track and Field**—designated by 'T' and 'F' with low numbers indicating a greater disability. This system is still evolving and reference is made to the older general classes as a starting point for functional classification. For example, a Class 2 cerebral palsy wheelchair athlete (general) would relate to a T30, T31, and F30 (functional) classification. A T42 standing track classification would include A2 and A9 amputee (general) classifications.

3 Team

Teams are made up of a number of competitors with individual disability scores which add up to a maximum score for a team. Examples:

- **Yachting**—Points are allocated to individual crew members based on hand function, movability, stability, vision, and hearing. Total points for a crew of three may not exceed 12 points. Points for an individual crew member may not exceed 7 points.
- **Wheelchair basketball**—Competitors with a high level of disability score 1, up to 4.5 points for competitors with a low level of disability. A team is allowed a maximum of 14 points on the court.
- **Wheelchair rugby**—Competitors are graded from 0.5—4.0 points and maximum 8 points are allowed on the court during play.

[1] P Gray 1997 In E Sherry, D. Bokor (ed) *Sports medicine problems and practical management* Ch 18. GMM, London

701

Introduction

Sport benefits children—they become fitter (higher VO_{2max}) and stronger (greater strength). Their participation in competitive and recreational sport is increasing. Injury may occur. It is important to be aware of the nature and cause of injuries, so that the benefits of sport and exercise can be maximized and injuries minimized. Children are *not* small adults and have their own physiological and developmental parameters (Fig. 21.1). They are less metabolically efficient than adults, but can significantly improve performance by improved economy of movement and are more prone to heat illness and to disturbances of bone growth from injury. *In general, child and youth sport is safe.*

An Australian (NSW) Sports Injury Survey of 15,525 high school students (aged 11–19 years) conducted over a 2-year period revealed that 54% reported at least one injury in the previous 6 months (males>females).[1] Most of the sports were 'fun' games and at the Club level (28%). The sports causing the injuries were rugby union (36%), rugby league (35%), gymnastics (34%), netball (33%), hockey (32%), Australian Rules football (31%), soccer (25%), horse riding (23%), martial arts (23%) and basketball (21%). *The most common injuries were bruising* (36%), muscle sprain (32%), joint injury (20%), bleeding (16%), fractures (11%), dislocation (8%); 5% were 'knocked-out'. The most common sites of injury were ankle (32%), knee (30%), finger (15%), leg (24%), back (4%), neck (4%), head (10%). 74% stopped activities for a day, 53% saw a doctor, and 29% lost time from school, 4% for over 2 weeks.

Other authors' experiences reveal that organized sport is no more or less dangerous that play in other childhood arenas, such as the home, school, and the street.

Age, size, and maturity of young athletes is a factor. As size and age increase (sports injuries increase with age and peak at 15–17 years),[1] the speed and violence of collision and contact is greater, resulting in a greater incidence of injury. One needs to be aware of the enormous variability of growth and maturation of children at a similar point in time. Sports programs that match children according to age alone, misunderstand this variability. Their injury patterns may differ in type and severity from adults (Fig. 21.2).[2] Boys are probably more prone to injury than girls, and any sex difference relates to the fact that girls usually choose less violent sports. As one would expect, the incidence of sporting injuries is related to the inherent violence of the sport itself, there being a much higher incidence of injury in football compared to tennis or swimming. *The following factors contribute to children's injuries*:

- recklessness
- foul or illegal play
- poor playing area/equipment
- inappropriate body size/strength for the sport or the opposition encountered in it
- lack of fitness or postural problems
- lack of/defective protective gear
- poor footwear/sports gear

1 Northern Sydney Area Health Service *NSW Youth sports injury report* July 1997 2 B Zaricznyi *et al* 1980 *Am J Sports Med* 5 318–24

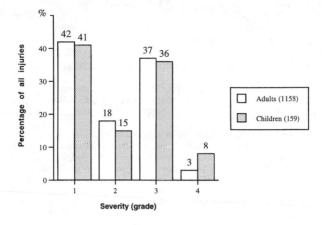

Fig. 21.1 Children's skiing injuries are more serious than adults.

- incomplete recovery from injury/inadequate rehab
- rules which place player at risk
- poor supervision
- lack of adequate warm-up
- parental influences

Such factors are amenable to change by *coaches, trainers, parents, teachers and sports physician.*

A child's readiness for sporting competition is decided by their motor skills level, social, sophistication and ability to follow instructions. It is well to remember that sporting ability **is not** accelerated by early starting.

Children do not appear to be at greater risk of head or spinal cord injury (factors of smaller weight, lower speeds or intrinsic properties of the immature spine). The incidence of such (catastrophic) injury is rare. Children than< 10 years have a relatively higher incidence of atlantooccipital or atlantoaxial injury, while those >10 years have a relatively higher incidence of subaxial spine injury.[3] *Note*: children have an excessive range of flexion/extension at C2–C3 level (>3mm above range of normal) and that Down's syndrome children have excessive atlantoaxial instability therefore no contact sports where >4.5mm of flexion/extension excursion).

2 E Sherry *et al* 1987 *Med J Aust* **146** 193–5 **3** L Micheli 1994 In LY Griffen (ed) *OKU sports medicine* IL p353. AAOS

Distribution of sites of injury in adults and children

Site of injury	Adult (n)	Adult (%)	Children (n)	Children (%)
Foot and ankle	65	6.0	65	1.0
Lower leg	144	10.0	37	23.0
Knee	353	31.0	48	30.0
Femur	27	2.0	11	7.0
Trunk	71	6.0	2	1.0
Neck and back	37	3.0	11	7.0
Head and face	143	12.0	21	13.0
Upper limb	348	30.0	18	11.0
TOTAL	1158	100.0	159	100.0

Comparison and frequency of the 5 most common injuries in adults compared

Injuries in adults	%	Injuries in children	%
Knee sprain	25.0	Knee sprain	28.0
Shoulder dislocation	5.0	Shoulder dislocation	12.0
Shoulder sprain	4.5	Shoulder sprain	9.0
Fractured wrist	3.5	Fractured wrist	5.0
Sprained wrist	3.5	Sprained wrist	5.0
Remainder	58.5	Remainder	41.0

Fig. 21.2 Children's skiing injuries are more likely to involve the lower limb and include shoulder dislocations.

Exercise testing/prescription

Fitness testing is now commonplace for children and endorsed by the American College of Sports Medicine (ACSM). A list of field tests in wide use include:

- *Cardiorespiratory endurance (useful; same indications as per adult)*
  - mile run/walk for time
  - half-mile run/walk (0.8km)for ages 6–7
  - steady state jog
- *Body composition*
  - skin fold measurements
  - body mass index
- *Muscular strength/endurance*
  - pull-ups
  - fixed arm hand
  - bent knee sit-ups or curl-ups
  - push-ups
- *Flexibility*
  - sit-and-reach-test
  - V-sit reach

Contraindications to exercise testing are: cardiac inflammatory disease, uncontrolled congestive heart failure, acute pulmonary disease, acute myocardial infarction, acute renal disease, acute hepatitis, severe hypertension, drug overdose (affecting cardiovascular response to exercise). (See Table 21.1 for exercises for some disorders.)

Exercise testing can utilize the Treadmill Test (follow the modified Balke Treadmill Protocol) and the cycle ergometer (but modify to fit children >8years or >125cm can use standard ergometer otherwise the McMaster Cycle Test as it has been extensively used to measure VO_{2max} in children; terminates when child is within 20% of baseline HR/BP).

Guidelines for exercise prescription

Children can safely use properly designed resistance training programs. The following guidelines from the ACSM are useful:[1]

- Remember that a child is physiologically immature
- Teach proper training techniques for whole of exercise program and proper breathing(no breath holding)
- Control speed of exercises to avoid sudden/ballistic movements
- Use at least 8 repetitions of weights and do not exercise to momentary muscular failure
- Gradually increase repetitions and then resistance
- Use one to two sets of 8–10 different exercises(with 8–12 repetitionss per set)and make sure all major muscle groups are included
- Use twice per week and combine with other forms of exercise
- Use full rage and multi joint exercises
- **Do not overload** muscles and joints of adolescents with maxium weights
- Monitor and supervise

---

1 W Larry Kenny (ed) 1995. Ch 11. Exercise testing and prescription for children, the elderly, and pregnancy. In: *ACSM's Guidelines for Exercise Testing and Prescription*. Williams & Wilkins, Philadelphia.

Table 21.1 Exercise for particular disorders[1]

Disorder	Purpose	Activities
Anorexia nervosa	Behavioral modification. Educate re lean vs fat mass	Those with low energy demand
Bronchial asthma	Build confidence, conditioning, ?reduce exercise-induced bronchospasm	Aquatic, intermittent, slow build up
Cerebral palsy	Increase maximal aerobic capacity, range of motion, ambulation, and control	Depends on current disability
Cystic fibrosis	Improve mucous clearance, train chest muscles	Jog, swim
Diabetes mellitus	Improve metabolic control and control body size	Equalize daily energy use
Hemophilia	Limit muscle wasting and intraarticular bleeding	Swim, cycle, avoid contact sports
Mental retardation	Improve self-esteem, socialization	Variety, low pressure
Muscular dystrophies	Improve muscle bulk and strength, maintain ambulation	Swim, wheelchair sports, calisthenics
Rheumatoid arthritis	Prevent contractures/muscle atrophy, augment daily functions	Swim, cycle, sail, calisthenics
Spina bifida	Build-up upper body, control obesity, increase aerobic capacity	Upper limb resistance training, wheelchair sports

1 W Larry Kenny (ed) 1995. Ch11, Table 11-3 p226 *ACSM's guidelines for exercise testing and prescription*. Williams & Wilkins. Philadelphia

Soft tissue injuries

These injuries (contusions, sprains, and strains) are the **most common** form of injury in the skeletally immature, and occur in the leg. A **contusion** is an injury to a muscle belly. A **sprain** is an injury to a ligament. A **strain** is an injury to junctional areas i.e. bone/muscle, muscle/tendon, or tendon/bone interfaces. These latter injuries have also been variously described as overuse injuries, overload injuries, or stress-related injuries.

Contusions

Are probably the most common injury in the pediatric athlete. The initial response to an injury is a hematoma associated with inflammation. This is then followed by muscle regeneration. When a muscle fiber is injured, the peripherally placed satellite cells, which lie between the basement membrane and the sarcolemma, retain some stem cell potential and are mobilized. These are the myoblasts that fuse to form new myotubes. The regenerating myotubes are very similar to embryonic myotubes, and these myotubes possess the cellular components necessary for formation of contractile protein. In a child with an intact basement membrane, complete healing can be expected. With the more severe injury or advanced age, less complete forms of repair with formation of increased amounts of connective scar tissue occurs.

    Treatment of contusions is initially rest, ice, compressionn, elevation (RICE). Isometric quadriceps exercises to start when the patient is able. Once quadriceps control has been regained, active range of movement is instituted. Shadow weight bearing is allowed, and once there is 90° of knee flexion, progressive resistance exercises can begin. Physical modalities (ultrasound, heat, and interferential) may be useful in influencing the rate of recovery. *Avoid passive stretching* of the muscles in any form, as tearing a healing muscle unit can produce more connective scar tissue. Such connective scar tissue can interfere with the muscle's ability to contract efficiently and move through a normal range of motion. A return to sports is dependent on the demonstration of full strength and full range of motion of the injured limb.

Myositis ossificans

Myositis ossificans traumatica is an unfortunate sequela of severe muscle contusion (see Chapter 11). Myositis ossificans refers to the phenomenon of new bone formation in muscle following injury. The quadriceps and brachialis have long been documented as the favored sites of this condition. It appears most often in the second and third decades, but a lesion in a 5-year-old following a motor vehicle accident has been reported. **Symptoms** include pain, swelling, and progressive loss of movement. Heterotrophic bone is visible radiologically seen about 3 weeks or can be detected earlier on bone scan. The treatment involves rest followed by active mobilization. **Passive mobilization is definitely contraindicated**. NSAIDs can be beneficial by suppressing new bone formation.

Overuse injuries (microtrauma)[1]

Overuse injuries are the result of unresolved submaximal stress in previously normal tissues. With increasing participation of younger athletes in sport, such injuries are now becoming more common. Apart from the intrinsic demands that such sport places on children, there are *anatomic considerations* for such injuries in children.

First: growing bone has a looser periosteum and tendinous attachments than mature bone. This means less force can produce traction overload.

Second: the epiphyses and the apophyses are weak links in the bone–tendon–muscle unit, as they are susceptible to tensile overloads.

Third: the differential growth patterns in the length of bones relative to muscles, results in decreased flexibility in the large muscle groups of the upper and lower extremities and back. This tightness affects muscle strength by interfering with the normal length–tension relationships. A tight and weak muscle is the most susceptible to overload injuries. Overuse complaints usually produce a mechanical type of pain (increases with activity and diminishes with rest). The pain may only be precipitated by strenuous sports activity, by limited sports activity, or occur with day-to-day activities. **Risk factors include**:

- Training errors (abrupt changes in intensity/duration/frequency of training)
- Musculotendinous imbalance of strength/flexibility/bulk
- Anatomic malignment of leg (LLD/rotational profile of hips/patella position/genu varus or valgus/flat feet)
- Footwear (poor: fit/cushioning/stiffness/support)
- Other disease(circulation/arthritis)
- Growth spurt (growing articular cartilage is probably less resistant to repetitive microtrauma than adult cartilage and during rapid longitudinal growth the soft tissues lad behind resulting in muscle–tendon tightness about joints, loss of flexibility, and proneness to overuse problems: especially with our current day larger and stronger children)
- Environmental (equipment/playing surface/weather/altitude)

The most common significant factors are training errors.

General types of overuse injury

Stress fractures

Not uncommon in children There is a direct relationship to age (children have fewer fractures than adolescents, who have fewer fractures than adults). 9% of these fractures occur in children aged less than 15 years, 32% in 16- to 19-year-olds, and 59% in those over 20 years. The tibia is the most common site of fractures accounting for approximately 50% of stress fractures. Upper extremity stress fractures have been reported, namely, in the diaphysis of the ulna, in the non-dominant arm of the tennis player, caused by the use of a two-handed back hand stroke; midhumeral stress fracture in a 15-year-old tennis player due to excessive service and overhead strokes; stress fractures have been seen around the elbow in throwing athletes; and stress fractures have been seen in the distal radial epiphysis of gymnasts.

1 LJ Micheli 1983 *Orthop Clin North Am* **14** 337–59

Note: Osteoid osteoma, subacute osteomyelitis, Ewing's sarcoma, and osteogenic sarcoma must be differentiated from stress fractures (perform x-ray).

X-rays are usually unhelpful in the diagnosis of these injuries, as in the early phases many stress fractures are radiographically silent. Technetium 99 bone scanning is positive about 12–15 days following the onset of stress fracture symptoms. Midtibial stress fractures have proved difficult to heal, and the majority tend to go on to complete fractures. Once the fracture is complete, non-union tends to occur and bone grafting is required to achieve union.

- *Tendinitis*. Occurs in children, although less frequently than adults. Usually at the apophysis. Exclude stress fracture/osteochondritis or nerve entrapment. Use 'relative' rest with RICE, early dynamic eccentric training, but **no** steroid cream in the young athlete. May consider surgical excision of aseptic necrotic area of tendon
- *Bursitis*. Use 'relative' rest and RICE
- *Joint problems*: osteochondritis dissecans and patellofemoral problems

Sites of overuse injuries

- *Spine*: with growth spurt (enhanced anterior growth of vertebral body tethered by posterior fascia) develop lordodsis and flexion tightness of hips and tight hamstrings coupled with hyperextension sports (gymnastics), causes posterior element failure (pars defect and/or disk rupture). Juvenile roundback and some cases of Scheuermann's kyphosis may have a similar etiology.
- *Shoulder*: problems of 'little leaguer's shoulder' (microfracture proximal humeral growth plate from repetitive throwing); impingement (?tight posterior shoulder capsule, ?hypertrophy of the humeral head from repetitive stress to the immature articular cartilage).
- *Elbow*: 'little leaguer's elbow' (osteochondritis of the capitellum/LBs in the joint/premature closure of the proximal radial epiphysis/overgrowth of the radial head/irritation of the medial epicondyle) (see Fig. 9.4).
- *Hip*: ?premature OA of the hip from subtle SUFE, 'snapping hip'(?flicking of fascia over greater trochanter/tenosynovitis of iliopsoas/?subluxing hip ± labral tear). Apophyseal pain at muscle avulsion.
- *Knee*: common, often the extensor mechanism (patella) with chondromalacia. Recently called the 'patellofemoral stress syndrome'. Osgood–Schlatter's disease. Osteochondritis dissecans.
- *Ankle and foot*: heel pain (os calcis apophysitis–exclude stress fracture). Tendonitis of tibial posterior or peroneal tendons.

Physical examination should include an assessment of the alignment of the involved limb (both angular, rotatory, and longitudinal alignment). Assess the range of motion within the joints and the flexibility around the joints. Ligamentous laxity needs to be assessed. Local tenderness with increased warmth and swelling are common manifestations of tendonitis, apophysitis, bursitis, or stress fractures.

Overuse injuries (microtrauma) (*cont*)

Micheli[1] recommends a growth chart to detect growth spurt and so need for flexibility work or decreased intensity of training. Investigations include x-rays bone scans and ultrasound. Treatment of overuse injuries involves six phases (Table 21.2).

Patient, parent, and coach education remains a significant component of management of overuse problems and focuses on training abuse and improper equipment. The long-term effects of chronic submaximal stress in skeletally immature athletes are still unknown.

1 LJ Micheli 1983 *Orthop Clin North Am* **14** 337–59

Table 21.2 Treatment of overuse injuries

1 Identifying the risk factor
2 Modifying the factors
3 Control of pain
4 Undertake progressive
5 Rehabilitation with emphasis on restoration of full flexibility, endurance and strength
6 Amaintenance program to prevent new injuries or a recurrence of the previous injuries

Fractures (macrotrauma)

Represent about 20% of sport related injuries in the skeletally immature, and tend to be more common in the upper limb. They should therefore **always be suspected** and need to be excluded. When **deformity** is present, the diagnosis is easy. In the **absence of deformity**, swelling, loss of function and localized bony tenderness are diagnostic. In the presence of bony tenderness, an x-ray is essential to plan appropriate management.

Sequence of ossification

Bone ossifies from a cartilaginous anlage. The **primary** center of ossification is in the diaphysis, and most of these are present at birth. The **secondary** centers of ossification, the epiphyses and the apophyses, appear at variable times after birth. Epiphyses occur at the end of long bones and are involved in longitudinal growth of the bone. **Apophyses** are at the sites of origin or insertion of major muscles or tendons, and are involved in circumferential bone growth.

Fractures in the skeletally immature can occur through the diaphysis, the metaphysis, the physis, or the epiphysis. Young bone is more porous than adult bone due to larger Haversian canals. As a consequence, when a force is applied to immature bone there is a longer plastic deformation phase before the bone fails. Thus 4 *different* fracture patterns can occur in the diaphysis and the metaphysis; namely, the torus or buckle fracture, plastic bowing, greenstick fracture, and the complete fracture (Fig. 21.3). The type of fracture produced depends on the duration of, and the force applied.

Anatomical realignment of fractures is obviously desirable, but during the healing process immature bone exhibits a greater degree of *remodeling* than is possible in the adult. Following an angulated fracture at the end of a long bone, the physis exhibits a spontaneous ability to change its inclination towards a normalization of the inclination of the epiphyseal plate. There is, however, an upper limit of angulation that can correct. In practical terms, with regard to the distal radius, complete normalization will take place after residual angulation of 20° or less. This process is exponential not linear, and at least 2 years of growth remaining is required for almost complete normalization. *The correction of angulation depends on longitudinal growth.* Therefore the closer the deformity is to the physis, and the longer the remaining growth, the more complete the correction.

Physeal fractures

Occurring through the growth plate have a peak incidence at the ages of 12 to 13. This coincides with the period of rapid growth. The separation usually occurs through the zone of cartilage transformation between the calcified and uncalcified cartilage. There is a high turnover of cells in this region, and the bone here has less resistance to shear and tensile forces than the adjacent bone.

Use the *Salter–Harris classification* (Fig. 21.4). This classification does exclude a number of less common events, and Peterson has formulated yet another classification of epiphyseal fractures which is more encompassing, in particular, type 6 lesion when the physis is missing (or perichondral ring injury).

Type 1 injuries are usually the result of shearing or torsional forces, or avulsion forces in the case of an apophysis. The commonest site of

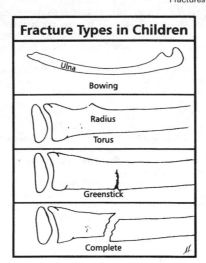

Fig. 21.3 Four types of fracture in children

injury is the *distal fibular physis*. Localized bony tenderness is diagnostic. The radiography usually appears normal. An ultrasound may demonstrate periostial elevation. These injuries require 3 weeks of cast immobilization. Movement and function return quickly, and complications are extremely rare.

Type 2 injuries most commonly involve the distal radial epiphysis with posterior displacement, and are frequently accompanied by a chip of bone off the ulnar styloid. Anatomical reduction is ideal, but as previously discussed, up to 20°of angulation can remodel. 5–6 weeks of immobilization is a well-moulded, short arm cast is required.

Children who present late with type 1 or 2 fractures in an unacceptable position, are best left alone. These fractures heal quickly and attempts at closed manipulation may result in further growth plate damage. Late corrective osteotomy may be required if remodeling fails to correct the deformity.

The most commonly seen type 3 fracture involves the distal tibial epiphysis (Tillaux fracture). Open reduction to anatomically restore the articular surface is essential. Growth disturbance is not a problem following this fracture, as the fracture occurs just prior to physeal closure.

The most commonly seen type 4 fracture involves the lateral condyle of the humerus. This injury requires open reduction and internal fixation. Left untreated, this intraarticular injury will produce joint stiffness and deformity, secondary to mal-position of the fracture. This can be associated with a non-union and progressive valgus deformity of the elbow. Ultimately, a tardive ulnar palsy can occur. With anatomic reduction and internal fixation, the long-term consequences are minimal.

Pure type 5 injuries are rare. Variable degrees of crush injury to the growth plate can accompany any physeal fracture, and it is for this reason that physeal plate fractures should be followed up during periods of growth to ensure that growth arrest and deformity has not occurred.

The site most at risk of physeal injury with incomplete or complete bony bars is the distal femur. (Lombarod and Harvey reported on 34 cases of distal femoral physeal fractures, and noted that one third developed varus or valgus deformity, and one-third had a leg length discrepancy greater than 2cm).[1] It is usually a Salter–Harris 2 fracture.

Pathological fractures

Childhood fractures can also occur in pathological bone (e.g. as unicameral bone cysts).

1 SJ Lombardo, JP Harvey 1977 *JBJS* **59A** 742–51

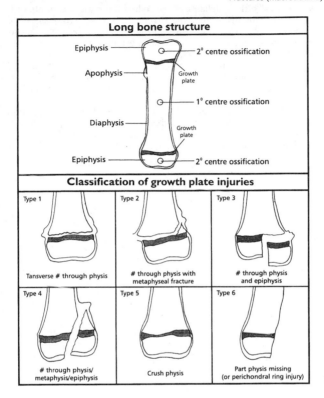

Long bone structure

Epiphysis — 2° centre ossification

Apophysis — Growth plate

1° centre ossification

Diaphysis — Growth plate

Epiphysis — 2° centre ossification

Classification of growth plate injuries

Type 1
Tansverse # through physis

Type 2
through physis with metaphyseal fracture

Type 3
through physis and epiphysis

Type 4
through physis/ metaphysis/epiphysis

Type 5
Crush physis

Type 6
Part physis missing (or perichondral ring injury)

Fig. 21.4 Salter–Harris classification of growth plate fracures.

Dislocations

Usually involve the patella or elbow. When the patient presents with these joints still dislocated, the diagnosis is easy. However, these dislocations often spontaneously *relocate*. In these cases the diagnosis must be based on clinical evidence, with a high index of suspicion.

Patellar dislocation—see below.

Elbow dislocations may be associated with a fracture of the medial epicondyle. The elbow can reduce with this fragment in the humer-oulnar joint. This requires open reduction and internal fixation of the displaced fragment.

The uncomplicated elbow dislocation requires sling immobilization and ice initially, followed by gradual mobilization as pain allows. **Physiotherapy is not required**. *Return to sport should be delayed until full elbow extension* has been regained (may take many months).

Hip and pelvic injuries

Are relatively rare in the young athlete. Table 21.3 classifies these injuries.

Of the skeletal injuries, apophyseal avulsion fractures and slipped upper femoral capital epiphysis would be the most common.

Apophyseal ovulsion fractures

Usually occur during the course of an extreme effort due to a sudden violent muscular contraction. The injury most often occurs in the adolescent athlete aged between 14 and 17. **Clinically** there is localized swelling, tenderness, and limitation of motion. The diagnosis is usually confirmed radiologically. **Treatment** is rest and analgesia initially, and movement is then increased as pain allows. As with all injuries, once a full range of active motion has been restored, then a resisted exercise program can be commenced, and a return to sport occurs after full strength of the injured areas has been achieved.

Note: *significantly displaced avulsion fractures* of the ischium may require open reduction and internal fixation.

Slipped upper femoral capital epiphysis (SUFE)

This is the **most common hip disorder** in the adolescent. Rarely does the slip occur in association with a discrete injury (an acute slip). Rather, there is a gradual microfracturing process of the physis under physiological loads (a chronic slip). Occasionally, there may be an element of both (an acute on chronic slip). This condition occurs in about 2 per 100,000 adolescents. It occurs 2.5 times more frequently in boys than girls. The mean age of presentation for boys is 13.5 years and for girls is 11.5 years. The condition is bilateral on initial presentation in 10–15%, and over time can occur in 25 to 35% of the individuals.

The adolescent may present with increasing anterior thigh and knee pain, associated with a limp. The pain may be aggravated by physical activity. **Clinically**, the leg may lie in *slightly more external rotation* and there is a loss of internal rotation of the hip in flexion (see Fig. 11.3). The diagnosis is usually confirmed on x-ray, but if not obtain a bone scan. **Treatment is operative**, with fixation by a single center cannulated compression screw, which stabilizes the epiphysis and encourages early closure of the growth plate.

In the assessment of 'sports injuries' in the child, congenital, developmental, infective, and inflammatory conditions always need to be considered. Therefore, Perthes' disease, developmental dysplasia of the hip, septic arthritis, and inflammatory synovitis should be excluded.

Table 21.3 Hip and pelvic injuries in the young athlete

Skeletal injuries
- *Apophyseal avulsion fractures*
  - iliac crest (abdominal musculature)
  - anterior superior iliac spine (sartorius)
  - anterior inferior iliac spine (rectus femoris)
  - lesser trochanter (iliopsoas)
  - Ischium (hamstring)
- *Growth plate injuries*
  - slipped capital femoral epiphysis
  - Salter–Harris physeal fractures
- *Nonphyseal fractures*
  - pelvic Fractures
  - iliac wing fractures
  - acetabular fractures
  - stable pelvic fractures
  - unstable pelvic ring fractures
- *Femoral neck fractures*
  - transcervical fracture
  - cervicotrochanteric fracture
  - intertrochanteric fracture
- *Hip dislocations*
- *Stress fractures*
  - femoral neck
- pelvic

Soft tissue injuries
- *Musculotendinous strains*
  - snapping hip syndrome
  - iliac apophysitis
  - osteitis pubis
- *Contusions*

Knee injuries

In the skeletally immature, pain in the front of the knee during or following sports, activity, is an extremely **common presenting symptom** to the sports doctor.[1] In an attempt to indicate the complexity of the problem and also to give a basis for rational treatment, Thomson proposed a classification based mainly on mechanical aspects affecting the patellofemoral joint (Table 21.4).

In the **traumatic group**, consider a direct blow to the patellofemoral joint, a traumatic dislocation, a fracture, and meniscal damage. In the **malignment group**, idiopathic subluxors and dislocators and torsional problems, muscle imbalance and bony abnormalities need to be considered. The **compressive group** includes 'the hamstrung knee' due to excessive tightness of the hamstrings. The **overuse group** includes Osgood–Schlatter's disease, Sinding-Larsen-Johansson syndrome, multipartite patellae, and plicae. The **degenerative group** are usually post-traumatic as a result of osteochondral fractures, secondary to patellar dislocation. In the **idiopathic group**, osteochondritis dissecans of the patella, and the small group of idiopathic primary chondromalacia of the patella.

Chondromalacia of the patella is not a clinical syndrome. It refers to the morphological change of the articular cartilage lining the retro-patellar surface. It may appear as a bulging, softening, fissuring, or fimbrillation of the smooth surface of the articular cartilage, and may progress to surface degeneration. Its diagnosis should be confined to macroscopic, arthroscopic, or microscopic observation of the articular surface.

The **history and physical examination are very important** in the assessment of *anterior knee pain patients*. The character, site, intensity and frequency of the pain, and also aggravating and relieving factors need to be considered. Catching, popping or giving way, particularly with rotation, suggests patellar subluxation or instability. On **physical examination**, the lower limbs need to be assessed in regions (Table 21.5). **First**, *above the patella*, looking for muscle weakness or contraction, and looking for excessive internal femoral torsion.

Note: *Hip pathology with referred pain to the knee should always be excluded.*

Second, *the patella itself*, looking at patellar height [a high patella (patella alta), a low patella (patella baja), or a laterally titled patella]. The laterally titled patella can also be associated with tight lateral retinacular structures. Excessive lateral patellar mobility with an apprehension sign also requires assessment. An effusion or crepitus suggests the possibility of retropatellar erosion. Crepitus, however, can be present with a normal retropatellar surface. Active flexion and extension of the knee allows assessment of patellar tracking.

Third, *below the patella*, looking for a laterally placed tibial tubercle, a valgus knee, internal tibial torsion, tight hamstrings. Skin changes or alterations in temperature may indicate a reflex sympathetic dystrophy.

Patellar malignment

Iis a *common source* of sports disability, particularly in sports requiring jumping or rapid changes of direction. The terms 'malignment' and 'instability' are commonly used interchangeably. *Malignment* is

---

1 LJ Micheli, TE Foster 1993 *Instr Course Lect* **42** 473–81

Table 21.4 Thomson classification of patellofemoral disorders

- Traumatic
- Overuse
- Malignment
- Degenerative
- Compressive
- Idiopathic

Table 21.5 Assessment of the knee

Above the patella	Muscle weakness contraction internal femoral torsion
The patella	Alta/baja/lateral tilt
Below the patella	Lateral tibial tuberosity/valgus/int. tibial torsion/tight hamstrings

an abnormal relationship between the patella and its associated soft tissue and bony surroundings throughout the course of knee motion. *Instability* is usually manifest only at *certain* points within the range of motion when abnormal alignment occurs.

During knee motion the patella follows a course of tilt, flexion and rotation (a toroidal path or J-curve) (see Fig. 12.7). Stability through this path depends on a complex series of interactions among joint congruity and static and dynamic stabilizers, both local and remote. *Static forces* that provide stability include primary knee joint patellofemoral congruity, the meniscopatellar ligaments, the medial and lateral tethers extending from the iliotibial band, vastus lateralis, and vastus medialis. *Dynamic forces* include the quadriceps groups, specifically the tethering effect of the vastus medialis obliquis. Femoral and tibial rotational abnormalities also affect patellofemoral orientation. The maximum amount of femoral anteversion or tibial torsion that can be compensated for, and tolerated without symptoms, is unknown, but appears to be significant in view of the large number of patients and femoral and tibial torsion, who are completely asymptomatic. *Anatomic factors* purported to predispose patients to patellar instability, include patellaalta, generalized joint hypermobility, increased Q-angle, increased femoral anteversion, increased external tibial torsion (last two are failure of remodeling from childhood), abnormal iliotibial band attachments, genuvalgum, genurecurvatum, femoral condylar hypoplasia, or dysplasia of the patella, or a combination of these. However, no one of these factors is always present in cases of patellar instability, and in some situations none of these factors are clinically obvious.

Patellar subluxation

Is a transient event in which the median ridge of the patella moves over the lateral edge of the lateral femoral condyle in predisposed patients when pivoting or twisting on a flexed knee. There is a popping sensation, anterior knee pain, and pain over the medial aspect of the knee (stretching of the medial patellar retinaculum). These patellae reduce spontaneously, and as the patella returns to the femoral sulcus, shear stresses are placed on the median ridge and medial facet of the patella, resulting in chondral fractures (with or without the release of chondral debris). This debris then acts as a synovial irritant and can produce an effusion. **The history is very important** as the physical examination may reveal an apparently normal knee, or an effusion and any number of the factors previously mentioned.

X-rays of the knee include AP, lateral, tunnel views and merchant views of the patellofemoral joint (the knee flexed to 45° outline the patella). Such views will assess bony contours, and height of the patella, and exclude osteochondral fragments. CT scanning is useful. **Treatment** initially is non-operative with an intensive quadriceps rehabilitation exercise program, lateral retinacular stretching and hamstring stretching exercises and the use of the S-knee splint. The small number of cases that fail to respond to these measures may benefit from arthroscopic lateral retinacular release.

Patellar dislocation

Is classified in Table 21.6.

724

Table 21.6 Classification of patellar dislocation

- Congenital
- Recurrent
- Habitual
- Traumatic

Congenital dislocation of the patella
The patella has never been dislocated (as in arthrogryposis multiplex congenita, Down's syndrome, or familial congenital dislocation of the patella).

Recurrent dislocation of the patella
The patella dislocated intermittently. The onset is usually in adolescence, and may be secondary to the underlying causes described.

Habitual dislocation of the patella
The knee dislocates with every flexion or extension of the knee. Dislocation in flexion needs to be differentiated from dislocation in extension. Dislocation in flexion is secondary to quadriceps contracture, and if one is able to forcibly hold the patella in the midline, the knee cannot be flexed more than 30°. Further flexion is possible only if the patella dislocates laterally. Dislocation in extension is usually due to patellar malignment. In terminal extension the patella moves laterally, such that it lies outside the normal toroidal path of the patella. As the knee flexes the patella may or may not engage the patellofemoral groove. If it does not, it then tracks laterally until it flicks back into the patellofemoral groove.

Acute traumatic dislocation of the patella

In acute dislocation differentiate the non-contact type from the contact type (was the patella pushed out of place as it came in contact with the ground or another player, or was it pulled out of joint by intrinsic factors related to the previously mentioned anatomical variations). **Treatment** is surgical (60% show evidence of osteochondral or chondral fractures). Arthroscopic lavage and debridement is to remove these debris. If there is no significant effusion or pain, and full range of movement, chondral damage is unlikely and an active physiotherapy program can be commenced. Following surgery, an intensive quadriceps rehabilitation exercise program is needed along with hamstring stretching. Cast or S-knee splint. **Surgical reconstructive procedures** for the management of patellar instability comprise of:
1 Proximal realignment by means of lateral release, medial reefing or combined lateral release with medial reefing
2 Distal realignment by means of the patellar tendon or tibial tubercle transfer, or semitendinosis tenodesis
3 A combination of 1 and 2.

Multipartite patella

The bipartite variant is the most common (also three or even four segments).[1] Often, an incidental x-ray finding. The reported incidence of bipartite patella ranges from 0.2% to 6%. It is uncommonly bilateral, and there is a strong male dominance of 9 to 1. There is pain in the superolateral quadrant of the anterior knee. **Examination** reveals asymmetry with an alteration of the contour of the superolateral quadrant (enlarged with associated tenderness), seen on x-ray. **Treatment** includes modification of activity, physiotherapy with lateral retinacular stretching and quadriceps strengthening, a short period of splint immobilization. If symptoms persist then surgical excision.

1 JA Ogden SM McCarthy P Jokl 1982 The painful bipartitie patella J Paediatr Orthop 2 263–269

726

Osgood-Schlatter's disease[1]

This is not a disease. It is a microavulsion of the patellar tendon from the anterior portion of the developing ossification center of the tibial tuberosity, due to repeated traction injuries (Fig. 21.5). The growth plate remains intact. It is an extremely common source of sports disability. Boys are more commonly affected (girls present between 11 and 13 years, boys between 12 and 15 years). Five times more common in adolescent athletes. Bilateral in 20–30%. **Diagnosis** is based on symptoms and physical signs. The pain is usually activity related (in association with running and jumping sports). There is swelling and prominence of the tibial tuberosity, associated with localized tenderness and significant hamstring tightness.

X-rays show soft tissue swelling with fragmentation of the tibial tubercle. **Treatment** to relieve pain and swelling (ice, oral analgesics, anti-inflammatory agents and physiotherapeutic modalities). Quadriceps strengthening and hamstring stretching are important as is activity modification but complete denial of sports participation is unnecessary (very occasionally a short period of cast immobilization). A *painful sequestrum* within the patellar ligament *will need to be excised.*

Sinding-Larsen–Johansson Syndrome[2]

This is an apophysitis of the inferior pole of the patella, occurring in pre-teen boys (Fig. 24.4). It is activity related and associated with jumping and running sports. There is point tenderness over the inferior pole of the patella. There are varying amounts of calcification or ossification of the inferior pole of the patella.

Distinguish from an acute patellar sleeve fracture (complete separation of the patellar tendon from the inferior pole of the patella). A sleeve fracture of the patella is defined as an extensive sleeve of cartilage that is pulled off the main body of the bony patella, together with a bony fragment from the distal pole. In such situations the patient would be unable to perform a straight leg raise, and radiologically there would be evidence of a patella alta. This lesion requires open reduction and internal fixation. **Treatment** as for Osgood–Schlatter's disease (symptomatic, with modification of activities, quadriceps strengthening, and hamstring stretching).

1 RB Osgood 1903 *Boston Med Surg* **145** 114–17   2 MF Sinding-Larsen 1921 *Acta Radiol* **1** 171–4

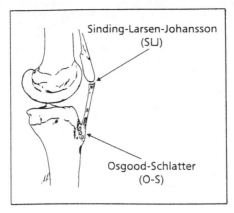

Fig. 21.5 Sinding-Larsen–Johansson syndrome is a traction apophysitis of the lower pole of the patella; Osgood–Slatter's is of the lower end of the patellar tendon.

The meniscus[1]

Meniscal injuries in children are now not uncommon. The exact incidence is not known. Injuries of the lateral and medial menisci occur with equal frequency, but if discoid meniscal injuries are eliminated, the medial meniscus is more often injured. The mechanism of injury is (as in adults) a decelerating contact or non-contact force causing a compressive load with rotation. There is pain, giving way, stiffness, swelling, and occasionally locking. One-third of patients have no significant findings on physical examination. In children, there is poor correlation between the physical findings and arthroscopic findings. The younger the child, the poorer the correlation. **Treatment** depends on the site and size of the tear (Fig. 21.6). Peripheral meniscal tears of less than 1cm are *stable* (less than 2mm of motion when probed) and heal with 4–6 weeks of immobilization. Tears between 6mm and 30mm are *unstable* (occur in red/red or red/white zone), and may heal because of the improved vascularity. Such are suitable for meniscal suture followed by 4–6 weeks of immobilization. Meniscal lesions not amenable to meniscal preservation require **partial meniscectomy**. Following partial meniscectomy an intensive quadriceps exercise program is undertaken and no sport for at least 4–6 months of graduated rehabilitation is required.

The discoid meniscus

The incidence of the discoid meniscus varies world-wide from 3% to 5% in Anglo-Saxons, to 20% in the Japanese. The cause is unknown; as a discoid configuration is not seen in any stage of fetal development. A *symptomatic discoid* lateral meniscus causes a snapping sensation over the lateral aspect of the knee. Otherwise they are incidental findings at arthroscopy. When **symptomatic treat by excision** of the unstable part and reshape to a normal crescentic shape.

1 RR Scroble *et al* 1992 *Clin Orthop* **279** 180–9

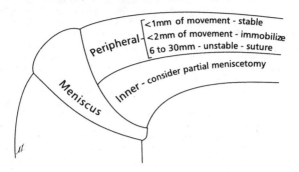

Fig. 21.6 The treatment of meniscal injuries in children depends on the site and size of the tear.

Anterior cruciate ligament[1]

The most common ACL injury in the child is an avulsion of the tibial spine. Myers and McIver describes three grades of tibial spine avulsion (type I fractures, non-displaced; type II, some elevation; type III, elevation with displacement and rotation).

Associated tears of the medial collateral ligament may occur. **Treatment** depends on the grade. Type I and type II injuries require casting with the knee in 15–20° of flexion for 6 weeks; type III requires open reduction and internal fixation. These injuries are associated with stretching of the anterior cruciate ligament prior to bone failure (knee laxity is identified by an increase in the Lachmann's sign, but functional instability is not a problem). *Substance tears of the anterior cruciate ligament in the skeletally immature* are being seen (previously thought to be rare as the tensile strength of ligaments is greater than that of the growth plate; also the capsular and cruciate ligaments are inserted within the epiphyses of the tibia and femur, only the insertion of the tibial collateral ligament crosses the tibial physeal plate). Anterior cruciate injuries are treated non-operatively in the child do no better than in the adult. Treatment remains controversial (as the surgical procedure must avoid damage to the physeal plates if there is significant growth remaining). Opinion differs as to when the growth plate can be breached. Some treat as in an adult if the child is within 2 years of skeletal maturity or there is less than 1cm of growth remaining (in distal femoral epiphysis). *If significant clinical instability exists* below this age range, then reconstruction using tubularized iliotibial band to provide both a lateral extracapsular reconstruction and an intracapsular reconstruction via the over the top position is successful.

1 AW Parker *et al* 1994 *Am J Sports Med* **22** 44–7

Osteochondritis dissecans

A lesion of uncertain etiology, rare under the age of 10 years, with a male predominance of 3 to 1, and a 20% incidence of bilaterally. 80% involve the lateral aspect of the medial femoral condyle, 20% involve the posterior aspect of the lateral femoral condyle. The patient **presents** with pain on activity and occasionally a clicking sensation. There is usually little on physical examination.

X-rays (AP, lateral, and tunnel views) usually define the lesion. MRIs may provide information on fragment healing or risk of separation. The **goal of treatment** is to prevent fragment separation with its associated risk of early knee osteoarthritis. *Treatment and prognosis is determined by age* (Table 21.7).

The *childhood group* usually heals spontaneously, and should be followed up with x-rays to bony union. The *immature group* can be observed for 12 months, and if they remain symptomatic and the lesion is ununited on x-ray, then arthroscopic Herbert screw fixation is recommended. For those patients under observation, complete cessation of sport is not justified. Activity modification within the limitations of symptoms is all that is required. The *junctional group* require immediate screw fixation, as there appears to be a greater chance of healing prior to the growth plate closure. If the lesion has not separated, then screw fixation alone can be performed. If the lesion has separated, then open surgery with bone grafting and fixation is required. In *the adult*, open surgery with grafting and fixation is recommended, or if a loose body is already present, then removal.

Table 21.7 Thomson and Gray classification of osteochondritis

	Age (years)
Juvenile	
Childhood	10–13
Immature epiphyses open)	13–16
Junctional (epiphyses closed)	16–18
Adult	
Mature (epiphyses closed)	>20

Ankle and foot problems

Ankle and food pain, secondary to congenital and developmental abnormalities, are not uncommon and often sport is the precipitating event. Consider the following conditions but do not forget acute injuries.

Tarsal coalition

Is a bony or fibrocartilaginous connection of two or more of the tarsal bones due to failure of differentiation and segmentation of the primitive mesenchyme. Calcaneonavicular and talocalcaneal coalitions are the most common. The **age of presentation** is 8–16 years. A family history may exist (autosomal dominant with incomplete penetrance). There is gradual onset of hindfoot pain, aggravated by running over uneven ground. **Clinically**, there may be peroneal spasm resulting in valgus of the hindfoot with pes planus deformity. Significant limitation of subtalar joint motion is present.

Calcaneonavicular coalitions can be **diagnosed** on a x-ray using a 45° oblique view. Talocalcaneal coalitions are difficult to see x-ray but are well imaged on CT. **Treatment** is initially symptomatic with rest and modification of activities. Relieving plaster casts may be required. Those who fail to respond to these measures may require surgery.

Calcaneonavicular coalitions are treated by resection of the bar with interposition of the extensor-digitorum brevis muscle. The results are very good. *Talocalcaneal* coalitions may be amenable to surgery. The size of the coalition that can be resected is unknown (up to 50% of the involved facet). In the symptomatic patient with an unresectable coalition, and arthritis in the talonavicular joint, triple arthrodesis is necessary.

Accessory navicular

Adolescents **present with pain and tenderness** over the medial border of the foot, aggravated by running or jumping sports or rubbing footwear. **Clinical examination** reveals a cornuate prominence on the medial side of the navicular, which may be tender and show pressure from footwear.

A x-ray will confirm the presence of an ossicle at the medial border of the navicular (controversy whether a stress fracture, or a separate center of ossification). **Treatment** is an arch support and modification of footwear. Acute pain, aggravated by weight bearing may require 6 weeks of cast immobilization. Rarely, excision of the lesion with tightening of the tibialis posterior tendon is required.

Osteochondroses

These are idiopathic disorders of enchondral ossification which occur during the years of rapid growth. Trauma may influence their development, particularly from sport.

Freiberg's disease

Involves collapse of the articular surface and subchondral bone of the metatarsal head (most commonly seen in the 2nd metatarsal, then the 3rd or the 4th). More common in females, and presents between 12 and 15 years of age. The adolescent **presents with pain** on weight bearing, particularly during toe off. **Clinically**, there is localized tenderness and swelling.

The **diagnosis** is confirmed by typical x-ray appearances of initially increased density, followed by collapse with flattening, and occasionally fragmentation with loose body formation. **Treatment** is rest and a metatarsal dome. Surgery to bone graft the collapsed head or remove loose bodies or realignment with dorsal osteotomy is occasionally required.

Köhler's disease

Is irregular ossification of the tarsal navicular, resulting in localized pain and x-ray narrowing and increased density of the navicular. The age of onset of this *completely reversible condition* is from 2 to 9 years. **Treatment** is symptomatic. Supportive casts for 6 weeks may be required. With time, the bone fully reconstitutes without long term-sequelae.

Severe's disease

Or calcaneal apophysitis is a common entity in the 9- to 11-year-old age group. The child may **present with heel pain**, particularly with running and a limp. **Clinically**, the calcaneal apophysis is very tender. The tendo-Achilles may be tight.

X-rays are not helpful because the calcaneal apophysis is frequently fragmented and dense in normal children. **Treatment** depends on the severity of the child's symptoms, and includes relative rest, calf stretching and strengthening exercises, and occasionally the use of a heel raise. It is a self-limiting condition with no adverse long-term sequelae.

Osteochondral lesions of the talus

Osteochondritis dissecans was used to describe lesions on the medial aspect of the talar dome. It is now believed that lesions on both the medial and lateral aspect of the talar dome are secondary to trauma. The site of the lesion is the end result of the force applied (lateral fractures produced by inversion and dorsiflexion, and medial fractures by strong lateral rotation of the tibia on a plantarflexed and inverted foot). Such lesions have been classified, see Table 21.8.

The **diagnosis** should always be considered where persisting ankle pain 6 weeks after an injury. **Investigations** include a x-ray and a CT to better define the lesion. If the x-ray is normal, and there is a higher index of suspicion, then a bone scan should be performed. If this is positive, then an MRI scan is useful. **Treatment** depends on the stage of the lesion:

- **Stages 1 and 2** lesions are immobilized in a cast for 6 weeks. Such lesions need to be followed to ensure that union is complete.
- **Stage 2a, Stage 3, and Stage 4** fractures may all require surgical intervention, and following arthroscopic assessment, either internal fixation or removal of the lesion may be indicated.

Table 21.8 Anderson classification of osteochondral lesions of the talus

Stage 1
- There is subchondral trabecular compression
- The x-ray is normal
- The bone scan is hot and the MRI is diagnostic

Stage 2
- Incomplete separation of the fragment*

Stage 2
- The formation of subchondral cysts*

Stage 3
- Unattached, undisplaced fragment*

Stage 4
- Displaced fragment*

* Seen on computed technology.

Somatization disorders[1]

These are syndromes where bodily complaints (e.g. knee locked in full extension—unusual in the absence of a dislocated patella) are an expression of underlying psychological stress (from competition anxiety, family concerns or developmental concerns/anxiety). Doctors and coaches need to maximize performance without compromising the development of a fully rounded individual.

1 JC Hyndman 1994 In M Harries *et al* (ed) *Oxford textbook of sports medicine.* p632, OUP, Oxford

Rehabiliation[1]

Same principles as for the adult, with following provisos:

- Children have a short attention span, feel vulnerable, do not think it is important and do not want to be different. Therefore, keep it short (define goals, e.g. 15–30min), simple (small number of exercises), fun, and motivate with promise of better performance.
- Must be pain-free next day, avoid pain-causing activities, do not predispose to further injury(no sport while limping), do not mask pain with modalities.
- Return to sport when muscle strength and endurance is 85–95% of normal, flexibility and ROM normal, proprioception and co-ordination normal, and cardiorespiratory fitness present.

1 A Smith 1996 In WB Kibler (ed) *ACSM's Handbook for the team physician* p428–31.

General warning

Treating clinicians need to be always aware that pain and tenderness
of a low grade may be the first presentation of a bone tumor in a
child. This needs to be borne in mind when treating overuse injuries
and stress fractures. Remember that Ewing's tumour may mimic
osteomyelitis with fever and constitutional symptoms of listlessness.

745

22 The older athlete
SUE OGLE, TOM GWINN

Introduction

There is a rapidly increasing number of older people in the world today. In an industrialized country everyone can reasonably expect to grow old, many very old (the 85-plus age group being the fastest growing segment of the population). The Third World is also ageing, in absolute numbers at an even faster rate.[1] People are becoming more health conscious and are exercising more. An unprecedented number of elderly (>65) athletes are donning their walking/jogging shoes, golf gloves, swimsuits, and gym gear in an attempt to keep fit. Many are participating in competitive sport (e.g. masters and seniors tournaments) so that seniors world records for track field and swimming have improved dramatically. This trend must be fostered as there is now evidence for the adage 'use it or lose it' (i.e. that exercise improves health and function in old age). Regular exercise also reduces mortality by up to 25% per annum and improves mood and well-being.[2] For many older participants sport is a major source of enjoyment of life and a focus of social interaction. Older athletes require not only encouragement but informed advice about type of exercise, nutrition, prevention, and management of injuries.

1 SJ Moritz, AM Ostfeld 1990 In WR Hazzard *et al* (ed) *Principles of geriatric medicine and eerontology* 2nd edn. 146–56. McGraw-Hill   **2** RS Parffenbarger *et al* 1993 *New Eng J Med* **328** 538–45

Physiology: ageing and exercise

Ageing, disuse, and disease

Reduced physiological reserve previously ascribed to ageing is now thought to be due to the complex interaction between true genetically determined ageing, disease (often subtle or subclinical), and disuse.[1] Preconceived societal notions about ageing may greatly reduce expectations of performance, disuse leading to premature inactivity, being more prevalent in women. The rate of ageing varies, the elderly are a heterogeneous group, no two 80-year-olds are the same, chronological age may not reflect biological age so that each person must be assessed individually.

Endurance aerobic capacity

Cross-sectional data shows that VO_{2max} declines in men and women at 1% per year; the fall in marathon performance is 13% per decade.[2] A non-linear curve is seen in logitudinal studies with a rapid decline in early adulthood in sedentary individuals followed by a less steep decline in later life.[3]

Studies have confirmed that with regular exercise the decline in VO_{2max} can be halved.[4] Also, in master athletes who maintain their competitive training over 10 years no decline in VO_{2max} (but no improvement) has been observed.[5] The decline in VO_{2max} is due to both central (cardiorespiratory) and peripheral (musculoskeletal) factors.

Cardiovascular

At rest, heart rate (HR) and cardiac output (CO) are normal in patients screened for coronary artery disease (CHD). There is, however, an increase in arterial stiffness with ageing leading to an increase in blood pressure (BP)and compensatory mild left ventricular hypertrophy. The ventricles are less elastic and filling is both slower and occurs via late atrial contraction.[6]

During exercise there is a marked reduction in maximal HR even in healthy subjects. HR max declines by 3.2% per decade [i.e. 10 bpm/10 years or roughly according to the equation: HR (bpm) = 220 − age (years)]. Cardiac output (CO) during exercise falls (20–30% by age 65) due to reduced myocardial performance, increased afterload and impaired β-adrenergic modulation.[7] In some healthy older individuals normal CO may be maintained by an increase in systolic volume during exercise (Frank Starling mechanism). Regular endurance exercise favorably alters lipid profiles with an increase in high density lipoprotein cholesterol (HDL-C) in elderly male runners, is protective for cardiovasular disease, and is associated with reduced mortality.[8]

Respiratory

Ageing changes include a decrease in elasticity of lung parenchyma, increase in fibrous tissue, reduced alveolar surface area, and a decrease in respiratory muscle strength and rib cage elasticity. There

1 WM Bortz 1989 *J Am Geriatr Soc* 37 1092–6   2 JF Fries 1980 *New Eng J Med* 303 130–5   3 ER Buskirk, JL Hodgson 1987 *Fed Proc* 46 1824–9   4 JM Hagberg 1987 *Fed Proc* 46 1830–3   5 ML Pollock et al 1987 *J Appl Physiol* 62 725–31   6 EG Lakatta 1990 *Eur Heart J* II 22–9   7 R Xiao, EG Lakatta 1991 *Rev Clin Gerontol* 1 309–22   8 M Higuchi et al 1988 *Clin Physiol* 8 137–45

is an increased resistance to airflow with reduction in vital capacity (30–50% by age 70) and increase in residual volume (40–50% by age 70), plus a slight reduction in PO_2, O_2 saturation and diffusing capacity. This reduced respiratory reserve causes no apparent problems at rest, but compared to the young, the ageing athlete will experience breathlessness at lighter workloads.[1]

Muscle

Maximum isometric strength is achieved in the third decade, levels until about the age of 55 or 60, declines by 10–15% per decade till age 75, then declines more rapidly at 1.8–4.1% per year.[2] The isometric strength of a 70-year-old has been estimated to be 50% that of a 20 year old. The extent to which these changes are attributable to disuse (sedentary lifestyle) is uncertain. Muscle strength followed longitudinally in active elderly men and women declines more slowly. The decline in muscle strength with ageing is multifactorial. Muscle size is highly correlated with strength. A 50% reduction in muscle mass has been demonstrated on CT scanning of arm and leg muscle size in young and elderly men. The lower extremity musculature declines at a faster rate than the upper extremity. Neuromuscular changes with ageing include:

- Slowing of central and peripheral motor latency.
- Decline in number and size of motor neurones.
- Degeneration of neuromuscular function.
- Reduction in number of motor units (50% by age 60). After age 60 motor units decline at 1–3% per year with a selective loss of fast motor units leading to a decrease in the number and size of fast twitch (type II) fibers and a relative increase in slow twitch (type I) fibers. Experimental evidence suggests that this is due to progressive denervation with increasing age of muscle fibers innervated by large motor neurones and their subsequent reinnervation from small motor neurones, a process that increases the proportion of type I at the expense of type II motor units. Muscles of elderly people also show reduced mitochondrial oxidase capacity; ultrastructural studies show an increased proportion of abnormal mitochondria with disrupted cristae.[3]

Exercise can modify these changes. Active elderly subjects show up to 70% greater strength compared to sedentary controls. Strength and muscle mass in an older adult can be improved with training. The training response should be similar to that seen in the young, variability observed is related more to intensity of training than to ageing factors.[4,5]

Cartilage

With ageing there is reduced water content and smaller proteoglycan subunits which contain more keratin and less chondroitin sulfate.

1 ML Nochomovitz, NS Cherniak 1984 *Geriatr Med* **3** 49–60   2 A Young 1992 In J Grimley-Evans, T Franklin Williams (ed) *Oxford textbook of geriatric medicine* 597–601. OUP   3 L Larsson *et al* 1978 *Acta Physiol Scand* **103** 31–9
4 JL Seto, CE Brewster, C. E. 1991 *Clin Sports Med* **10** 401–2   5 G Grimby *et al* 1992 *J Appl Physiol* **73** 2517–23

This results in cartilage with less tensile strength. Joints, especially knee, hip, ankle, and facet may be at more risk of developing osteoarthritis. However, studies of runners have shown no evidence of premature osteoarthritis. In fact running may be protective in healthy persons but for those with degenerative arthritis an alternative form of low impact exercise should be advised.[1]

Menisci, discs, ligaments, and tendons

In the meniscus there is a reduction in both water content and non-collagenous matrix leading to degeneration of the central core. This increases susceptibility to horizontal tears with the potential for the development of osteoarthritis.[2] The water content and proteoglycan subunits decrease in the intervertebral disk with ageing. After 40, the nucleus pulposis becomes increasingly fibrillar, losing its gel form and capacity for shock absorption. However, disk degeneration although common in old age, is not invariable.[3] Ageing tendons and ligaments lose elasticity—a combination of reduced water content and altered collagen and elastin fiber cross linkage. The elderly athlete is more susceptible to sprains and strains which can be avoided by regular stretching to maintain joint range of motion.

Bone

Maximal bone mass is reached at about the age of 30 and is stable for around 10 years. Thereafter, cortical bone mass declines at 0.6% per year and trabecular at 0.7% per year (probably from an earlier age). The smaller the bone mass accumulated during skeletal growth the greater the risk of fracture in later life.

There are two distinct phases of bone loss: (1) a protracted slow phase in men and women resulting in similar losses of cortical and trabecular bone, and (2) a transient accelerated phase after the menopause in women that results in a disproportionately greater loss in trabecular bone.[4] By age 70 in men 20% cortical and 35% trabecular bone mass and in women 35% cortical and 50% trabecular bone mass has been lost. Determinants of bone loss are genetic and hormonal but also include modifiable lifestyle factors such as diet (especially calcium) and exercise. Skeletal stress from weight bearing exercise stimulates osteoblast function thereby increasing bone mass. Bone density has been shown in cross-sectional studies to be greater in athletes compared to sedentary controls. Prospective studies demonstrate that postmenopausal women enrolled in a regular exercise program gain bone, whereas controls loss of bone.

Homeostasis: nervous and renal systems

Neuronal loss with ageing is variable, 10–60% by 70 years but is less with stimulation.[5] Common cognitive changes are:
- Good long-term memory.
- Poor short-term memory.
- Difficulty focusing concentration under stress (during the game).

1 Lane *et al* 1990 *Am J Med* **88** 452–9 **2** P Ghosh *et al* 1987 *Clin Orthop* **224** 52 **3** LT Twomey, JR Taylor 1987 *Clin Orthop* **224** 97 **4** L Riggs, J Melton 1992 In J Grimley-Evans, T Franklin Williams (ed) *Oxford textbook of geriatric nursing* OUP p405–11 **5** R Katzman, R Terry 1991 In R Katzman, J Rowe (ed) *Principles of geriatric neurology, contemporary neurology series 38* p18–59 F. A. Davis, Philadelphia

- Harder to learn new tasks (during coaching). 25–30% have dementia but this should not preclude supervised exercise (e.g. with a partner).
- Reaction time slows. Nerve conduction velocity is reduced by 15% at 70. Impaired vibration sensation and pain perception predispose to injury.[1]
- Loss of vision, hearing, and balance (40% women >70 fall annually) mean precautions with traffic and uneven surfaces are important.

  Sleep architecture alters with ageing:
- More time to fall asleep
- Less stage 4 deep sleep
- More brief awakenings.[2] The elderly often need to sleep longer to feel rested after exercise

A number of factors predispose the elderly to dehydration during exercise:

- Impaired hypothalmic thermoregulatory control
- Reduced thirst sensation
- Reduced glomerular filtration rate (GFR)[3]
- And a reduction in total body water (TBW). The elderly must drink routinely before, during, and after exercise, break-up work-outs, and limit activity in the heat of the day

Altitude

Research suggests that older climbers may have a reduced incidence and severity of acute mountain sickness. This condition is commonly experienced by individuals who ascend above 3000 meters. Symptoms include anorexia, nausea, vomiting, weakness, headache, and insomnia within several hours of arriving at altitude. A potentially life-threatening complication is pulmonary edema, but in general, the symptoms are self-limiting. Ageing is associated with a reduced PaO_2, and the ageing athlete is unable to deliver the same volume of O_2 to working muscles compared to the young. At high altitude the partial pressure of O_2 in the atmosphere is less so that less O_2 is available to capture and be carried to the tissues. This compounds older athlete's physiological disadvantage, creating a greater challenge. However, fitness rather than age correlates with the older athlete's ability to tolerate exercise at altitude.[4]

Skin

The skin provides a barrier against trauma, infection, UV irradiation, heat, and cold and is an energy storage site.[5] Changes seen in the ageing skin which compromise these functions are due as much to sun damage as to physiological factors. Overall, the skin is thinner and more fragile. Blisters are more common. Renewal of the epidermis is slower, leading to delayed healing. The dermis is less cellular and less

1 MA Tucker *et al* 1989 *Age and Ageing* **18** 241–6   2 WC Dement *et al* 1982 *J Am Geriatr Soc* **30** 25–50   3 JW Rowe *et al* 1976 *J Gerontol* **31** 155–633   4 AC Balcomb, JR Sutton 1986 In JR Sutton, RM Brock (ed) *Sports medicine for the mature athlete* p213–24. Benchmark Press   5 AK Balin, Kligman (ed) 1989 *Ageing and the skin*. Raven Press, New York

vascular and there is less subcutaneous tissue, thus less insulation especially in elderly women. Sweat gland numbers and function are reduced. Meissner's and Pacinian corpuscles—the cutaneous end organs responsible for pressure, vibration, and light touch sensation—decrease to approximately one-third of their initial density between the 2nd and 9th decades. The resulting increase in pain threshold may contribute to skin injury. There is diminished T cell function, Langerhans cell die, and after 50 years melanocytes decline at 2% per year making the aged more susceptible to infection neoplasm and UV damage. Ageing athletes can minimize risks by wearing hats, protective clothing, sun screen, sun avoidance (exercise before 10am and after 4pm), and good footwear. Sores that are slow to heal or moles that change must be seen by the doctor.

The older athlete
Physiology: ageing and exercise

Psychological factors

Benefits

Older athletes are less tense, depressed, angry and confused, have greater vigor, a more positive attitude, and higher self-esteem. Reasons given by older athletes for competing are:

- to belong to a group exercise such as walking and swimming, maintains muscle mass enabling older people to retain their independence thereby postponing frailty. This has economic advantages and also contributes to self-esteem[1]
- to enhance mood
- fitness. From regular aerobic exercise, even low intensity

Stresses

Ageing competitors almost always have more financial, professional, social, and family obligations than the young. This may mean suboptimal training, hurried warm-ups, and increased risk of injury. As an ageing athlete begins to lose his/her competitive edge there may be denial, anger then acceptance (typical grieving process). These mature athletes need to be reassured that they can still bring skill and wisdom to the game and be an inspiration to the young. Many do this by remaining involved in their sport as trainers and officials. Although some world class athletes become world class masters, many do not—perhaps because of earlier exhausting training schedules causing 'burn-out' or previous injuries. A positive attitude towards ageing is an important determinant of success for ageing both in general and in competition.[2]

1 RJ Shepard 1993 *Geriatrics* **48** 61   2 S Ungerleider *et al* 1989 *Percep Motor Skills* **68** 607–17

Exercise programs

Assessment

History

This should include:

- *Past/present medical problems*: especially recent myocardial infarction, bypass surgery, pacemaker.
- *Medications*: especially chronotropic and inotropic drugs.
- *Risk factors* for cardiovascular disease: obesity, hypertension, high cholesterol, smoking, diabetes, family history.
- *Nutritional status.*
- *Previous injuries.*

Stress testing:

The American College of Sports Medicine (ACSM) guidelines[1] suggest stratification into 3 risk categories:

1 Apparently healthy, not >1 symptom/sign*/ or risk factor:
   - exercise < 60% Vo_{2max}—without screening
   - exercise > 60% Vo_{2max} – women >50 – men >40—stress test
2 Higher risk: 2 or >2 symptoms/signs and/or risk factors:
   - exercise <60% Vo_{2max} (+ no symptoms)—without screening
   - exercise > 60% Vo_{2max} all ages—stress test
3 Known cardiac/pulmonary/metabolic disease:
   - all subjects require stress test under medical supervision to assess functional capacity.

*Note: symptoms/signs include: chest pain or discomfort suggestive of ischemia, shortness of breath or dizziness, syncope palpitations, tachycardia.

Musculoskeletal evaluation

- *Muscle strength* testing in the legs is important as most injuries in the older athlete involve the lower extremities—especially knees, ankles, feet. Quadriceps strength can be tested by using your hand as resistance—the older athlete should be able to generate enough force to lift 50% of their bodyweight. The same is true for ankle plantar- and dorsi-flexion. If in doubt, strength can be checked with an isokinetic dynamometer by a physiotherapist who can provide remedial strengthening exercises based on a 10RM (repetition max) program.
- *Flexibility* at the ankle and hip should be checked. A minimum of 10° dorsiflexion at the ankle is required before participation in walking or jogging. Tendon Achilles stretching may improve range; if not, a pair of running shoes with a good heel can accommodate for up to 10° of the missing range. The hip should have at least a 60° arc of motion; if not, remedial stretching should be prescribed.
- *Deformities*, such as hallux valgus, genu valgus, femoral anteversion, leg length discrepancies, and obvious joint deformity should be noted and appropriate exercise programs devised to promote muscle balance and stability around the joint (e.g. knee: 60/40 quadriceps/hamstring strength ratio). Arthritis does not preclude running, but swimming, rowing, or cycling may be more appropriate.

1 ACSM 1978 *Med Sci Sports Exercise* **2** 433-2

759

Exercise programs (*cont*)

Sensory testing

Check hearing and eye sight including color discrimination; a warning about traffic may be required. Light, touch, and pain in the feet should be tested and if needed advice given about shoes and regular podiatry. Soft accommodating orthoses are better accepted than rigid orthoses used in younger athletes.

Endurance exercise prescription

This should include:

- Intensity
- Mode
- Duration
- Frequency
- Progression

Intensity of exercise required to induce training (ACSM recommendations) can be measured in two ways:

1 VO_{2max} (50–80%)
2 HR max (60–80%)

Athletes should be taught to feel their own carotid or radial pulse during exercise and calculate their own age-corrected %max HR:

$$\%\text{max HR} = \frac{\text{HR observed as bpm} \times 100}{220 - \text{athlete's age}}$$

These measures can be applied at any age. However, many older people exercising will have cardiac arrhythmias (e.g. atrial fibrillation) which preclude the use of a heart rate test. A functional assessment, such as walking speed and distance or number of flights of stairs climbed, before breathless may be more useful.

MML: maximum MET level (45–85%)

The MET (metabolic equivalent unit) is defined as consumption of 3.5ml O_2/kg bodyweight/min. The work intensity of different activities in METs can be read off tables (see Table 22.1); this allows the athlete to choose an activity most suited to his/her target MET level. One MET of activity burns approximately one kcal/kg/h of activity. A 70kg individual engaged in an activity requiring 10 METs would expend approximately 70 kcal/hr.

Rhythmic activity using large muscle groups is preferred; some weight bearing (to prevent osteoporosis) is also recommended. Older people starting an exercise program should be commenced at a low intensity with very gradual build-up.

To promote **good health**, a program designed to expend >2000kcal/week is sufficient and may comprise:

- *daily activity* (not necessarily continuous) such as walking, climbing stairs, active gardening for a minimum of 60min (uses approx 1250kcal/week), plus
- *exercise sessions* 3 times per week involving major muscle groups in repetitive activity, as in fast walking, swimming, or cycling, (jogging or aerobics in those without osteoarthritis) for 30–45min each session (uses approx 750kcal/week).

To maintain **fitness**, ACSM guidelines suggest:

Table 22.1 Metabolic equivalent unit (MET)

Activity	MET
Level walking 4km/h	3.0
Running 8km/h	8.4
Running 13km/h	10.2
Swimming 30m/min	10.0
Tennis	6.0–10.0
Golf	5.1
Cycling 24km/h	7.0

Exercise programs (*cont*)

- Aerobic training with intensity 50–80% VO_{2max}, at a frequency of 3–5 sessions per week and a duration of 20–60min continuously, combined with
- strength (resistance) training based on one set (8–12 repetitions) of 8–10 exercises that include all major muscle groups, at least twice per week.

Healthy older individuals can tolerate endurance training at relatively intense levels with few injuries, speed being a more important determinant of injury than intensity.[1] Safe stretching for older people with emphasis on lower limbs especially with coexisting neurological disease (e.g. Parkinson's disease) is essential. The following should be included:

1 hip extension—prone lying
2 hamstring stretch—sitting on bed or floor
3 quadriceps, tendon Achilles

Adduction and abduction are optional. A progressive slow non-ballistic stretch ('stretch and creep technique') for 30–60s, 1–2 times daily is preferred.

Maintenance

Major goals:

- improve endurance capacity and increase strength
- minimize injury
- enjoyment

Secondary goals:

- better sleep
- more energy
- social interaction
- raised self-esteem
- enhanced qualify of life

Improving compliance:

- season proof
- safe (traffic, pollution, assault, UV exposure)
- injury-free (treat prior conditions, contain inflammation quickly, more time to recover,
- cross training to maintain fitness after exercise injury
- realistic goals (start slow)
- feedback (diaries, charts, document progress)
- proper equipment/clothing/footwear
- more time to loosen up and recover
- adequate hydration
- exercise with friend/partner.[2,3]

1 P Ghosh *et al* 1987 *Clin Orthop* **224** 52   2 G Grimby *Acta Med Scand* **711** (Suppl.) 233–7   3 KM Gorman, JD Posner 1988 *Clin Geriatr Med* **4** 181-92

Injuries

Etiology

Exercise-related injury in the aged can result from current training, earlier injuries causing trouble in later life. Of major influence are underlying ageing changes, especially reduced compliance, and the nature of the exercise; elderly people engage in less high impact and contact sport. Common causes of exercise-related injury in the aged are listed in Table 22.2.[1,2]

Overuse syndromes account for 70–80%. This type of injury tends to progress slowly, may be ignored, neglected or self-treated by the elderly athlete who often presents late. Sites of injury resemble those in the young, the knee being by far the most common, followed by the foot and lower leg (Table 22.3). Reduced strength and flexibility in the lower limb leading to reduced shock-absorbing capacity probably accounts for knee and foot problems in the older athlete. Overuse superimposed on tissue degeneration cause shoulder, tendon, and ligament problems. With bone demineralization, older people may be more susceptible to stress fractures—sometimes uncommon sites such as os calcis, neck of femur or metatarsals, as well as the tibia (common in younger athletes).[3]

Diagnosis

In 80% of cases a good history and examination are sufficient. Useful questions: Are your symptoms:

- aggravated by activity?
- exaccerbated by a pre-existing condition?
- precipitated by sudden changes in intensity or trauma?

Diagnosis may be more difficult in the old as osteoarthritic symptoms are common, injury/disease can present with atypical symptoms and traumatic injury such as internal joint derangement is uncommon, therefore unexpected and may be missed or ascribed to osteoarthritis. Careful examination is important. Special tests (plain x-ray, CT, bone scan, blood chemistry, or arthrogram) may be useful in selected individuals. Specialist consultation should be necessary in only 10–15% of cases. A *proactive approach to diagnosis is important* so that treatment can begin early as injury and inactivity pose a greater threat and healing takes longer in the old. Comprehensive evaluation and the decision to refer for specialist opinion should be based on symptoms, not age. *Remember*, pain is not a normal accompaniment of ageing.

Treatment

Since the majority of injuries are due to overuse, older athletes are most often managed conservatively.

1 Rest, ice, compression, elevation (RICE)
2 Drugs
   - *Adverse drug reactions* (ADR) more common, as the elderly[4]
     – consume more drugs
     – altered drug handling
     – may have impaired homeostasis/subclinical disease.

1 GO Matheson *et al* 1989 *Sci Sports Exercise* 21 379–85   2 KE DeHaven *et al* 1986 *Am J Sports Med* 14 218–24   3 MB Devas 1970 *J Roy Coll Gen Pract* 19 34-8   4 PA Atkin, SJ Ogle 1996 *Adverse Drug Reactions Toxicol Rev* 15 109–18

Table 22.2 Sports injuries in the elderly

Diagnosis	No.	%
Tendinitis	181	23.0
Patellofemoral pain syndrome	79	10.0
Osteoarthritis	73	9.3
Muscle strain	69	8.8
Ligament sprain	64	8.1
Plantar fasciitis	47	6.0
Metatarsalgia	45	5.7
Meniscal injury	39	5.0
Degenerative disk disease	34	4.3
Stress fractures/Periostitis	29	3.7
Unknown	26	3.3
Morton's neuroma	22	2.8
Inflammatory arthritis	20	2.5
Multiple diagnoses	16	2.0
Vascular compartment	10	1.3
Bursitis	10	1.3
Adhesive capsulitis	8	1.0
Rotator cuff tear	5	0.6
Subcromial impingement	4	0.5
Achilles tendon rupture	3	0.4
Spondylarthritis of C-spine	2	0.2

Table 22.3 Sites of sports injuries in the elderly

Location	No.	%
Knee	237	31.0
Foot	139	18.0
Lower leg	78	10.0
Shoulder	68	8.8
Ankle	63	8.1
Lumbosacral spine	43	5.6
Multiple sites	43	5.6
Elbow	34	4.4
Hip/Pelvis	31	4.0
Upper leg	20	2.6
Neck	11	1.4
Wrist/Hand	7	0.9

Injuries (*cont*)

- *Pharmacokinetics*
  - absorption, hepatic metabolism, plasma protein-binding—no clinically significant change
  - renal clearance nonsteroidal antiinflammatory drugs (NSAIDs) and antibiotics impaired
  - distribution: reduced total body water (TBW) or muscle mass relative to fat means that fat soluble drugs (diazepam) have a reduced concentration after a given dose, are widely distributed in fat and thus take longer to excrete when stopped.
- *Pharmacodynamics*
  - receptor sensitivity is reduced for some drugs (beta blockers) and increased for others (benzodiazepines, morphine)
- *Particular drugs*
  - NSAIDs cause gastrointestinal bleeding
  - codeine can cause nausea, constipation, and confusion
  - paracetamol given regularly (1gm, 4–6 hourly) for pain may be more suitable
  - morphine can cause nausea, constipation, and confusion; much smaller doses (2.5–5.0mg, 4–6 hourly) required
  - benzodiazepines should be avoided as they cause drowsiness, confusion, ataxia, falling, and postural hypotension
- *Principles for drug prescribing in the aged*
  - start low, go slow
  - be aware other medications (stop, if possible)
  - new symptoms may be an ADR
  - regular review

3 Therapy for injuries in the old takes longer.[1] Start rehabilitation early and plan to treat for twice as long in those >60 and for three times as long for those >75. Decrease activity by 15–25% until symptoms disappear. Similarly return to activity should be in increments of 15–25% over 3–6 weeks. Physiotherapy is useful including ultrasound, stretching, and gentle manipulation such as Maitland's mobilization.[2] Exercises ideally to be performed at home but with support to aid motivation and compliance can be prescribed. Muscle strengthening (agonist–antagonist) exercises, such as quadriceps and hamstring exercises in knee injury, can be taught to and performed by the elderly

4 Bracing/orthotics may play a role for such problems as Achilles tendinitis, posterior tibial tendinitis, plantar fasciitis and ankle instability

5 Local corticosteroid injection should be considered (10%)

6 Surgery may be required rarely (2–4%)

Prevention

Strategies for the prevention of injury in the older athlete have been touched on already and are summarized in Table 22.4.[3]

Protective clothing is important as the aged are more sensitive to thermal stresses. The risk of hypothermia can be reduced by covering the head (one-third of the heat lost from the body is via the head). Also, layered clothing offers maximal insulation and specialized

1 MB Brown 1989 *Clin Sports Med* **8** 893–901 2 GD Maitland 1986 *Vertebral manipulation* 5th edn. Butterworth 3 AJ Ting 1991 *Clin Sports Med* **10** 319–25

Table 22.4 Strategies for prevention of injury in the older athlete

- Regular program of exercises and range of motion activities to maintain muscle mass and flexibility
- Adequate warm-up and cool-down
- Sensible program of exercise with adequate rest
- Protective clothing and good footwear
- Avoid the heat of the day
- Reduce weight bearing exercise for those with arthritis
- Safe environment for those with vision and balance problems (e.g. static bicycle)

thermal (e.g. polypropylene) clothing helps keep the body dry and reduces skin irritation. In extreme heat, especially when UV irradiation is high, a broad-brimmed hat should be worn and the trunk and shoulders covered. Shoes for the older athlete should have maximum shock absorbing capacity. Most cushioning is provided by the heel. Degeneration of the heel fat pad may occur in the old. Shoes should be replaced after about 400–800km (250–500 miles) of running on a surface equivalent to asphalt. Resoling of shoes (where only the outer sole is replaced) is not recommended. Running surfaces vary in their stiffness. Turf, dirt, and wooden tracks are. more compliant than asphalt and concrete, and therefore have decreased impact forces.

Sports-related injuries

Swimming

Relative weightlessness reduces stress on degenerative joints. Lower limbs are relatively spared except for the patellofemoral joint (knee flex >70° during kick in swimming). Shoulders support a repetitive load with overhead stroke action which may exacerbate soft tissue irritation and collagen deterioration to produce subacromial bursitis or supraspinatus tendinitis. Swimming may aggravate arthritis in the shoulder joints contributing to spur formation and cuff impingement or tearing. Bicipital tendinitis and rupture of the long head of the biceps may develop either suddenly or insidiously.

Running

Most injuries are caused by overuse and impact under torsional load. Back and lower limb injuries predominate. Bone injuries include stress fractures (neck of femur, tibial shaft and plateau, calcaneus, metatarsals) as well as lower back and disk injuries. Cartilage damage is seen particularly in joints with previous articular or meniscal tears; genu varum or valgum may accentuate osteoarthritic joint problems. Muscle strains, especially of glutei, hamstrings, and quadriceps are common, as are tendon injuries including tendinitis of the tendon Achilles, iliotibial band, patellar or posterior tibial tendons and bursitis over the greater trochanter. In racket sports (tennis, squash), knee injury in older players commonly involves tear in the posterior horn of the medial meniscus when age-related structural degeneration is present. Disruption of the extensor mechanism of the knee ascends from the tibial tubercle as age increases. The usual cause is eccentric overload to the extensor mechanism with the foot on the ground and an obstacle preventing full extension (as in a stumble or stubbing the foot). Fracture of the patella and/or rupture of the quadriceps tendon may result. Sudden dorsiflexion of the foot while running with the foot extended or not quickly released from the ground may overstretch or rupture the tendon Achilles. Older players making a sudden start to chase the ball may tear the medial head of the gastrocnemius due to the impact of the forefoot in toe off.

Golf

Cervical and lower back pain frequently result from forward flexing of the cervical spine and rotation of the body during the swing, when the head is steady and eyes locked on the ball. Management involves strengthening the abdominal muscles, long trunk extensors, and shorter paraspinal groups. Encourage use of isometric neck exercises. Shoulder pain in older golfers often reflects degenerating collagen and reduced blood supply which has resulted in rotator cuff impairment. Less frequently, instability and posterior shoulder pain may indicate a tight posterior capsule. The swing of right handed golfers, especially in dudded shots, may aggravate back of neck pain from left lateral and right medial epicondylitis.

Cycling

Compression syndromes (carpal tunnel, Guyon's canal, cubital tunnel) and inflammatory conditions (subacromial bursitis, lateral epicondylitis, de Quervain's stenosing tenovaginitis) are more prevalent in older cyclists. Cervical and lower back pain may cause problems, which if combined with degenerative disk disease or arthritis, may prevent older cyclists from continuing with this sport. Fractures incurred in falls typically involve clavicle, forearm, and wrist. Static cycling may prove useful where balance has deteriorated or environmental factors present problems.

Rowing

Stresses spread through the body by repetitive use of upper and lower limbs in the sculling position can lead to extensor tenosynovitis in elbow and wrist, stress fractures of the pars interarticularis and ribs, mechanical and discogenic lower back pain/radiculopathy, and in the lower limbs to patella and ankle sprains.

Downhill skiing

The majority of injuries in older skiers result from collisions and falls rather than overuse. Patellofemoral degenerative joint disease exacerbated by posture with knees flexed and the quadriceps mechanism contracting concentrically and eccentrically is more prevalent in older skiers. Contributing factors include prior cartilage damage, muscle atrophy, and low compliance of soft tissues/tendons/ligaments. Predominant fractures affecting older skiers involve neck of femur, tibial plateau, proximal humerus, greater tuberosity avulsions, and Colle's. Predisposing factors include osteopenia in post-menopausal women. The twisting, rotating, and impact forces of skiing may produce anterior cruciate and medial collateral ligament tears and meniscal tears about the knee. The ubiquitous 'skier's thumb' (rupture of the ulnar collateral thumb ligament) is also seen after hyperabduction of the thumb in older skiers (use S-Thumb splint, Johnson and Johnson), to prevent and to treat incomplete tears (see Fig. 10.3). Management involves strengthening quadriceps and vastus medialis obliquus, stretching of quadriceps, and hamstrings. Reduce level of activity to be consistent with fitness level. Encourage older skiers into cross country rather than downhill/slalom skiing.

Continence

Urinary incontinence is common in elderly women—10–20% >65 years.[1] Bladder capacity falls from 600ml to around 450ml in the elderly. After micturition there should be no residual urine though the bladder tends to empty less efficiently as we age. There may also be less central nervous system (CNS) control and a loss of pelvic floor integrity in women after childbirth and the menopause.

During exercise the leakage of small amounts of urine usually indicates genuine stress incontinence (GSI). GSI is more common in women who have had four or more children. It is due to pelvic floor weakness and descent of the bladder neck. Pelvic floor exercises taught and supervised by a specially trained physiotherapist and/or surgical culposuspension (bladder elevation) is successful in up to 80% of cases.[2] Urodynamic evaluation should be performed prior to surgery. Prescription of estrogen—either HRT or topically—may be useful.

Leakage of larger amounts of urine during exercise may be due to detrusor instability. The detrusor or bladder wall muscle is a large involuntary smooth muscle supplied by cholinergic parasympathetic efferent fibers via sacral nerve roots (S2,3,4). Detrusor instability may be caused by disease of the nervous system, local bladder pathology or poor bladder habits. Accompanying symptoms are urgency, frequency, nocturia and the voiding of small volumes of urine. After examination to exclude underlying pathology behavioral retraining of the bladder by a nurse continence adviser is recommended. The first step is to establish regular bowel motions as constipation exacerbates the problem. Then a bladder diary is opened; this records:

- fluid intake (should be 8 glasses per day)
- time and amount urine voided
- urge
- precipitating factors (e.g. exercise, coughing).

- From this can be established bladder capacity and pattern of voiding. The person is then taught to 'hold on' and the diary gradually improves. Studies indicate a 70–80% success rate.

- Anticholinergic drugs, which inhibit detrusor action, such as oxybutynin 2.5–10mg daily or imipramine 25mg–50mg, at night, have limited usefulness as anticholinergic side-effects are common.

1 NM Resnick, SV Yalla 1985 *New Eng J Med* **313** 800–5   2 PD Wilson *et al* 1987 *Br J Obstetr Gynaecol* **94** 575–82

Nutrition

- A good diet is important for athletic performance and for general health and should not be overlooked by the doctor.[1]
- Caloric need decreases for those over 75 years (1800kcal for men, 1400kcal for women). However, the older athlete should maintain the same mix of food groups as that of younger athletes (carbohydrates 50–60%, protein 10–20%, fat not >30%). If involved in endurance training, carbohydrates need to be increased to 60–70% of the diet. Adequate protein (containing essential amino acids) is essential and vegetarian diets commonly need to be supplemented.
- Vitamin supplementation is only useful if dietary intake is inadequate. Iron is particularly important in distance runners. Older athletes, especially women, should ensure daily intake of 1500mg of calcium for bone integrity. This may be difficult to achieve without supplementation as calcium is poorly absorbed.
- Dehydration is more common in the elderly. Drinking water before, during, and after exercise helps control core body temperature and reduces risk of dehydration (a cause of muscle cramps).

1 CL Rock 1991 *Clin Sports Med* **10** 445–57

Conclusion

More people are reaching old age and many older people are exercising. The observed physical changes with ageing are compounded by disuse as inactivity is still common among the aged. The benefits of regular aerobic exercise are now well documented and include: physical (reduced mortality), psychological (elevated mood), and social (less isolation). Injury, especially overuse injuries occur but can be treated and prevented.

The doctor's responsibility is to encourage exercise/activity for older people to increase their overall health and sense of well-being. Provision of pre-exercise evaluation, prescription of an exercise program, diagnosis, and management of injuries plus counselling about prevention and nutrition is essential for all older athletes.

Addendum. Muscle weakness and high resistance training in frail old people

GREG BENNETT, TOM GWINN

Introduction

Lean body mass in aged master athletes is maintained into the 7th decade after which it declines (1). Most of these athletes are participating in endurance training and not resistance training. These are individual examples of very active elderly athletes participating in resistance training in whom little loss of muscle mass is observed over an extended period. On the other hand, the typical 80-year-old will demonstrate a 30–40% decline in the voluntary strength of the muscles of the leg, arm, and back compared to subjects aged 30 years. A significant portion of older people will experience much larger declines than this average and can be said to define the 'frail elderly'. The marked loss of muscle strength in the frail elderly not only results in a barrier to participation in recreational pursuits, but also presents a major hindrance to their ability to perform basic activities of daily living (ADL).

Several common interrelated factors which often coexist to produce reduced physical activity include: undernutrition (2), depression, social isolation, and muscle weakness (3). Reduced physical activity exacerbates these factors thereby creating a vicious cycle of progressive inactivity and accelerated muscle weakness (3). Muscle weakness is well correlated with impaired mobility and ability to perform ADLs and predicts poor health outcomes, institutionalization, and impaired ADLs. In the last few years, several studies have demonstrated the value of resistance training in frail weak older people. Most exercise programs prescribed to very old people, especially the physically frail usually consist of 'gentle exercises' and walking. It is well known that high resistance training of younger adults results in marked increases in muscle strength and mass. This brief review examines the efficacy and feasibility of applying such regimens to the frail elderly in order to enhance their ability to perform ADLs.

Prevalence of muscle weakness

Muscle weakness that is sufficiently marked to result in functional impairment is unfortunately quite common in elderly populations. The Framingham cohort of free-living older people over 75 years reported large proportions unable to lift 4.5 kg using their upper limbs (4). According to a 1984 survey of 70–74-year-olds conducted in the USA, 23% of men and 27% of women had difficulty walking 0.4km and 23% of men and 40% women had difficulty lifting or carrying a load of only 11.4kg (5). A study of >80-year-olds in three US populations found that the majority of subjects were unable to undertake heavy housework. Inability to climb stairs was found in 10–15% of men and 12–31% of women. Inability to walk across the room ranged from 12–23%. The rural population performed much better than the two urban ones (6).

Relevance

In association with advancing age is an increased incidence of persons who experience locomotion problems in activities, such as ambulation, rising from a chair, and ascending stairs. These mobility problems in turn are often associated with a decreased capacity to perform ADLs such as shopping, and cooking, cleaning, etc. As mobility restrictions become more profound, institutionalization (e.g. hostel or nursing home) may be required.

Laukkanen *et al* studied 2000 random samples from a central Finnish population and found that those with maximal knee extension strength below the total mean were significantly more likely to die within the 2-year study time than the group with strength above the mean (**7**). In Guralnik's study of more than 2000 persons aged 71 and over, three activities involving the lower extremity were assessed (walking speed, timed rise from a chair, and standing balance) to produce an overall measure of each individual's lower limb capacity rated on a 12 point summary scale (**8**). When this population was followed up it was found that the results of the summary scale were strongly predictive of the incidence of nursing home admission (see Fig. 1) and mortality over the next 2.5 years. Individuals with scores in the 25th percentile were approximately 3 times more likely to be admitted to nursing home than those in the 75th percentile.

The findings of Guralnik are consistent with the observations that deteriorating lower extremity function (**9**), requiring help or aid for mobility (**10**), and low ADL status are significant predictors of nursing home admission (**11–12**). Mobility in seniors is related to the strength of the muscles of the lower limb: knee and leg extensor strength is strongly associated with walking speed, chair rising capacity, dynamic balance, and stair climbing speed (**13–16**). Associations of muscle weakness with falls and fractures have repeatedly been reported (**17–21**). In Australian elderly populations, reduced strength of the leg muscles has been specifically related to the incidence of nursing home admission among residents in hostel care (**22**) and increased risk of osteoporotic fracture (e.g. older Australian males who have a strength deficit of the knee extensors of 1 standard deviation or more below the mean have more than double the risk of hip fracture) (**23**).

Causes of muscle weakness (24,25)

Biological changes ageing and disuse.

Many changes in muscle function and composition that have been described in various otherwise healthy populations of older people have been attributed to ageing *per se*. It is important, however, to note that these changes have been documented in populations of relatively sedentary older people. On the basis of these studies, it is not possible to separate the effects of long-standing underuse of muscle from the changes associated with healthy optimal ageing. A decline in muscle mass and strength occurs in both sedentary and endurance athletes with age. On the basis of a small number of individuals studied who have maintained resistance training well into old age, it may be that muscle mass may decline to a relatively minor degree on the basis of ageing alone. The muscle architectural and microscopic changes of disuse and average ageing are very similar.

Undernutrition

Has been documented to occur in 20–65 % of older people. Based on animal and human studies protein calorie malnutrition is associated with altered morphology (reduced fiber area, selective fiber atrophy,

777

and disorganized myofibrils), reduced oxidative capacity, and decreased performance. Many of these changes resemble changes documented as age related. The potential for nutritional supplementation to reverse changes has not been studied extensively as yet.

Diseases and drugs

Common diseases affecting muscles include electrolyte disorders (most commonly diuretic induced Na or K depletion or drug-induced inappropriate antidiuretic hormone excretion). Acute or chronic infections may produce altered muscle metabolism and performance as well as increasing muscle catabolism and causing reduced nutrient intake through anorexia. Corticosteroids cause proximal myopathy with chronic usage. Hypogonadal disorders, hypopituitarism and thyroid diseases may present with muscle weakness. Hormone deficiency disorders respond to replacement therapy.

People with chronic neurological diseases such as stroke, parkinsonism, chronic spinal stenosis, and chronic musculoskeletal disorders often have secondary muscle weakness due to disuse in addition to primary muscle weakness.

Effects of high resistance training

Research since the late 1980s has consistently demonstrated that high resistance weight training results in large increases in the muscle strength of older subjects. For example, Table 22.5 summarizes the results of weight lifting programs for the leg extensor muscles. While the training outcomes are clearly variable (i.e. increases in strength ranging from approximately 25% to more than 170%), it would not be unreasonable to expect 70% increase in strength for a 70-year-old person as a result of performing a high resistance training program. It is significant to note that all these studies have used high relative training intensities, with subjects training with weights of between 65–90% of their maximal capacity (65–90% of 1 repetition maximum, RM). None of these studies have reported the incidence of any serious misadventures associated with performing these exercises, and programs are usually reported as being enjoyable with low drop-out rates.

Efficacy

One important question is whether lower limb strength training increases indexes of mobility in older subjects. Several studies have demonstrated very significant gains in strength in very frail institutionalized residents. Fisher *et al* noted improvements in subjects whose initial muscle force averaged only 50% aged matched controls (**37**). One of the best studies was by Fiatarone and coworkers demonstrated in a randomized study of 100 frail elderly subjects of average age 87–90 years within a residential setting, that high resistance strength training 3 days per week is effective in increasing functional capacity (**2**). Of the subjects in this study, 83% required a walking aid, 66% had fallen during the previous year. Many subjects suffered multiple chronic diseases; most commonly a history of osteoporotic fracture (44%), arthritis (50%), pulmonary disease (44%), and hypertension (35%). Cognitive impairment was found in over 50%, and 35% met criteria for depression. After 8–10 weeks of

Table 22.5 Summary of results of high-resistance training of the lower extremity in older people

Study (Ref. no.)	No. (Exp/Ctrl)	Av. age (yrs)	Duration (weeks)	Muscle group or movement	Training intensity	Strength increase (%)	Drop-outs (%)	SAE
(26)	14	63	12	knee ext/leg press	70–90% 1 RM	23	0	None
(27)	13/6	70	12	knee ext/leg press	65%–75% 1 RM	93	19	None
(2)	25/25	87	10	knee ext/leg press	80% 1 RM	167	6	None
(28)	10	90	8	knee ext	80% 1 RM	174	10	None
(29)	12	65	12	knee ext/flex	80% 1 RM	107	0	None
(30)	11	71	12	knee ext	80% 1 RM	44	0	?
(31)	23/12	60	16	knee ext/leg press	5–15 RM	43	0	None
(32)	76/66	68	40	leg press	80% 1 RM	22	16	None
(33)	21/19	60	52	knee ext/leg press	80% 1 RM	66	3	None
(34)	18/18	67	26	knee ext/flex	80% 1 RM	21	17	None
(35)	16/6	68	52	knee ext/leg press	75% 1 RM	95	12	None
(36)	28/27	80	12	knee ext	70–75% 1 RM	34	11	None
Average		71				74	8	

exp, experimental group; ctrl, control group; ext, extension; flex, flexion; 1 RM, 1 repetition maximum.

779

high intensity strengthening exercise the knee and leg extensor strength increased in these subjects approximately 170% and 30%, respectively. These changes were associated with significant increases in habitual walking velocity (8–15%), stair climbing capacity (23–34%), balance ability (48%), and overall level of physical activity (17–51%). Some of these large responses probably reflect altered patterns of motor unit recruitment, but increases of muscle mass from 12% to 17% have also been demonstrated by objective radiological techniques (**2**, **25**, **32**, **33**).

In contrast, mixed training programs which include only low resistance high repetition and aerobic training, produce modest or no improvement (**38**). For example, Mulrow *et al* describes a 4-month mixed program combining range-of-motion, strength, balance, transfer, and mobility exercises for frail nursing home residents. The intervention resulted in no significant changes in strength or in any of the other primary outcome measures (**39**).

In Fiatarone's study, nutritional intervention with exercise vs exercise alone showed a trend to improved muscle strength which did not reach significance. Total protein intake was not reported. Meridith et al found benefit from the daily ingestion of a supplement that added 0.33g/kg of protein and 33kJ/kg of food energy to the usual diet (**40**).

Adverse effects

As demonstrated in Table 22.5, high resistance training is associated with little in the way of adverse effects. Some authors have noted reductions in bodily pain and no adverse effects exercising arthritic knees. Other authors report reduced arthritic symptoms. Patients require a period of supervised acclimatization and build-up before high resistance commences. This period should be approximately 1–2 weeks. *It is important to note* that low adverse effects relate to the relatively low maximal strength of weaker elderly subjects. Hunter *et al* found that younger subjects suffered more adverse symptoms than older subjects (**30**).

Safety in chronic active medical conditions

In general frailty and arthritis present no barriers to resistance training. Significant numbers of subjects with ischemic heart disease, cardiac failure, and pulmonary diseases were trained in Fiatarone study without ill effect. This is not surprising given that mean arterial blood pressure elevations during training did not exceed 150mmHg. Benn *et al* for double leg press which is comparable to that found climbing stairs (**41**). Blood pressure elevation related to resistance exercise is very short lived in comparison to aerobic endurance training.

Other benefits

High-resistance training in older people reduces the rate of bone loss (**42**), improves insulin sensitivity (**43**), significantly reduces depression, and modestly increases VO_{2max}. Improvements in VO_{2max} in one study was independent of increased spontaneous activity.

Exercise prescription

Training regimens currently recommended to improve strength in frail older people are essentially identical to that for younger health adult who have had no prior experience of high resistance training. Disabled older people may require assistance and encouragement to use resistance equipment because of disability and fear.

Definitions

The intensity of resistance exercise is defined by the number of contractions that can be performed in a continuous sequence until fatigue is induced and no further lifts can be performed. Generally, it should take 2–5s to lift and lower the weight with 2s rest between lifts. A weight that can be lifted 10 times followed by fatigue is termed 10 RM (10 repetition maximum). The higher the RM the lower the weight for an individual. The highest weight a person can lift is 1 RM.

Classic dose–response experiments by Richard Berger in the 1960s helped define the optimum weight training program for college-aged males. His work and that of others identified an intensity range of between 8 RM to 12 RM, times 3 sets, to produce optimal gains in strength. 2–3min rest is taken between sets. From the evidence in Table 22.5 one, it appears that this regime is equally effective in older people. It is generally recommended that training be on non-consecutive days. Every 2 weeks the 1RM should be retested so that an appropriately higher resistance is used in order to maintain the same training stimulus.

Younger people usually require 1 week build-up to a full training stimulus of about 80% 1 RM. In frail old people a supervised build-up period of about 3 weeks is required to avoid muscle pain following exercise, to familiarize them with the equipment and to monitor any atypical responses. Commencing at a weight of 60–70% 1 RM is appropriate.

Introduction (*cont*)

References

(1) T Kavanagh *et al* 1988. Health and sociodemographic characteristics of the Masters competitior. *Annals Sports Med* vol 4 no 2 55-64

(2) MA Fiatarone *et al* 1994 Exercise training and nutritional supplementation for physical frailty in very elderly people. *N Engl J Med* 330 1769–75, 1994

(3) WM Bortz 1982 Disuse and ageing. *JAMA* **248** 1203–8

(4) AM Jette, LG Branch The Framingham Disability Study: II. Physical ability among the ageing. *Am J Public Health* **71** 1211–16

(5) MG Kovar, AZ LaCroix Ageing in the eighties: Ability to perform work-related activities. Data from the supplement on ageing to the NHIS, United States, 1984, *Advance data from Vital and Health Statistics*, No 136 (DHHS Publication No PHS 87-1250). DHHS, Hyatsville, MD

(6) J Coroni-Huntley *et al* Established populations for epidemiological studies of the elderly. *Resource data book* (NIH Publication No 86-2443). US Public Health Service, National Institute in Ageing, Washington, DC

(7) P Laukkanen *et al* 1995 Muscle strength and moblity as predictors of survival in 75–84-year-old people. *Age Ageing* **24** 468–73

(8) JM Guralnik *et al* 1994 A short physical performance battery assessing lower extremity function: Association with self-reported disability and prediction of mortality and nursing home admission. *J Gerontol* **49** M85–94

(9) FD Wolinsky FD *et al* 1993 Changes in functional status and the risks of subsequent nursing home placement and death. *J Gerontol* **48** S93–101

(10) MA Cohen *et al* 1986 Client-related risk factors of nursing home entry among elderly adults. *J Gerontol* **41** 785–92

(11) P Narain *et al* 1988 Predictors of immediate and 6-month outcomes in elderly patients. *JAGS* **36** 775–83

(12) MA Rudberg MA *et al* 1996 Risk factors for nursing home use after hospitalisation for medical illness. *J Gerontol* **51A** M189–194

(13) EJ Bassey *et al* 1992 Leg extensor power and functional performance in very old men and women. *Clin Sci* **82** 321–217

(14) DM Buchner *et al* Evidence for a non-linear relationship between leg strength and gait speed. *Age Ageing* **25** 386–91

(15) MA Fiatarone *et al* 1994 High intensity strength training in nonogenarians. *JAMA* **263** 3029–34

(16) MA Hughs *et al* 1996 The role of strength in rising from a chair in the functionally impaired elderly. *J Biochem* **29** 1509–13

(17) DM Buchner, EB Larson 1987 Falls and fractures in patients with Alzheimer-type dementia. *JAMA* **257** 1492–5

(18) AJ Campbell *et al* 1990 Examination by logistic regression modelling of the variables which increase the relative risk of elderly women falling compared to elderly men. *J Clin Epidemiol* **43** 1415–20

(19) GS Sorock GS, DM Labiner 1992 Peripheral neuromuscular dysfunction and falls in an elderly cohort. *Am J Epidemiol* **136** 584–91

(20) ME Tinetti 1987 Factors associated with serious injury during falls by ambulatory nursing home residents. *J Am Geriatr Soc* **35** 644–8

(21) H Whipple *et al* 987 The relationship of knee and ankle weakness to falls in nursing home residents: an isokinetic study. *J Am Geriatr Soc* **35** 13–20

(22) SR Lord 1994 Predictors of nursing home placement and mortality of residents in intermediate care. *Age Ageing* **23** 499–504

(23) T Nguyen *et al* Prediction of osteoporotic fractures by postural instability and bone density. *Br Med J* **307** 1111–15

(24) MA Fiatarone, WJ Evans 1993 The etiology and reversibility of muscle dysfunction in the aged. *J Gerontol* **48** 77–83

(25) AP Goldberg *et al* 1996 Exercise physiology and ageing In EL Schneider, JW Rowe (ed) *Handbook of the biology of ageing.* London

(26) AB Brown *et al* 1990 Positive adaptations to weight training in the elderly. *J Appl Physiol* **69** 1725–33

(27) SL Charette SL *et al* 1991 Muscle hypertrophy response to resistance training in older women. *J Appl Physiol* **70** 1912–16

(28) MA Fiatarone *et al* 1990 High-intensity strength training in nonagenarians. *JAMA* **263** 3029–34

(29) WR Fontera *et al* 1988 Strength conditioning in older men: skeletal muscle hypertrophy and improved function. *J Appl Physiol* **64** 1038–44

(30) GR Hunter *et al* 1995 The effects of strength conditioning on older women's ability to perform daily tasks. *J Am Geriatr Soc* **43** 756–60

(31) BF Hurley BF *et al* 1995 Effects of strength training on muscle hypertrophy and muscle cell disruption in older men. *Int J Sports Med* **16** 378–84

(32) N McCartney *et al* 1995 Long-term resistance training in the elderly: Effects on dynamic strength, exercise capacity, muscle and bone. *J Gerontol* **50A** B97–104

(33) CM Morganti *et al* Strength improvements with 1 yr of progressive resistance training in older women. *Med Sci Sport Exerc* **27** 906–12

(34) JF Nichols *et al* 1993 Efficacy of heavy-resistance training for active women over sixty: Muscular strength, body composition, and program adherence. *J Am Geriatr Soc* **41** 205–10

(35) G Pyka *et al* 1994 Muscle strength and fiber adaptations to a year-long resistance training program in elderly men and women. *J Gerontol* **49** M22–7

(36) L Wolfson *et al* 1996 Balance and strength training in older adults: Intervention gains and Tai Chi maintenance. *J Am Geriatr Soc* **44** 498–506

(37) NM Fisher *et al* Muscle rehabilitation: Its effect on muscular and functional performance of patients with knee osteoarthritis. *Arch Phys Med Rehab* **72** 367–74

(38) KA Vitti *et al* A low-level strength training program for frail elderly adults living in an extended attention facility. *Ageing Clin Exp Res* **5** 363–9

(39) CD Mulrow *et al* A randomised trial of physical rehabilitation for very frail nursing home residents. *JAMA* **271** 519–24

(40) CN Meridith CN *et al* Body composition in elderly men: Effect of Dietary modification during strength training. *J Am Geriatr Soc* **40** 155–62

(41) Benn *et al J Am Geriatr Soc* 44 121–5

(42) AS Ryan *et al* 1996 Resistive training increases insulin actin in postmenopausal women. *J Gerontol* **51A** M199–205

(43) AS Ryan *et al* 1994 Effects of strength training on bone mineral density: hormonal and bone turnover relationships. *J Appl Physiol* **77** 1678–84

23 The female athlete

JENI SAUNDERS, SAMEER VISWARATHAN

Introduction[1]

We have come a long way from the time that Baron Pierre de Coubertin considered 'women's sports are against the laws of nature'. At the 1996 Atlanta Games nearly 50% of the Australian Team were female. Women are now encouraged to participate in regular sporting activity. However, a number of health concerns specific to the female athlete have been described.

1 G Bryant *et al* 1997 The Female Athlete In E Sherry, D Bokor (ed) *Manual of sports medicine* Ch 17, 243–64. GMM, London

Gynecological concerns

Menstrual cramps

Menstrual cramps (dysmennorrhea) occur during menstruation. The pain is abdominal and can range in severity from mild to severe. The pain is characteristically worst at the start of the cycle. Pathophysiologically, the pain is thought to be due to ischemia in the myometrium during uterine contractions and is mediated by prostaglandin release by the endometrium. Severe symptoms may decrease athletic performance. Exercise may have a beneficial effect on dismenorrhea by the effects of β-endorphins on the uterus. **Treatment**: obtain a complete menstrual history and inquire about the severity of symptoms. For moderate to severe dismenorrhea, ketoprofen, naproxen sodium, or ibuprofen, taken 24–48h prior to the onset of menses, and for the duration of the discomfort, may be helpful as they work by limiting the release of prostaglandins. The oral contraceptive pill (OCP) reduces the severity of symptoms. Mild dismenorrhea may be treated with mild analgesics or even nothing.

Premenstrual tension (PMT)

PMT refers to physical and emotional symptoms (Table 23.1) which begin with the onset of ovulation and decrease in intensity with the progression of menstruation. As with dismenorrhea, exercise may actually dampen the symptoms of PMT. This is thought to be due to the effects of β-endorphins acting centrally or due to a decrease in the pulse frequency of gonadotropin releasing hormone (GnRH). **Treatment**: the OCP can be used. The OCP can, however, cause an exacerbation of symptoms in some women. Pyridoxine (vitamin B_6, 200–600mg/day) has been found to be effective in reducing fluid retention, breast tenderness and depressive symptoms. Diuretics can be used to treat fluid retention, but care must be taken to prevent dehydration and must not be prescribed for competitive sport (banned by the International Olympic Committee).

Table 23.1 Symptoms of PMT

Emotional	Physical
Mood cravings	Headaches
Anxiety	Fluid retention
Depression	Bloating
Irritability	Breast soreness
Insomnia	Breast enlargement
Alteration in libido	Appetite changes

From G Bryant *et al* 1997 The female athlete. In E Sherry, D Bokor (ed) *Sports medicine problems and management* Ch 17. GMM, London p246

Contraception

Choice of a contraceptive agent depends on the athlete's fertility, medical history, and coital frequency. Choices include diaphragms, condoms, and intra-uterine devices (IUD). Barrier methods (e.g. condoms) which do not affect the normal hormonal balance of the body or alter athletic performance are to be preferred. They also prevent the transmission of sexually transmitted diseases. Condom usage should be encouraged to prevent transmission of genital herpes, genital warts, hepatitis B, and HIV. Spermicidal (containing nonoxynol-9 and menfegol) creams improve the efficacy of condoms as a method of contraception. With respect to athletes, a diaphragm can be in place during training or competition and must be left *in situ* for at least 6h after the last sexual encounter. A smaller size diaphragm can be used if uncomfortable for the athlete during training periods. Other options include cervical caps and sponges impregnated with spermicidal creams.

IUDs can be used for athletes who have completed child bearing and have regular sex. IUDs are also more reliable than barrier methods. Complications arising from IUDs include an increased risk of pelvic infection and resulting subsequent infertility. In addition, heavier bleeding and increased cramping has been associated with IUD usage. Other contraceptive options include 'natural' methods (rhythm method, basal temperature and mucous viscosity status) but may be unreliable in females with menstrual irregularities.

The oral contraceptive pill

There are two types. The combination pill which usually contains ethinyl estradiol and a progesterone such as levonorgestrel. The other preparation is the progesterone-only pill (minipill). The combination preparation acts by inhibiting the hypothalamus–pituitary system and causes anovulation. The progesterone-only pill acts by making the cervical mucus thicker and impenetrable to sperm. The combination preparation is available in monophasic, biphasic, and triphasic formulations. In addition the OCP can be prescribed in low dose (decreased side-effects) or high dose preparations. Side-effects can include weight gain, fluid retention, breakthrough bleeding, carbohydrate metabolism changes, adverse clotting factor changes and changes in platelet function. Beneficial effects of the OCP include reduced premenstrual symptoms, reduced breast volume changes, and decreased menstrual flow (hence reducing menstrual iron deficiency anemia). The OCP can preserve bone density in women with chronic amenorrhea. The OCP is also associated with a reduced incidence of endometrial and ovarian cancers, as well as reduced incidence of benign breast lesions, pelvic inflammatory disease, ovarian cysts, and ectopic pregnancies. The OCP is associated with lessening of symptoms of endometriosis and a reduction in the incidence of pelvic inflammatory disease and ectopic pregnancies. The effect on athletic performance (detailed in Table 23.2) appears to be minimal.

Contraindications (2–3% of the female population):

- Pregnancy
- Endogenous depression
- Otosclerosis
- Smokers over 35 years of age
- Undiagnosed abnormal uterine bleeding

Table 23.2 The oral contraceptive pill in athletes

Beneficial effects	Side effects
Reduced dismenorrhea	Water retention
Control of the menstrual cycle	Altered glucose retention*
Estrogen source for amenorrheic athletes	Possible decreased VO_{2max}
Reduced blood loss and hence reduced risk of iron deficiency anemia	

*Progestin component.

From G Bryant *et al* 1997 The female athlete. In E Sherry, D Bokor (ed) *Sports medicine problems and practical management* Ch17 p247 GMM, London

Contraception (*cont*)

- History of thromboembolic events
- Estrogen-dependent cancers (breast and uterine cancer and liver hepatomas)
- Active liver disease
- Intestinal malabsorption
- Hypertension (moderate and severe)
- Diabetes with vascular complications
- Cardiovascular disease

Relative contraindications include:

- Epilpesy
- Hyperlipidemia
- Sickle-cell Anemia
- Migraine
- Oligomennorrhea
- Varicose veins

Menstrual cycle and performance

Studies are beginning to indicate that at an élite level of competition, hormonal alterations due the ovulatory menstrual cycle may be of some impact. Athletes have felt that the premenstrual phase or the menstrual phase of the cycle coincides with a decrease in performance. Dysmenorrhea and the premenstrual syndrome may also contribute adversely to athletic performance. However, further study is needed in this area as Olympic medals and athletes have obtained world records at all stages of the cycle.

Control of the menstrual cycle for athletes

Athletes who wish to avoid having their menses during competitive events can use monophasic OCPs. A withdrawal bleed can be induced by stopping the pill 7 days before a competitive event, and then started again at the end of the menstruation or after the event. An alternate method is to induce a bleed by taking progesterone for 10 days, stopping 10 days prior to the athletic event. Skipping the 7-day sugar tablet and beginning the next packet prevents the withdrawal bleed and is another method of controlling menses.

Relationship between exercise and the menstrual cycle

The relationship between menstrual cycle disorders and exercise has been established. There is a wide spectrum of menstrual cycle disorders including delayed menarche, and menstrual dysfunction.

Delayed menarche

The onset of menses (menarche) can be considered delayed if there are no periods by age 16. The average age of menses in Australia is 12–13 years. Of the athletes with delayed menarche, there are two groups. One group being athletes, who exercised intensely before menarche and the other group which did not. Factors contributing to delayed menarche include:

- Intense exercise
- Low bodyweight
- Genetic component

The physiological mechanism involves the hypothalamic axis being affected by a combination of the above factors. Delayed menarche may confer an athletic advantage due to slower rates of maturation causing delayed closure of the epiphysial plates. These results in longer legs narrow hips and less body fat, which might be advantageous in certain sports.

Menstrual dysfunction

Includes oligomenorrhea (irregular menstrual cycle length ranging from 35 to 90 days), amenorrhea (absence of menstrual bleeding), chronic anovulation and shortened luteal phase. Important sequelae of menstrual dysfunction include:

- Reversible infertility.
- Skeletal demineralization[1] (which might be rapid and not completely reversible). This might manifest as stress fractures and premature osteoporosis. Major bone loss occurs early (first 2 years) and seems to affect trabecular bone more than cortical bone.

1 G Barrow, S Saha 1988 *Am J Sports Med* **16** 209–15

- Endometrial hyperplasia (with increased risk of adenocarcinoma of the uterus in females with unopposed estrogen seen in chronic anovulation).
- Increased cardiovascular disease associated with the low estrogen levels (similar to postmenopausal women not receiving estrogen).

Oligomenorrhea and secondary amenorrhea

Oligomenorrhea (irregular menses) and secondary amenorrhea (cessation of spontaneous menstruation for at least 6 months after normal menstrual cycles had been established) are examples of menstrual dysfunction that is relatively common with a 5% incidence in the general population. Overall, the incidence in the athletic community is 10–20% with a peak incidence of 50% in endurance athletes.

Etiology of amenorrhea: the role of the hypothalamic–pituitary–adrenal axis is crucial in menstrual dysfunction. Intense exercise is associated with increases in catecholamines, cortisol, δ-endorphins, and decreases in prolactin, LH, and FSH concentration. Intense activity has been implicated in the activation of the adrenal axis, which in turn suppresses the pulse generation of GnRH. This inhibition leads to decreased gonadotrophin release and hence amenorrhea. Common causes of secondary ammenorrhea include pregnancy, psychological stress, thyroid disorders, polycystic ovaries, medications, drugs, pituitary tumors, and eating disorders.

Abnormal luteal phases

The luteal phase is a 14-day long period between ovulation and the onset of menstrual bleeding. Classically, in athletes the luteal phase is shortened and associated with lower than normal progesterone levels. The cycles may however be normal due to longer follicular phases.

Anovulatory cycles

Can occur despite normal estrogen levels. In athletes, low progesterone levels due to changes in LH pulsatility during the luteal phase can cause these anovulatory cycles.

Sequelae of abnormal luteal phases and anovulatory cycles

The main effect is infertility or suboptimal fertility. There is also the theoretical risk of adenocarcinoma due to the inadequate endometrial protection afforded by the low progestrone levels.

Contributing factors to menstrual dysfunction

- **Exercise level:** decreased exercise results in the restoration of the menses in athletes who had amenorrhea. Exercise is thought to act as a stressor which causes the release of hormones that affect the hypothalamic–pituitary axis.
- **Low body fat**: it was previously thought that a critical body fat percentage was required for normal cycling. However, considerable variability has since been noted in individuals. Increase in body fat has been associated with the return of menses in several cases.
- **Diet**: calorie restricted diets have been associated with irregular

menses. However, it is not clear if the menstrual irregularity is due to the low caoric intake or the resultant low body fat.

- **Psychological stress**: arising from the environment and family has been associated with menstrual irregularity.

Treatment: The principle concern must be to exclude non-exercise related causes of menstrual dysfunction. Thus, pregnancy, polycystic ovaries, pituitary and thyroid conditions, psychological stress, and medication-related menstrual irregularities must be excluded. Delayed menarche warrants investigation if no menstruation has occurred by the age of 16. It is also important to exclude endocrine, gynecological, and genetic causes here.

History and examination

- Changes in weight
- Secondary sexual characteristics
- Virilization
- Pregnancy
- Visual acuity and visual fields
- Pelvic examination (which may include transabdominal ultrasound)
- Prolactin and TSH levels, pregnancy tests (human chorionic gonadotrophin)
- Provera (medroxyprogesterone acetate) challenge test. Presence of estrogen will cause a withdrawal bleed. No bleed indicates, low estrogen levels, or anatomical pathology
- FSH/LH levels. Low FSH/LH levels is seen secondary to intense exercise or pituitary/hypothalamic tumors. High FSH/LH levels might indicate ovarian failure or ovarian resistance
- Family history
- Sexual history
- Medications including use of OCP
- Nutritional history

Treatment

- Reduction in exercise and an increase in body fat
- Optimum nutrition and appropriate calcium intake (1200mg/day)
- Cyclic estrogen/progestin in women with low estrogen levels. Estrogen supplementation can be in the form of OCP or HRT (hormone replacement therapy which is composed of 0.625mg estrogen for days 1–25 and medroxyprogesterone acetate 5mg for days 14–25)
- Estrogen supplementation is contraindicated in women with a history of deep venous thrombosis, breast/endometrial cancer, or abnormal liver tests
- Counseling, education, and a multidisciplinary approach

The female triad[1]

This refers to a condition which features disordered eating, amenorrhea, and osteoporosis. True prevalence is unknown and probably under reported. There is, however, an established link between disordered eating and intense exercise, which is classically seen in athletes for whom a lean physical appearance is a competitive factor. It is not known if the athlete begins high levels of exercise to help to decrease body weight, or if the obsessive nature of the exercise attracts those individuals to whom are predisposed to eating disorders. Thus, figureskaters, gymnasts, divers, and long distance runners seem to be prone to this illness. (See Fig.23.1.)

The disordered eating pattern can range in a continuum of severity with the most severe condition being anorexia nervosa (defined in DSMIV). Bulimia (binge eating), unnecessary dieting, and/or purging can all be features of this condition. Weight control practices can include purging, laxative usage, diuretics, and diet pills. Conversely, these behaviors usually lead to a decreased athletic performance. In some cases disordered eating lasts only as long as the competitive season. **Treatment**:

- Recognition of disordered eating pattern.
- Multidisciplinary approach
- Correction of the 'body dysmorphic' syndrome. Improvement of self-esteem
- Psychiatric and psychological consultation and therapy
- Cognitive/behavioral therapy.

1 A Nattiv *et al* 1004 *Clin Sports Med* **13** 405–18

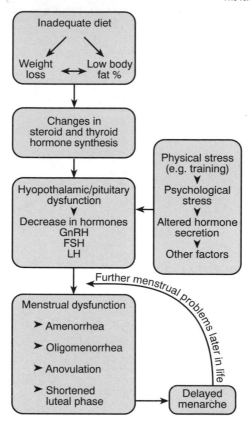

Fig. 23.1 Proposed mechanism for the mechanism of exercise-associated amenorrhea.

Menstrual hygiene

There is no known ill effect to training during menstruation and tampon usage is popular amongst athletes.

Pregnancy and its impact on the female athlete

Exercise can be conducted during pregnancy. However, this should be at mild to moderate level. High levels of activity may be possible in a highly conditioned athlete. In most cases, pregnancy is not an appropriate time to begin a new intensive exercise program or sport.

Important factors to consider about exercise during pregnancy[1]

Overheating: Studies have shown that maternal temperatures greater than 39°Celsius are associated with neural tube defects (particularly failure of the neural tube 25 days post conception). Maternal hyperthermia is also associated with intrauterine growth retardation, intrauterine death, and other abnormalities. **Recommendation**: Advice should be provided indicating that exercise should be avoided during the hottest part of the day, and in addition loose light clothing should be worn. Mothers should be encouraged to maintain an optimal fluid intake. Increased internal plasma volume may help fetomaternal heat transfer and dissipation.

Exertion levels: intense exercise during pregnancy might adversely affect fetal oxygenation. During exercise in excess of 80% of maximum heart rate may result in the diversion of uterine blood flow to exercising muscles. Hypoxic effects on the fetus are usually minimized due to the fact that uterine blood flow is maximal in the area of placental attachment. Despite this, changes in fetal heart rate have been observed during exercise (tachycardia and bradycardia). There is an additional risk of premature labour. Although not common, this is thought to be due to an increase in noradrenaline levels which may lead uterine irritation and hence premature labour. **Recommendation**: exercise levels to be maintained below 60% of maximal heart rate. Each period of exercise should not be longer than 45min including an adequate warm-up and cooling-down period. Exercise routine should be resumed gradually over the 4–6 week postpartum period. Ensure adequate diet, as pregnancy requires additional 300kcal/day.

Risk of injury: during pregnancy, changes in bodyweight and shape may cause an alteration in the mother's center of gravity. Hence, the mother is at risk of losing her balance and having a fall. A fall could cause damage to the placenta. In addition, during a pregnancy ligamentous laxity in the joints can develop increasing the chances of injury. A common complaint during pregnancy is lower back pain. This is thought to be due to circulating estrogen and relaxin. Attention to posture, and muscle strengthening exercises (for the abdomen and back) should be commenced. Avoid even mild abdominal trauma. Non-weight bearing exercises (cycling, swimming) are useful. Do not exercise in supine position after first trimester (as cardiac output is reduced).

Contraindications to exercise in pregnancy

Medical conditions such as cardiovascular disease, respiratory disease, infectious disease, anemia, endocrine disorders, and obesity.

802

---

1 American College of Obstetricians and Gynecologists 1994 Exercise during pregnancy and the postpartum period *Technical Bulletin* No.189. ACOG, Washington, DC

Obstetric complications in past history such as prior miscarriages, prematurely, and intrauterine growth retardation

Current obstetric status

Factors including cervical incompetence, preterm rupture of membrane, preterm labor, persistent second to third trimester bleeding, hypertension, and intrauterine growth retardation are contraindications to intense exercise during pregnancy.

Symptoms when exercise should stop[1]

- Bleeding
- Any 'gush' of fluid from the vagina (premature rupture of membranes)
- Unexplained abdominal pain
- Excessive fatigue, palpitations, chest pain
- Persistent tachycardia after exercise.
- Uterine contractions(>6–8/h: query premature labour)
- Severe headaches and/or visual disturbance; unexplained faintness or dizziness
- Dyspnea
- Reduced weight gain(<1.0kg/month during the last two trimesters)
- Increasing edema.

Benefits of exercise[2]

- Psychological and physical well-being
- Less weight gain
- Less back pain from improved posture
- Tendency for shorter labour and reduced time to recover.
- Improves digestion and reduces constipation
- Reduces 'post partum' belly
- Greater energy reserves

Post-partum Exercise

The basic rule of thumb should be to reintroduce exercise gradually. Factors including ligamentous laxity and weight gain may predispose to injury. For the first 6 weeks post partum, exercise such as walking is recommended. Weight lifting and strenuous exercise is generally not advisable for the first 6 weeks post partum after a normal vaginal and 12 weeks after a Caesarean section. Attention should be paid to fluid intake during exercise and optimal nutrition.

1 LA Wolfe et al 1989 Sports Med 8 273–301 2 W Larry Kennedy et al (ed) 1995 ACSM's guidelines for exercise testing and prescription 5th edn p238 Table 11.7. Williams & Wilkins, Philadelphia

The menopausal athlete

Menopause is defined as the cessation of menstruation. This generally occurs when the woman is about 50 years of age. It can, however, occur earlier or later than this age. Menopause is a stage of decreased estrogen production and as such the two major concerns to a menopausal athlete are:

1 Osteoporosis
2 Cardiovascular disease

Osteoporosis

This illness results in the reduction of bone mass (osteopenia) and hence fractures due to minor trauma. This is an illness seen overwhelmingly in females. **Risk factors** for osteoporosis include:

- Athletic amenorrhea
- Slim build
- High consumption of caffeine, tobacco, and alcohol
- Family history
- Caucasian race
- Nulliparity
- Older age
- Corticosteroid use
- Lack of weight bearing

Fractures in the wrist, hip, and the vertebral column are common in women with osteoporosis. It also tends to affect trabecular bone compared to cortical bone. **Investigations**:

- Bone density studies (dual energy x-ray absorptometry, DEXA)
- Qualitative computed tomography

Treatment: the major factors determining the course of the illness is the peak bone mass attained and the rate of loss. Hence, the aim of treatment would be to maximize peak bone mass prior to menopause and then reduce the rate of bone loss. Peak bone mass is achieved at about 25 years of age. After this the amount of bone produced is eclipsed by the amount of bone mass being resorbed.

Exercise

Weight bearing exercise can reverse bone loss or reduce the rate of loss, which might occur during disuse. Exercise has been shown to increase mineralization of cortical and trabecular bone. Dynamic muscular pull is thought to have a positive effect on bone mass. This is indicated in women who supplement aerobic exercise with weight training, having greater spinal bone mineral densities than women who do not use weight training or those who are sedentary.

Calcium intake

In combination with estrogen has been shown to be effective in the reversal of bone loss. Diets rich in calcium (dairy products, green leafy vegetables, and fish) have been shown to be effective in restoring bone mass in ammenorrheic athletes.

Hormone replacement therapy (HRT)

Cn have the dual effect of preserving bone mineralization and decreasing the risk of cardiovascular disease. Estrogen is thought to modulate calcium metabolism with the effect of increasing dietary calcium absorption and reducing calcium loss. A 50% reduction in the incidence of hip and arm fractures as well as an 80% reduction of vertebral compression fractures have been observed in women who have taken estrogen in the perimenopausal period.

The **therapy** consists of estrogen (0.625mg daily) and medroxyprogesterone acetate (10mg daily) for days 1–2 of the calendar month. The progesterone component reduces the risk of endometrial cancer, which has been attributed to the effect of unopposed estrogen. The progesterone component is associated with withdrawal bleeds and side-effects, which can lead to noncompliance. In women who have had hysterectomies, an estrogen-only preparation is recommended. In osteoporotic athletes who are already using HRT, the bisphosphonates can be useful.

Coronary heart disease

Increased incidence of CHD is seen in postmenopausal women. This is thought to be due to the lack of estrogen and its cardioprotective effects. **Management**: Aerobic exercise can increase cardiovascular fitness, which results in a lower blood pressure and favorable blood lipid profiles. Favorable lipid profiles (i.e. HDL increase and decreased serum triglycerides) lower the risk of ischemic heart disease. HRT has also been shown to decrease the risk of myocardial infarction.

Guidelines to safe exercise for the menopausal athlete

Prior to the commencement of exercise, the menopausal athlete should complete a thorough medical examination. Significant points to be elicited in the **history** must include:

- Exercise history
- History of any cardiovascular disease
- History of any other medical illnesses which might influence further exercise patterns
- Prior and current medications
- Investigations that might need to be performed may include an exercise ECG, blood tests (screening for Hb, glucose, and lipids), depending on the medical history of the patient.

Advice for commencement of an exercise program should include an initial moderate pattern of exercise. The general guidelines being to attempt 30min of exercise 3 times a week at 40–60% of maximal heart rate (220 minus age). The exercise program should also include a warming-up and cooling-down period. This should improve cardiovascular fitness. If any symptoms such as chest pain, severe shortness of breath were to occur the patient should be advised to stop immediately and seek medical attention. As fitness attained the exercise intensity can be elevated to 70% of maximal heart rate.

Nutrition

Of primary importance is the *prevention of iron and calcium deficiency*.

Iron deficiency

This is a common condition in female athletes (20—30%). Iron loss can occur via menstruation, iron poor diet, gastrointestinal loss, sweat, and urine. The deficiency can occur with or without anemia and with or without pseudoanemia. Pseudoanemia describes a condition peculiar to endurance runners and represents a physiological adaptation. Plasma volume expands and the hematocrit can drop. Iron deficiency can progress in three stages to an iron deficiency anemia. The first stage being iron depletion. This represents a depletion of body stores of iron in the liver, spleen and bone marrow. The next stage is an iron deficiency erythropoeisis. A fall in serum iron levels causes an increase in total iron binding capacity. The last stage is an iron deficiency anemia (Hb<120g/L).

The effect of iron deficiency on the athlete depends on the stage of depletion. Anemia due to iron deficiency has been shown to decrease performance and associated lethargy and tiredness (due to lower clearance of lactate levels). However, athletes with low ferritin alone have not been shown to have had their performance affected. However, low ferritin levels can lead to anemia and must therefore be followed. **Investigations**:

- Full blood count (anemia indicated by low Hb and hematocrit)
- Iron studies. Serum ferritin will indicate iron stores. Levels below 50mg/L indicate absent iron stores.

Treatment is indicated if iron stores are low and the athlete is symptomatic. As well as specific dietary advice, iron supplementation is necessary. If there is no anemia then do not use a slow release iron as it will not be absorbed. Make sure the iron is taken in the absence of cereals and coffee. The use of a vitamin C preparation at the same time will enhance the absorption. The athlete should be advised to eat lean red meat at least 3 times per week. Consultation with a sports dietitian is necessary if the athlete is vegetarian. Up to 15mg *per day* of iron supplementation may be indicated for 6 months to replenish body stores. Vitamin C supplementation may be considered as it increases iron absorption. OCP to combat menstrual loss

Calcium deficiency

Calcium is an essential component in bone health and in the prevention of osteoporosis. In amennorrheic athletes, intakes of 1500mg/day, and 1200mg/day for women with normal menstruation is recommended. Maximum bioabsorption of calcium occurs after a meal due to stimulated gastric juices.

Breast injuries

Discomfort during exercising is a common complaint. During the premenstrual period, fluid retention may cause breast tissue to swell. This may contribute to the discomfort. Nipple injuries can occur due to rubbing with clothing during exercise. This injury is often seen in males as well. Traumatic injuries to breast tissue are seen in contact sports such as martial arts. **Management**: large breasted women often find a well-fitted sports bra to be comfortable. Generally, larger breasted women use a bra which limits breast motion, lifts, and separates the breasts. Smaller breasted women often use pullover 'compression' bras, that compresses the breast against the chest wall. Applying petroleum jelly on the nipple prior to exercise or taping it before sport can prevent nipple injuries. The use of plastic 'cup' protection or the use of padding can prevent breast trauma.

Musculoskeletal injuries[1]

Studies indicate that injuries appear to be more sport-specific than gender-specific. However, certain injuries have been noted to occur commonly in women.

Shoulder injuries

Rotator cuff injuries especially when the arm is placed overhead and pronated repetitively.

Knee injuries[2]

Anterior cruciate ligament injuries appear to be common in women involved in sport which involves jumping or pivoting such as soccer and basketball. Patellofemoral pain is also noted to be frequent in women. This is attributed to laterally placed patella and the wider pelvis of females.

Iliotibial band tendinitis

Pain is felt at the point where the tendon passes over the greater trochanter. Females are thought to be more prone due to their greater pelvic span and the greater prominence of their greater trochanter. More commonly occurring problems tend to appear at the distal end of the iliotibial band where it crosses the lateral femoral condyle. This is called 'iliotibial band friction syndrome' and occurrs most commonly in runners and cyclists.

Pes anserinus tendinitis

The pes anserinus tendon is the common insertion of the gracilis, semitendinosus, and sartorius muscles on the medial proximal tibia. It can become inflamed if there is excessive external rotation of the lower limb which can occur in some individuals due to the increased Q-angle at the knee. It is best treated by strengthening the lower trunk-stabilizing muscles and the use of a foot orthoses to correct excessive foot pronation.

Ankle impingement

This injury appears to be due to forced plantarflexion causing irritation of the posterior ankle capsule, and trauma to the os trigonum, as well as posterior tibial tendinitis. This injury is common in gymnastics, dancing and diving.

Stress fractures

Amennorheic women have an increased incidence of stress fractures (up to 4fold). Primarily, cancellous bone appears to be affected. Women on the OCP have fewer stress fractures.

Other injuries

Spondylolysis, vertebral body apophysitis (due to flexion-extension motion of the spine), and foot disorders such as bunions, corns, and calluses occur and must receive appropriate treatment.

1 K Clarke, W Buckley 1980 *Am J Sports Med* **8** 187-91   2 J Powers 1979 *Clin Orthop* **143** 120–4

Other issues

- *Genital injuries*: vulval injuries (bruising or lacerations) can occur due to falling astride.
- *Cancer and exercise*: athletes appear to have a lower rate of breast and reproductive system cancer due to later menarche and early menopause.
- *Performance-enhancing drugs*: Anabolic steroids can have potentially damaging side-effects and are banned from international competition. Side-effects can include virilization (hirsutism, baldness, increased size of the clitoris), and hypertension.
- *Gender verification*: molecular biology techniques such as PCR techniques to detect the SRY gene of male DNA or Barr body detection in cells can be used.
- *Stress urinary incontinence*: this can occur in multiparous women. However, nulliparous women have also been noted to suffer occasionally. Treatment can involve pelvic floor exercises, control of fluid intake prior to exercise, or surgical correction of abnormal anatomy.

Conclusion

Women take part in many more sports than ever before. Data is available on established sports such as swimming and running; but less on new sports such as rowing and bodybuilding.

The problem of the female triad is troubling. It is the question of how to maximize performance without causing serious health problems. Training programs should be based on sound scientific principles. The future is promising—men's and women's world records are converging (as women's progression is more rapid). Figure 23.2 shows the predicted times for the 200m and 1500m events (already women outdo men on long distance swimming)[1].

1 G Bryant *et al* 1997 In E Sherry, D Bokor (ed) *Sports medicine problems and practical management* p246 Fig 3. GMM, London

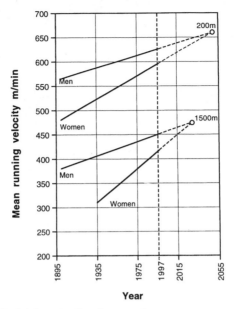

Fig. 23.2 Predicted running times in men and women

Part V
Organization

24 Protective equipment in sport

JOHN ESTELL

Introduction

Protective equipment in sport aims to avoid or minimize injury. In general, there is little controlled evidence of the effectiveness of many types of protective equipment, but many of the principles are based on extensive experience. Sport should be both enjoyable and safe for the participants and this chapter deals with issues of safety in sport related to protective equipment.

Each sport has its own rules and regulations for participation and play, and included in the rules there is usually a section on permitted and restricted aids or devices. Some of the protective devices are considered minimum requirements to allow participation in the sport (such as a helmet for all cycling events) while others will be recommended but optional (e.g. mouthguards in contact sports).

Ideally, protective equipment should satisfy the following criteria: provide adequate protection from injuries, be comfortable to wear, affordable, and if appropriate carry an approval of the relevant sporting body. Specifically, it should not be used as an offensive weapon, should not provide a target for opposition, and should not impair joint function, field of vision, or reaction time.

Technical issues include the intended life of the equipment eg. sporting helmets should clearly indicate whether it is for single impact or multiple impacts. The helmet should not produce dangerous fragments if damaged. Any helmet should be securely fastened but allow easy removal and should not impair thermal regulation. It is obvious that any protective equipment should not increase the risk, occurrence or severity of injury through its use either to the wearer or an opponent (1).

Some simple common sense approaches are better than all of the protective braces and splints currently available. Protective equipment is not a substitute for training, preparation, and acclimatization to the sporting environment.

It is recommended that people competing in a sport should train on a regular basis in all of their protective equipment to become accustomed to its weight, restrictions and overall 'feel'. In this way players are not exposed to risk of injury through inappropriate use, or inexperience with the equipment that is being used for protection from injury.

This chapter will first review the more general protective techniques then review, by body region, some more specific protective equipment and devices.

Reference

(1) J Bloomfield *et al* 1992 Injuries to the head eye and ear. *Textbook of science and medicine in sport* 2nd edn Blackwell Science

General protection

Clothing

Most sports have a particular uniform or dress code. Some sports clothing is designed to minimize heat loss and the risk of hypothermia e.g. snow skiing, underwater diving. Other sports have clothing which has high protection qualities e.g. fire-proof suits for motor racing. Clothing should generally be appropriate for the prevailing environmental conditions and should protect against thermal injury (either hypo- or hyperthermia).

Sun protection

Sunscreens have been shown to reduce the long-term development of skin cancers (1) and should be used in combination with other barriers such as hats, long sleeve shirts, and sunglasses to minimize sun exposure on the sports field. For many outdoor sports, sun and ultraviolet exposure may be high and unrecognized on overcast days e.g. fielding in cricket. Reflected rays from water or snow and ice all have the potential to burn the skin and a high sun protection factor sunscreen should be applied to all exposed skin.

Taping

The use of elasticised or rigid adhesive tape to restricts excessive, or potentially harmful motion at a joint while still allowing a desired range of motion. It is most commonly used over moderate sized joints such as the ankle, thumb, and wrist. Boxers may use tape over their hands and wrists before applying boxing gloves. However, the application of tape over the skin of a joint does not strengthen that joint but merely provides additional skin proprioceptive feedback, and thus an unstable joint may require a more rigid form of bracing or complete rest from the sporting field until injury recovery has been completed. The *two indications for which taping* is used are:

1 *Prevention*—taping is used as a preventative measure for sportspeople competing in high risk activities without an underlying structural weakness (e.g. ankle taping in basketball players)

2 *Rehabilitation* where taping is used as a protective measure for a structurally weak joint during the recovery and rehabilitation phases of injury tissue repair.

Rigid (non-elastic) tape is most often used for restricting undesired movement at a joint. However, it has been shown that the tape holds its position and provides the desired proprioceptive feedback only while the adhesive is dry and in firm contact with the skin. This varies between 15min and 50min, depending upon the nature and intensity of the sport and the forces applied through the tape (2). Tape should ideally be applied to skin which has been shaved at least 12h beforehand to minimize skin irritation. An adhesive skin spray can be applied to assist with tape adhesion in a sweaty individual.

The principle underlying rehabilitative taping is that injured ligaments should be maintained in a shortened position to minimize risk of re-injury. For prevention, taping should aim to maintain the ligaments in an anatomically neutral position. Tape should be of an appropriate width with overlap of the preceding layer of tape. Care must be taken to ensure no creases or folds occur in the tape as this will predispose to skin irritation and blisters. Circulation and nerve compression can be a complication of taping which is applied too tightly, while the tape will be ineffective if is applied too loosely. When removing tape it is best done with a pair of tape scissors and moistening the tape may make it easier to remove. With regular application the skin may become sensitized to the tape adhesive and an allergy may develop. The cost of regular application of adhesive tape becomes quite prohibitive if large amounts are required. In general, taping is labour intensive and therefore more expensive that the use of bracing (splints).

Bracing (splints)

Where long-term joint protection is required, braces may be more practical and inexpensive than taping. They have the advantage of being easier to apply and less painful to remove and are less likely to cause local skin irritations. The problems of braces are problems with sizing and fit of the brace, movement of the brace if not a perfect fit, the additional weight of the brace, and risk of brace failure. The simplest braces are heat-retaining neoprene sleeves that are commercially available for most of the joints of the body. This type of brace helps to retain heat in an inflamed or stiff joint but offers little mechanical support across the joint. As braces become more specialized the cost, size, and weight of the brace tends to increase, and the support or restriction of abnormal or unwanted movement at a joint also becomes more controlled.

References

(1) E Azizi *et al* 1984 *Isr J Med Sci* **20** 569–77
(2) T Viljakka 1986 *Acta Orthop Scand* **57** 54–8

Head and neck

Helmets

The role of a helmet is to absorb the forces and decelerate the blow at the point of impact, distribute the focal impact over a larger area, withstand surface abrasion and to protect the bone and soft tissues of the head from injury. The use of helmets, however, increases the size and mass of the head. This may result in an increase in brain injury by a number of mechanisms. Blows that would have been glancing become more solid and thus transmit increased rotational force to the brain. These forces result in shearing stresses on neurones which may result in concussion and other forms of brain injury (1).

Helmets should be sports-specific to be most effective. There are a number of potential risks of inappropriate helmet use in sports. An ineffective helmet may provide the wearer with a false sense of security, encouraging risk-taking and worsening the chance of injury. Poorly designed helmets may obscure peripheral vision.

As helmet requirements vary greatly between sports and there are a number of types of helmet, the demands of an individual sport must be considered, and then an appropriate helmet configuration, shock absorbing material, and outer surface should be used. Athlete preference, and protection requirements may account for some of the variations in helmet design within a sport. The use of helmets is mandatory in some sports (such as motorized sports), recommended in others (cricket), optional in some sports (rugby union), and illegal in a few (soccer).

The ideal protective headware should provide adequate protection from injuries, be light in weight, be comfortable to wear, be affordable, should not impair field of vision, and should not impair reaction time. All helmets must be securely fastened but easily removable. The helmet must not produce dangerous fragments if damaged, it must not increase the risk of cervical spine injury. These factors should be reflected in its endorsement by the relevant sporting or standards association approving its use in the designated sport. The helmet should clearly indicate whether it is intended for single or multiple impacts, it should not provide a target for opponents and it should never be used as an offensive weapon.

Motorsport helmets are composed of a hard outer shell (usually made of fiberglass or polypropylene) with a large amount of internal padding. This padding is full contact to ensure a snug fit of the helmet and prevent twisting of the helmet over the head. Helmets for motor sport need to withstand high velocity impacts and are thus designed as single impact use, which means they should be discarded and replaced following an accident. These type of helmets have the largest helmet weight and strong cervical muscles are required to wear a helmet such as this and withstand the high gravitational forces applied in motorsports.

There are a number of different styles of helmet but the type offering the most protection is the full-face style, which includes a low protective bar across the jaw and also provides some support to the upper cervical spine. This type of helmet contains a built-in faceshield usually of clear perspex of polycarbonate to protect the eyes and face from flying debris or insects. Another style of helmet is the open-face type which offers little protection to the face, and the profile of the helmet is higher on the head. For this reason the open-face helmet offers no support for the upper cervical spine in the event of a crash. All motorsport helmets are securely fastened under the lower jaw with an adjustable chinstrap and are compulsory equipment.

Cycling helmets are also designed to withstand a single impact and have been shown to markedly reduce the incidence of head injury in wearers (**2**). There are four basic types of helmet classified according to their construction. They are the hard shell, racing shell, soft shell and hard shell with vents. The hard shell and racing shell have a smooth outer shell of injection moulded plastic or fiberglass and a softer inner lining. Contact with the head is primarily around the brim of the helmet so that an air space exists between the crown of the head and the helmet lining. The smooth outer lining helps with reduction in air resistance and so these models are preferred by competitive cyclists. The soft shell and hard shell with vents have an overall similar shape to the hard shell helmet but the major construction material is the polystyrene or polypropylene inner. This type of helmet offers less protection against penetrating injuries, but is more comfortable, as it allows air to circulate and heat to be dissipated more rapidly than the hard shell helmets. For these reasons this type of helmet is preferred by recreational cyclists. Cycling helmets are secured under the lower jaw with a chinstrap that must be correctly adjusted to ensure a snug fit. The wearing of cycling helmets is compulsory in some countries (e.g. Australia). Today, however, the majority of bicycle commuters and recreational cyclists world-wide have no legal enforcement (e.g. China). The need for head protection in cyclists, particularly children, cannot be overemphasized. (Fig. 24.1.)

Basketball, softball, and cricket helmets have a different type of construction and purpose. These helmets are all designed as multiple impact helmets. Their primary function is to protect the head from being struck by a ball or batting implement. In baseball and softball the use of a helmet is compulsory for the batter and for running between bases. The helmet is usually constructed of injection moulded plastic or fiberglass with a double earflap. This helmet is not necessarily secured under the lower jaw but fits snugly to the head via the ear protection. In cricket, the helmet is optional for the batting team but often worn when batting against fast bowlers. This helmet is secured under the lower jaw and most often has an attached face-shield made of either carbon steel, aluminium, or perspex. This type of helmet is also optional, but recommended, for players fielding in positions closer to the batter or batsman.

American football helmets are compulsory for players in all positions. The helmets are composed of an outer shell of hard resilient plastic, and an inner lining of either foam pads or air-filled cells. The helmet covers all of the head from the eyebrows in front, over the crown of the head to the upper neck. The helmet is completed in front by a facemask made of either aluminium, carbon steel, or a resilient plastic. Additional pads anchor the helmet to the cheeks and side of the face, and a chinstrap securely fastens the helmet to prevent any movement.

Ice hockey helmets are similar to American football helmets but have a narrower profile, flatter crown, and a closer facemask. They are also composed of a lighter plastic and have less interior padding. This makes the helmet much lighter in weight that a football helmet. Helmets with facemasks and fastened chinstraps are compulsory in ice hockey and have been demonstrated to reduce the incidence of head and facial trauma (**3**). In **Field hockey**, only the goalkeeper wears a helmet and this is of a similar construction to the ice hockey helmet. These helmets are designed as multiple impact helmets but must be inspected regularly for cracks or faults at which time they must be replaced.

Amateur boxing headgear is compulsorily worn for all sparring (training) sessions as well as competitive bouts. This headgear is composed of a pliable leather of plastic outer encompassing a soft foam cushion. The headgear is contoured to the shape of the head and curves across the bony prominences of the eyebrows and cheek bones. There is evidence that the headgear minimizes the number and severity of lacerations sustained in this sport.

Rugby league and rugby union use a lightweight headgear of similar construction to the boxing headgear but with less facial coverage. This helmet is fastened under the jaw with a three-piece fastener to allow it to release if the helmet is forcibly pulled out removed from the head of the wearer. This helmet is optional, but increased numbers of children and adolescents are wearing this protective device since its introduction only 15 years ago. While this helmet has protective properties in regard to lacerations there is little protection from concussive episodes. (Fig. 24.2.)

Protective eyewear

The majority of eye injuries occur in a small number of sports, usually the result of bodily contact, or accidental contact with a ball, shuttlecock, or implement. Many people require glasses or contact lens for visual acuity in daily living but may neglect to wear them on the sports field. The perfect eye protector for sport should be able to prevent ocular injury without creating other injuries or restricting the field of vision. It should be comfortable, securely mounted on the head, have a strong, preferably single-piece frame into which are securely mounted lens (prescription if necessary) of proven impact resistance, such as polycarbonate. However, polycarbonate cannot be used for high correction prescriptions, so that in this circumstance the ideal solution is to wear corrective contact lens with plain eye protectors for safety (**4**).

Contact lens are not protective in any circumstances and hard contact lens are potentially unsafe. Glass lens in prescription glasses are similarly unsafe for there is risk of trauma to the orbit or the eye. Some open eyeguards are available which have been shown in studies to offer no more protection to the eye than wearing nothing at all (**5**).

Goggles are used by swimmers to protect eyes from chemical irritation caused by chlorination of the water in pools. Although these goggles are optional they are highly recommended to minimize eye irritation. They are usually constructed of a clear or tinted plastic and contoured to the face. They are held in position by elastic straps around the head to minimize movement when diving into the pool.

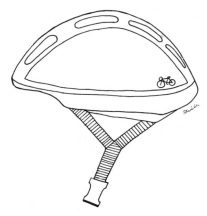

Fig. 24.1 Bicycle helmet

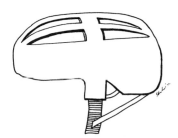

Fig. 24.2 Rugby league helmet

Faceshields

Are used in conjunction with helmets in many sports to reduce the risk of accidental injury to the face, mouth, and eye by implements, balls, or body parts. The actual construction of the faceshield varies between sports but essentially the function of the faceshield is to provide an obstruction to deflect an object or prevent it from striking or hitting the face. This is usually accomplished with a series or bars or grid network interlacing across the face with gaps between the bars small enough to prevent a ball penetrating. The facemask may be permanently attached to a helmet, such as is the case with American football or ice hockey helmets. Masks are used alone as a piece of protective equipment by baseball catchers and home-plate umpires.

Fencing and similar sports use faceshields with a fine mesh to prevent the foil or épée from contacting the face. This type of faceshield is used as a standard piece of safety equipment in these sports. The facemask is incorporated into a hood which fits over the head to hold the faceshield in position. One problem with this type of faceshield is that it quite markedly restricts the field of vision of the wearer but as this sport is conducted with face-to-face combatants this has minimal impact on the sport.

Ear protection

Should be worn in a number of sports with high noise, risk of trauma or injury to the ear, or as a protective barrier to prevent damage to the ear and hearing mechanism. The major types of ear protection can be divided into a number of subcategories.

Ear plugs can be worn as a barrier to prevent water entering the external ear canal in sports such as swimming and underwater diving. They are usually composed of either paraffin wax that can be moulded to conform to the meatus of the external canal or water-proof foam that fits the meatus. This second type allows more sound to enter the ear but is also not as waterproof as the waxy type. Ear plugs can also be used to reduce noise entering the ear, and are often used underneath helmets in motor racing.

Ear muffs are worn to minimize the noise entering the ear in sports such as rifle or pistol shooting. They are an essential protective device in noisy sports to minimize hearing loss associated with explosions occurring at a close range to the head.

Elastic tape is used by football and rugby players to hold the ears to the side of the head to prevent lacerations behind the ears. A second benefit of taping the ears to the side of the head is a reduction in the frequency and severity of auricular hematomas which may compromise cartilage perfusion, leading to collapse of the pinnas. This is referred to colloquially as 'cauliflower ears'. The ears should be protected from extreme cold as they are subject to frostbite. The is particularly important in alpine sports such as skiing and mountain climbing. Simple insulation either by a hooded jacket or ear muffs is usually all that is necessary.

Specific **ear protection caps**, manufactured from a firm plastic, with a soft foam inner, are worn by competitors in wrestling. This cap is designed to prevent or minimize trauma to the ear. The caps are secured in place by three straps which join the cup for each ear across the occiput, anterior to the crown of the head, and underneath the lower jaw. The ear cups are perforated with a series of holes to allow normal hearing.

Mouthguards

In body contact sports it is highly recommended that players wear a mouthguard. Mouthguards help to absorb and dissipate forces from a direct blow, protect the oral soft tissues from laceration, and give direct protection to the teeth. A properly designed and fitted mouthguard may also protect the mandible from fracture and could protect the wearer from concussive episodes. A mouthguard should cover the occlusal surface of the upper teeth and extend almost to the upper aspect of the gums. This ensures there is a barrier between the lips, buccal mucosa, and the teeth. The mouthguard should ideally extend beyond the last tooth on each side to ensure optimum fit and coverage. Ill-fitting mouthguards can cause ulceration of the soft tissues, and fail to provide the protection the wearer assumes they are obtaining (6). There are four basic types of mouthguards that satisfy some or all of the above criteria.

Stock or off the shelf mouthguards are made from a rubber compound or plastic and come in limited sizes. The mouthguard is retained in the mouth by clenching it between the upper and lower teeth but this type offers the least protection against concussion and dental injury.

Mouth-formed guards are composed of a firm outer shell with a softer rubber liner. These can be heated (usually by boiling) then fitted in position and bitten into when warm. This has the effect of improving the fit, contour, and comfort of the guard and is better than the Stock model in its protection of teeth.

Custom-made mouthguards are manufactured by a dentist or orthodontist using an accurate plaster cast of the individual's teeth. This mouthguard is made of a resilient thermoplastic material. Because this guard is cast on an accurate plaster mould of the teeth, comfort, fit, and sport-specific modifications can be made very easily and accurately.

Bimaxillary mouthguards are manufactured to cover both the upper and lower teeth and are usually worn following a jaw fracture or similar trauma to provide additional protection. The design of this guard is to lock the jaws into a predetermined position which makes breathing and speaking more difficult than with the other type of guard.

There is a large variation in the cost of the different types of mouthguards related to the degree of customized fit. However, the advantages of the customized mouthguards justify the additional cost. Mouthguards should be stored if a perforated plastic box to avoid build-up of mould. Before and after use they should be thoroughly cleaned with a disinfectant and rinsed.

Neck protection

There are no proven, practical and efficacious devices for protecting the neck from musculoskeletal injury. The best protection an athlete can have is strong musculature of the neck, obtained through appropriate training and desist from participation when suffering any neck injury. Neck injuries should be carefully assessed with functional x-rays and CT or MRI scans if indicated before return to sport.

In *baseball and softball* a throat guard extending below the catchers facemask is a compulsory piece of protective equipment, which is designed to protect the anterior throat structures (e.g. larynx, carotid vessels) from injury by direct contact with (usually) the ball.

In *American football*, a neck orthosis is available which fits underneath the shoulder pads, and extends up the sides and back of the neck, like an upturned collar, to provide a rigid support on to which the helmet sits. This orthosis is designed to minimize neck movement and unload some of the forces applied by a direct impact upon the helmet. It does not in any way protect the neck from injury, nor does it stabilize an injured neck.

Protection of the neck from further injury following trauma is achieved by application of a rigid cervical collar and head and neck support, but does not permit participation in sports.

References

(1) National Health and Medical Research Council 1994 Football injuries of the head and neck. *Report of NHMRC Committee 1994*
(2) Finvers K *et al* 1996 *Clin J Sport Med* **6**: 102–7
(3) T Murray, L Livingston 1995 *Paediatrics 1***95** 419–21
(4) N Jones 1993 *J R Coll Surg Edin* **38** 127–33
(5) M Easterbrook Eye protection in racket sports: An update. *Phys and Sport Med* **15** 180–82
(6) M Porter, M O'Brien M 1994 *J Ir Dent Assoc* **40** 98–101

Upper limb

Shoulder

Shoulders can be protected from direct injury by energy dissipation devices, or form excessive movement by taping or braces.

Shoulder pads are used in a number of body contact or collision sports to minimize the trauma of a direct impact on to the superior, anterior or lateral aspects of the shoulder joint (Fig. 24.3). Shoulder pads are usually composed of a soft padded material but in some sports this may be supplemented with a more rigid casing or insert. This is the case in ice hockey and American football. The fundamental design principle behind these protective devices is that they spread the impact over a larger area and prolong the time over which body collision occurs by cushioning of the impact. This minimizes trauma to the site of impact decreasing bruising and injury severity.

Range of motion restriction devices or braces are used to minimize any excessive or abnormal motion at the shoulder. They are commonly used by athletes following a dislocation or subluxation of the glenohumeral joint, or in athletes with ligamentous laxity, to stabilize the joint. These braces are designed to limit abduction and external rotation for the shoulder and thereby minimize the incidence of anterior dislocation or subluxation, by not exposing the athletes shoulder to this potentially unstable position. As always, enhancing the stability of a joint involves a trade-off, with range of motion being limited. This may compromise an athletes ability to perform at his/her sport. Posterior and multidirectional instability of the shoulder have not yet been successfully addressed by brace manufacturers.

Arm

Protection for the upper arm is focused on minimizing contact or collision type injuries. Most shoulder pads have an extension of the padding material down the anterior and lateral aspects of the upper arm to minimize tissue damage from direct trauma. Isolated arm pads or sleeves can be worn as additional protection for the arm.

Elbow

Similarly, there are two major types of elbow protection; impact minimizing elbow pads, and range of motion restriction devices.

Elbow pads are worn in contact sports to protect against abrasions from the playing surface, and to cushion impacts upon the elbow. They are also used in recreational sports such as skate boarding and in-line skating to protect the elbows from a fall. Some may be as thin as a stretch material sleeve while others will have a bulky foam pad attached or enclosed within the pad to provide impact absorption.

Elbow restriction braces are used in the rehabilitation phase following traumatic injury to the elbow, such as occurs with a dislocation or hyperextension. These injuries occur in contact and collision sports but may also occur in any athlete falling awkwardly on to an outstretched arm. The brace is designed to limit movement of the elbow joint to a safe range and thereby prevent re-injury. These braces are large or bulky, and not functional or legal in the majority of sports **(11)**. The most common use of bracing about the elbow is for 'tennis elbow'. The bracing used is often an elastic strap applied to the proximal region of the forearm, just distal to the elbow joint. Most braces employed for tennis elbow are counterforce braces,

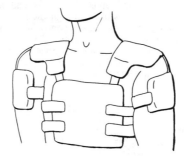

Fig. 24.3 Shoulder pads

which theoretically control muscular forces and direct potential overloads to healthy tissues and through the brace itself. Effective counterforce bracing does not alter agonist–antagonist muscle balance and does not restrict range of motion. The brace does constrain the full muscular expansion thereby diminishing the force a muscle can generate, and also 'broadens' the area of the common extensor origin by dispersing pressure from the area of injury.

Forearm

The use of forearm guards in a preventative role is uncommon except for a few sports. In archery, a leather guard may be used on the leading arm to prevent the string recoil from striking the forearm. In contact sports, competitors may use padded forearm guards to minimize impacts or when returning from forearm fractures for additional strength and security. One problem associated with forearm and wrist guards used by in-line skaters is that there is an increased risk of a fracture occurring at the proximal termination of the brace. Although wearing of forearm guards may reduce the incidence of distal forearm fractures, the overall incidence may remain similar to the unprotected rate, due to more fractures occurring at the midshaft level, associated with the termination of the brace (**12**).

Wrist

All wrist braces span the distal forearm, carpal bones, and heel of the hand. Most wrist orthoses are functional braces that protect the wrist region but allow some normal wrist motion to occur, so that participation in sport is minimally impeded. The materials commonly used for wrist orthoses are neoprene, thermoplastic, or adhesive tape, or a combination of the three.

Hand

Gloves are a very common piece of protective equipment worn in a large number of sports for a variety of different reasons. Gloves are worn to provide additional grip on a smooth ball or implement (e.g. golf or Australian Rules football). They can be worn to protect the skin from abrasions in the case of skate boarding or abseiling. Some gloves are designed for impact dissipation, such as those used in cricket by batsmen, or in ice hockey. Baseball, softball and cricket wicketkeepers use purpose-specific gloves to catch the ball and protect the hands from damage by repetitive, high speed impacts. Cyclists use a palm glove to provide some padding over prominences on the hand (such as the hook of hamate, pisiform, and base of first metacarpal) to prevent nerve compression and provide additional grip. Gymnasts use a modified glove with a dowel insert to provide additional grip on the bars. This device also protects the palm of the hand from developing blisters, excessive callosities, and trauma to existing callosities. Ski gloves are worn to insulate the hand and fingers from the cold in alpine terrain. Boxing gloves are the weapon with which the combatants fight, and are essential to the sport.

Fingers and thumb

Gloves will provide a great deal of the protection necessary for the fingers and thumb. However, there are a few circumstances in which a protective brace or 'buddy tape' will be used. Buddy taping is the use of adhesive tape to a splint a finger to its neighbor, to provide support. It is most commonly employed following trauma to one of the interphalangeal joints of the fingers. A finger extension splint may be worn by an athlete who has sustained a rupture (complete or incomplete) of a finger extensor tendon. The brace may permit the athlete to compete while immobilizing the affected joint or finger.

Gamekeeper's or skier's thumb is treated (when incomplete tear or after surgical repair of complete tear) with S-Thumb splint (Johnson and Johnson Medical) (see Fig. 10.3).

References

(1) L Giffin (ed) 1994 Orthopaedic knowledge update. sports med. *Australian Academy of orthopaedic surgeons.* 93–105
(2) S Cheng *et al* 1995 *J Trauma* **39** 1194–7

Trunk and abdomen

Chest

Protective equipment for the chest, sternum, and ribs is used in a number of sports. Most protective devices worn on or about the chest are designed for impact resistance; either from collision with another player, or impact from a ball or implement. It has been demonstrated tragically in children's baseball that impact of the ball on the chest during a vulnerable period in the cardiac cycle can precipitate a cardiac arrhythmia leading to death (1). It is for this reason that protective padding or devices should be worn in sports which pose this risk. Some protection is worn as part of the playing equipment underneath the team uniform, while some are strapped over the playing apparel. In some sports, such as football, the padding used in shoulder pads extends to cover a large portion of the anterior and also posterior thoracic cage. Sternum guards, which protect the superficial bone of the sternum from impact injuries, can be worn separately or incorporated into a set of shoulder pads.

In cricket, players may wear a thick protective padding that protects the lateral ribcage from impact with a ball. This is worn beneath the playing apparel and held in place with a strap that encircles the chest. The catcher in a baseball or softball game wears a chest pad over the uniform that extends to or below the lower abdomen. This is composed of a thick, stiff padding to dissipate the impact of a ball and distribute forces.

Field hockey and ice hockey goalkeepers also wear a chest protector which may extend below the abdomen, because of their risk of being struck by the ball (or other players) while protecting the goal.

Abdomen

There are very few protective devices designed to protect the abdominal region of the body. Some sports which wear protective suits (such as motor cycle racing or fencing) have in-built protection for the abdomen but it is not a specific feature of these suits. One exception is a kidney belt which is usually a wide elastic strap with attachments that has affixed to its inner surface two curved stiffened pads that protect the loin region and theoretically dissipate contact. This belt is recommended for those who have only one functional kidney, or for use in high velocity sports, such as motor cycle racing, where there is potential for high speed trauma. Another protective device commonly used is that worn by weight lifters. It consists of a wide leather belt that encloses the abdomen and lumbar spine to provide counterforce and decrease the risk of herniation of intraabdominal and retroperitoneal structures, through muscles and connective tissue, as a consequence of extremely high intraabdominal pressures. Corsets, flak jackets, or lumboabdominal binders may be worn in some athletic pursuits to control thoracolumbar, lumbar, or lumbosacral movements. These devices help to support the abdominal and lumbar spinal region but do not provide adequate rigid support to an unstable or weak spinal segment. All players with spondylolysis, spondylolisthesis, stress fractures, or spina bifida occulta need to be identified and thoroughly evaluated before entering the sporting arena.

Groin

A number of different types of protective equipment are available for the groin and pelvic region. Cyclists wear 'nix' or padded cycling shorts to provide additional cushioning to the perineal area. It is common for long distance cyclists to suffer from saddle soreness through being on a bicycle seat for a prolonged period. The cushioning of chamois leather helps to reduce chaffing and provide some padding between the cyclists ischial tuberosities and the bicycle seat.

Stretch shorts are worn by other sports people and they may contain padded inserts to protect bony prominences such as the greater trochanters or iliac crests, and also large muscle groups subject to contact trauma such as the quadriceps (Fig. 24.4).These shorts are worn by football players of many codes, and have been shown to be effective in reducing the incidence of thigh hematomas (2). Stretch shorts of a similar style are worn by some players with muscle strains in the inguinal and adductor regions to retain warmth in the muscles after the warm-up and stretching program has been completed.

A groin protector or 'box' is worn by cricket batsmen and close fieldsman. This is a solid contoured polypropylene shell with a soft cushion about its outer rim. It is worn inside the undergarments to protect the genitalia from direct injury through being struck by the hard cricket ball. Similar devices are worn by the goalkeeper in hockey and the catcher in baseball.

References

(12) B Maron *et al* 1995 *N Eng J Med* **333** 337–42
(13) B Mitchell 1995 *Proc Austral Conf Sci Med in Sport 1995*

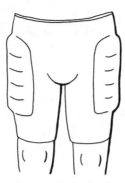

Fig. 24.4 Stretch material shorts with thigh pads

Lower limb

Hip

The hip joints are not able to be externally protected but the greater trochanters can be protected by padding worn inside stretch shorts. Some shorts may be worn to retain heat in warm muscles, but there are few other protective devices or pieces of sports apparel for specific use about the hip.

Thigh

The thigh is subject to trauma in contact sports and padding can be worn either as inserts in stretch groin shorts, or strapped on to that region of the lower limb. In cricket, thick thigh pads can be worn underneath the playing apparel to protect the thigh from contact by a ball. Ice hockey players wear pants that are well padded to minimize impact trauma from other players, the ice, and the puck. Field hockey goalkeepers wear large leg pads that may extend above the knee to cover a portion of the anterior thigh. Stretch material and neoprene sleeves are also available for retaining heat in the quadriceps and hamstring muscle groups following a muscle strain or contusion.

Knee

The most economic and functionally significant sports related injuries occur to the knee. Knee injuries occur commonly result in prolonged time lost from participation, and interfere with daily activities. Because of the high economic cost, as well as athletic cost of knee injuries, much research has been conducted into different protective knee braces, which aim to prevent or minimize the severity of injuries occurring at this joint. Knee braces fall into one of the following three categories.

Prophylactic knee braces are designed to distribute applied loads away from the ligamentous structures of the knee joint. The brace is either a lateral bar with a polycentric hinge and an extension stop, or, plastic cuffs with polycentric hinge. The function is to unload the medial collateral and anterior cruciate ligaments to reduce knee ligament injuries. These braces are not suitable for use in all sports and results of studies are conflicting and support the benefit of these braces only at low speed, non-physiological loading rates, that is, at speeds much lower than those encountered on a sporting field.

Functional knee braces are designed to provide stability for knee joints with ligamentous instability. They attempt to restrict abnormal translational movements at the knee joint by applying leverage in a specific direction to control motion. To combat brace movement and provide the control required for a specific purpose, a custom-fitted brace is essential. Studies into functional braces, while documenting a subjective benefit, have failed to demonstrate objective improvements in the frequency of episodes of instability.

Rehabilitative braces are used to control motion and rotation of the knee after ligament injury, or after surgical repair or reconstruction. (Fig. 24.5).They theoretically allow adequate ligament healing while the knee joint continues to work within a protected arc. These braces may be worn in high-risk sports, such as downhill snow skiing, to provide additional protection to a repaired or reconstructed knee ligament.

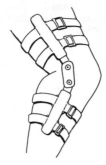

Fig. 24.5 Polycentric hinged knee brace

Patellofemoral braces are designed to diminish symptomatic lateral patellar subluxation and displacement. They are usually constructed of a neoprene or elastic sleeve with a strapping system or buttress pad to minimize lateral movement of the patella (Fig. 24.6). Protective knee pads are also available for in-line skaters and skate board riders which are constructed of a hard plastic shell with elastic straps to hold them in position. These pads are designed to minimize contusions and abrasions to the anterior knee surface, and may have absorbent foam to act as a cushioning medium.

S-Knee splint can be adjusted for patellar problems or the ACL/MCL deficient knee.

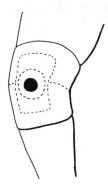

Fig. 24.6 Knee patellar support

Lower leg

Shin pads are a common piece of protective equipment that are worn in a large variety of sports. The size and shape of the pads tends to vary in relation to the specific demands of the sport (Fig. 24.7). Most shin pads have a hard plastic shell with a lining of absorbent foam or cushioning that overlies the anterior border of the tibia. Some sports utilize a larger pad, strapped over the playing apparel, that may extend from the ankle to well above the knee joint. This is the case with field hockey goalkeepers and cricket batsmen and wicketkeepers. In studies of shin pad efficacy it has been demonstrated that the force is distributed along the lower leg, and injury from focal impacts are reduced in those wearing the pads (1).

Ankle

Injuries account for a high proportion of athletic injuries, typically ligament sprains from excessive inversion. Taping is frequently used as prophylaxis during sports. A large variety of ankle braces are available that aim to control the abnormal or excessive movements of the ankle joint without excessively restricting ankle joint function. The most common athletic ankle injury is the inversion sprain with lateral ligament laxity and instability a possible long-term consequence. Ankle braces have control of inversion as the primary functional requirement of the bracing device. Again, a variety of different models are available which perform this task. They may be elasticised, lace-up, with or without lateral support splints. As high-top boots or footwear help to support the ankle within the lace-up body of the shoe, this simple piece of protective equipment may help to minimize the severity, frequency, and number of ankle inversion injuries. S-Ankle splint (Johnson and Johnson Medical) is a dynamic splint for lateral ligament injuries where the tibiotalar joint is tilted into funtional valgus and dorsiflexion.

Foot

The major piece of protective equipment for the foot is good quality, appropriate, and sports-specific footwear. Various shoe inserts and orthotics are available that can be used in conjunction with other bracing devices to achieve optimum foot and ankle alignment. Steel-capped shoes are a commonly worn piece of safety equipment used in the workplace, but are less commonly worn in the sporting arena. Blisters, corns, bunions and neuromas are common podiatric problems that may require specific attention, but which can be accommodated in correct footwear and judicious use of padding, orthotics, adhesive tape, or use of commercial products such as artificial skin.

In conclusion, well-designed, purpose constructed protective equipment should reduce and minimize the risk, occurrence, and severity of sporting injury for participants and officials. This increased safety in sport allows the athlete continued participation, increased competitiveness, and enjoyment in their chosen sport.

Reference

(1) C Bir *et a.* 1995 *Clin J Sport Med* **5** 95–9

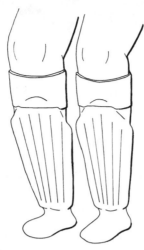

Fig. 24.7 Shin pads

25 Organization of sporting events

MEL CUSI

The team physician

Introduction
The medical care of sports teams and events is one of the most challenging in sports medicine. It requires both specific sports medicine skills, general medical knowledge, knowledge of the specific sport covered, communication and management skills not usually required in everyday sports medicine practice. The interface of sports medicine and organization requires knowledge of three areas:

1 Administration and management, liaison with other persons/bodies involved in the same event or team
2 Sports medicine
3 The specific sport being covered

Medical care[1,2]
The medical care of a sports team is a very enjoyable yet challenging aspect of sports medicine for a variety of reasons. It provides the opportunity of practicing both preventive medicine and treatment of acute and chronic injuries within the context of a team situation, both on and off the field, an educational role and the chance to learn other skills depending on the size of the off-field team.

Requirements
Good all-round knowledge of general and sports medicine is required, as team members will present both with sports injuries and general medical conditions, both acute and chronic. The team physician needs to have the ability to work within and fit into the organizational structure of the team. It is important to understand that in this situation the doctor's role is one of support: to assist team members to play to the maximum of their ability at all times.

The sports medicine team
The team physician heads the sports medicine team, which may comprise a variety of paramedical professionals, such as physiotherapists, masseurs, physical trainers, podiatrists, dietitians, and sports psychologists.

Communication
The team physician is often in a privileged position within the general team structure. He or she needs to be a good communicator with all: selectors, administrators, coaches and managers, players, opposing teams physicians and the other members of the sports medicine team.

Specific ethical issues arise in the context of team care, such as the early return to competition following an injury, confidentiality with other players, team management, and the media. The team physician needs to be familiar with these issues when they arise.

Role
Of the team doctor is wide ranging. He/she holds the ultimate responsibility for the diagnosis and management of medical and injury problems within the members of the team. This includes preventive aspects such as immunization, and specific strategies to minimize the risk of injury throughout the season. Areas of responsibility include:

1 P Brukner, K Khan 1993 In *Clinical sports medicine* p654–6. McGraw-Hill, Sydney   2 BG Sando 1992 In J Bloomfield *et al* (ed) *Textbook of science and medicine in sport*, Blackwell Scientific, Melbourne

- Pre-season screening of all athletes
- Establishment of preventive measures
- Injury assessment and management
- General medical management
- Nutritional aspects
- Communication with other team members

Pre-season screening

Most team sports have a discrete playing season. The pre-season screening begins at the end of the previous season. A complete review of injury and health status of each athlete in the team should be carried out immediately after the last game of the season. Appropriate treatment, including surgical procedures, should be carried out at this stage, and appropriate rehabilitation programs instituted during the off-season.

Content

At the commencement of training for the new season a full medical assessment of all players should be carried out. This is particularly important in the case of new players to the club. This assessment should cover the following aspects:

- **General health**
  - Past history of illness and medications. Special emphasis to be made on diseases such as asthma, diabetes, epilepsy and infectious diseases
  - Immunization status
  - Nutritional status. Food intake diary
  - Neuropsychometric tests: DSST (Digit Symbol Substitution Test). This is particularly relevant for contact sports and management of concussion[1] (see Chapter 5)
- Musculoskeletal screening
  - History of previous injuries, especially those that are sports related
  - Large joints examination. Test for generalized ligamentous laxity
  - Biomechanical assessment. This includes assessment of gait and of posture (and lumbar function)
- Fitness testing. This may cover:
  - Bodyweight and/or skin folds (7 sites)[2]
  - Aerobic fitness (VO_{2max} or shuttle run)
  - Plyometric strength (vertical jump)
  - Strength, flexibility, and proprioception. Isokinetic muscle testing may be useful
- Digit Symbol Substitution Test

Purpose

The purpose of the pre-season screening is several-fold:

- to detect any injuries or factors predisposing to injury
- to implement rehabilitation strategies to treat any existing injuries
- to establish preventive programs, either on an individual basis or as a routine for all team members
- to develop a database that will assist in injury prevention in future

1 R Richards *et al* 1979 *Med J Aust* 2 470–4   2 M Moore 1983 *Physician sports med* II 6

Prevention and management

Prevention strategies

Early in the season, or even the pre-season period, is often the best time to establish educational activities for the benefit of players and other team members in several aspects of sports medicine. Areas that can be covered are:

- the role of sports medicine
- warm-up and stretching routines
- the importance of early diagnosis and treatment of injuries, both acute and chronic (overuse). The RICE regime (acronym for rest, ice, compression, elevation)
- nutrition aspects. Role of carbohydrates, importance of fluid replacement
- drug use and doping regulations. Consult the team doctor before taking any over-the-counter drugs

General medical management

The establishment of baseline data is important for the management of medical conditions if and when they present in the course of the season. A good general medical history is the best baseline. The team physician needs to liaise with the individual player's family doctor with regards to general medical conditions. This is particularly relevant in the case of chronic conditions such as asthma, diabetes, epilepsy, and allergies.

Nutritional aspects

Nutritional requirements for high performance in sport are specific to the type of sport. The presence of a dietitian would be beneficial to establish a baseline and also adequate nutritional habits and understanding of energy requirements. Iron and calcium deficiencies, the former more often in female athletes, are often encountered in élite athletes, who need to be monitored in this regard. Fluid replacement and carbohydrate loading strategies (pre-game meal in particular) should be instituted. When traveling with a team, all meal arrangements are the responsibility of the team doctor with regard to their content.

Communication with other team members

- *Sports medicine team.* It is the responsibility of the team physician to ensure a good working relationship with all the members of the sports medicine team (physiotherapist, physical trainer, massage therapist, dietitian, etc.). A united supportive professional team provides confidence in a good recovery strategy following injury.
- *Athletes.* A good relationship with each individual athlete is paramount. An easy and confident approach will help the team physician gain the confidence of the athletes. Confidentiality must be maintained and the players appreciate that the doctor's main concern is the welfare of the players as individuals.
- *Management.* Coaches and managers need to be informed of all relevant facts, with the consent of the individual players. In the case of injuries, particularly when they are severe, a conservative and non-alarmist attitude will help gain the respect and confidence of all involved.

Equipment and facilities

Medical room

Appropriate facilities are essential for the adequate functioning of the sports medicine team, and the team physician in particular. Although space may be at a premium, a medical room should be made available at training and competition venues. It should be independent from the rest of team facilities to ensure privacy and confidentiality when necessary. It should be easily accessible to stretchers and ambulances, well lit and kept clean and functional. The room should have a good light source, a couch, running hot and cold water, appropriate equipment, and medications (*see Appendix A*). It is the responsibility of the sports medicine team to ensure that adequate first aid equipment is available at training and competition venues. Stretchers, basic resuscitation equipment (such as an Air-Viva), bandages, splints, and crutches and a container with an adequate supply of ice are essential. Many clubs purchase an ice making machine to meet the requirements. A telephone should be available and a list of emergency telephones next to it (road and air ambulance, nearest hospital, doctor, etc.).

It may be useful to make a 'wish list' of medical and surgical equipment and classify all items as 'must have', 'should have', or 'would like to have' priorities to be obtained as budget and physical space permit.

Medical kit

This will vary according to the circumstances. Several kit lists are included in *Appendix B*. Traveling with a team on a long tour will require more equipment and material than a simple 'away' game (*Appendix B*).

Record keeping

It is essential to maintain regular clinical records of all patient encounters. This is simply a matter of good clinical practice and is also essential for medico-legal purposes. It is particularly relevant when several members of the sports medicine team treat any particular individual. Individual records should contain a complete medical and injury history of each players, including immunizations, allergies, and treatments.

Ethical issues

Confidentiality

The medical condition of a player should not be discussed with other team members. Team members of professional sporting teams should be informed that information regarding illness and injury will be reported to the coach. Availability to play and time factors before an injured player is able to train or play are facts that coaches need to know.

Medical insurance

It is the responsibility of the team physician to secure adequate registration and malpractice insurance cover in the areas where he will be looking after a team, both at home games, away games, and on tour.

Ethics

A statement has been issued by the International Olympic Committee Medical Commission on medical ethics related to sports medical care. It covers most situations that may confront a team physician.

Coverage of a home game

Assessment of injuries in the field

In the event of injury to a player during a game, it may be possible for the team physician to run on to the field to assess the injured athlete. This should be done efficiently and safely for the player, to minimize the interruption in play. The goal of this first assessment on the field is to decide whether the player is able to continue in the game immediately or needs to be taken to the sideline for further assessment and treatment. This can be done with the TOTAPS technique, designed to answer two questions:

1 Is the player fit to continue?
2 Does the player require further medical attention?

T–Talk

- 'Where does it hurt?'
- 'How did it happen?'
- 'What did you feel?'
- 'Do you feel weakness, numbness?'

O–Observe

- Look for deformity
- Look for swelling
- Always compare with the opposite side

T–Touch

Feel for:

- Tenderness
- Swelling
- Deformity
- Abnormal movement

A–Active movement

- Invite player to move actively injured limb. If unable, the injured player needs to be removed from the field of play

P–Passive movement

- Gently and slowly
- Stop if pain or restriction
- Only go on if there is a full range of pain-free, non-restricted, passive movement

S–Stand

- Ask player to stand unaided
- Then walk
- Then jog on the spot
- Then run

Should the player not be able to continue in the game, transport from the field can be made by different means: assisted or unassisted walk, chair lift, stretcher, Jordan frame, or spinal board. Assessment and treatment can be continued on the sideline or the player can be transported to the medical room or to hospital. **Follow-up.** After the game every player should be checked for injuries and appropriate follow up arranged. This may require referral for imaging investigations, treatment (physiotherapy, etc.), and/or a follow up medical appointment. It may be useful to run an injury clinic at a convenient location on a fixed day of the week for this purpose.

Traveling with teams

The sports medicine services need to be well organized when a team travels away from home. This section will use as a model a medium size sporting team on a tour to a distant location that will last several weeks. Large multisports teams, such as Commonwealth and Olympic national teams require more complex organization from all points of view, and will not be covered here, although the principles are outlined below. Sports medicine coverage can be organized in three separate stages.

Planning stage

Several factors need to be addressed prior to departure:

- *Assist in the planning* of the tour's itinerary; 2 days should be allowed for recovery from long distance travel across several time zones.
- Knowledge of the region or regions to be visited. This includes climate (temperatures, humidity, anticipated rainfall, specific health risks such as water supplies, parasites, infections common to the area, etc.), altitude, air pollution, diet customs, water supplies, and local medical services available.
- *Knowledge of the tourists' state of health and athletes' fitness to play*. This is usually done days or weeks prior to departure depending on the nature and length of the trip. Medical clearance is usually required before selection of athletes is completed. If immunizations are required to travel to certain destinations they should be carried out in advance to prevent reactions or complications occurring on tour. The team physician should know all current medications of intending tourists, and ensure that adequate supplies exist for the duration of the tour. IOC-banned substances should not be available to athletes unless permission to use them for specific purposes has been obtained.
- *General advice on travel*: air travel, time zone changes, jet lag and travel fatigue. It is useful to prepare general guidelines for travellers. Melatonin has been advocated for the prevention of jet lag,[1,2] but it is not available in every country. Guidelines would include the following items:
- rest before setting out on a long journey. Avoid fatiguing pre-departure activities, such as functions and parties
- drink large amounts of fluids during flights. Avoid carbonic drinks, alcohol, and caffeine-containing beverages
- avoid tight-waisted and constricting clothing. Loose-fitting garments are best suited for air travel
- move around in the aircraft, avoid sitting for long periods of time if at all possible
- arrange a light exercise session/training on arrival to destination
- avoid going to sleep during daylight on arrival, wait until nightfall before going to sleep
- *Required equipment and medical supplies* for the entire length of the tour. A kit list is given in *Appendix B*.

860

1 *BMJ* 1996 **312** 1242, 1263   2 *Physician Sports Med* **24** 17–18

Traveling stage

When touring, the team physician's responsibilities include:

- *Diagnosis and treatment* of all injuries and medical conditions of all members of the touring party: athletes, coaches and administrators alike.
- *Deciding on such matters as evacuation to home base* if a member of the touring party is unfit to play for the rest of the tour or requires complex treatment.
- *Treatment of sporting injuries.* This includes both acute injuries sustained in the course of the tour, and more often, continuing management of chronic minor musculoskeletal ailments that athletes 'carry'.
- *The quality and type of food.* This should be arranged at the various accommodation venues on arrival. The content of the diet should be verified and appropriate instructions issued to the hotel management and kitchen staff. Food should be plentiful and varied, to ensure a healthy diet and prevent boredom caused by repetitive menus (see Chapter 16). Supply of fluids (bottled water or bottled 'sports drinks') for general consumption and use at training and playing venues is also best arranged with hotel staff.
- *General practice experience* is useful, as the majority of medical encounters are of a general medical nature.

Accommodation

- Living quarters should be close to training and competition venues. Long delays in travel to and from venues may result in boredom or anxiety of team members and be detrimental to performance.
- Room comfort is assisted by adequate ventilation and temperature control, heating, or air conditioning. Extra bedcovers may be required.
- The doctor should have a separate room in the accommodation area in which to consult and store equipment and supplies, or a sleeping room to himself, where consulting can take place. A consulting room is often shared with the physiotherapist's work room.
- Although the doctor should be reasonably available at all times, it is best to set specific times to operate 'clinics'. These clinics should be held after each game and at least on a daily basis to assess the progress of injured players.
- There should be the capacity to isolate a team member with a temporary infectious condition, to prevent the spread of infection.
- Personality and sleep patterns should be considered in the distribution of room-mates.
- Entertainment of team members is important as there is often leisure time between training sessions, competition and official off-the-field functions.

Debriefing

At the end of the tour a report should be prepared on the activities of the sports medicine team, identify possible problem areas, and offer suggestions for future tours. A list of useful contacts, medical facilities, and services in the region should be made for future reference.

Single day mass participation event: triathlon

Race cover

The provision of medical coverage is a necessary aspect of the organization of large endurance sports events. Organizing the medical care of a large mass participation endurance event is a challenging task for a sports medicine practitioner. Medical knowledge needs to combine with leadership and management skills to ensure safety for athletes and spectators alike.

General

The aim of the medical coverage of an endurance mass participation sporting event is, first, to provide immediate optimal treatment of medical problems that present in the course of the event, thus relieving the burden on the local public services. Second, the medical services can be utilized to treat spectators in the case of a disaster or major emergency arising.

Single sports and multisport events

Fun runs, long distance ski and skating races have been popular for many years. Triathlons are a combination of swimming, cycling, and running. Athletes change their apparel between the different legs in the transition areas, usually located in a centralized spot. Multisports events make the medical coverage more challenging, as it has to cover both land- and water-based legs. This results in more complex logistical requirements.[1]

Medical director

Has the overall responsibility for the organization of all medical personnel and facilities, and to oversee all safety issues. He/she should be involved in the planning stages of the event to help plan the time of the year, location, and timing of the event to optimize climatic conditions, and the route, to avoid unnecessary hazards to participants and spectators on the day of the event. This is not possible in some cases, as these parameters may be already set.

The medical director is responsible for organizing the appropriate number of medical staff for the event and bears overall responsibility for the organization of paramedical staff, first aid stations, medical tent (or field hospital), its facilities and supplies. He/she should have knowledge of and input into drink stations for the event. Depending on the size of the event the medical director may choose to have a medical committee to assist him/her in this task.

An Olympic triathlon [1.5km (0.94 miles) swim, 40km (25 miles) cycle, and 10km (6.25 miles) run] will be used in this text as the base for our recommendations, because of the more complex logistics involved in a multiple sports event. Single sports events can be organized along similar lines. Three phases can be identified:

1 the planning stages, before the event
2 the coverage of the actual race itself
3 debriefing, follow-up, and experience gathering after the event

The planning stages

The medical director of a triathlon should ideally be a member of the organizing committee. As in all areas of sports medicine, the medical coverage should keep a low public profile: it is not the main event, but

1 DG Robinson 1994 *Triathlon Australia: Medical and safety guidelines* personal communication: to be published

an ancillary service. Its importance, however, cannot be over-emphasized, for the sake of competitors' safety.

The purpose of the medical director's involvement in the planning and organizing stages is several-fold:

– to ensure a safe, optimal course, bearing in mind the logistic requirements of medical facilities and personnel along the course, the transition areas, the medical tent at the finish line, and the removal of injured athletes/spectators.

– to establish channels of communication between race director and medical director both during the planning stages and on race day; and to establish appropriate links with the local or nearest public hospitals and emergency services for evacuation of casualties and optimal treatment of those referred to hospital. An estimate number of expected casualties can be given once the course, the number of competitors and the climatic conditions are known.[1]

– to provide education/instructions to athletes on all matters medical and paramedical that will assist to improve their physical preparation for the event and reduce risk of injury.

– to set up, train, and co-ordinate the medical and paramedical team and facilities.

The course

Swim leg

- Race organizers should take into account tidal changes and variations as well as local environmental conditions before setting on a specific course for the swim leg.

- Entry and exit points are particularly important. Dangerous objects should be removed: rocks, glass, and other debris.

- Separate entry and exit points for marshals' and (para)medical craft, with independent routes for evacuation of injured athletes: they should never cross the swim course.

- The presence of any marine animals which could cause stings or injuries to swimmers should be identified if possible on race day, and athletes be given prior warning.

- Water temperature guidelines for length of course and use of wetsuits. The length of the swim leg is usually set by the type of race being held [1.5km (0.94 miles) for Olympic distance triathlons]. Maximum swim course lengths in given water temperatures are given in Table 25.1.

- These guidelines may be considered conservative, especially if the majority of athletes are acclimatized to cold water swimming. Their aim is to minimize the likelihood of hypothermia (Table 25.1)

- Water temperature should be recorded at least one meter (3 feet) below the surface in no less than 5 different locations along the swim course, with an appropriate thermometer.

- The maximum temperature at which a wetsuit should be worn is 21°C for élite athletes and 25°C for junior age groups.

- Rescue craft should patrol the swimmers to effect rapid rescue in case of need. Surf rescue boards/skis are useful. Power boats should be of soft material ('rubber duckies') and have covered propellers

1 R Richards *et al* 1984 *Med J Aust* **141** 805–8

- Number of craft: there should be adequate space in the total surface are of all boats on the course to evacuate the majority of the swimmers in the event of a disaster
- There must be clear visibility of all swimmers at all times. The race should be postponed in the event of fog covering the course

Cycle leg

- The course must be clearly signaled for competitors and spectators alike. 'Witches' hats', barriers, etc. should provide enough space to accommodate a large number of competitors. Personnel may be required to indicate the direction of the course to athletes should there be any possibility of confusion.
- General road traffic should be minimized. Ideally, the road should be closed to other traffic. If the roads used are not closed to general traffic, RACE IN PROGRESS signs should be displayed by patroling vehicles.
- There should be no crossover traffic between cyclists and runners. This is especially important near the transition zones.
- Mobile vehicles should be patroling the course. They should be in contact with the medical tent/medical director.
- Drink stations should be set up every 10–15km (6.25–9.4 miles).
- Two first aid stations should be set up (every 15–20km, 9.4–12.5 miles) next to the drink station. They should have a shaded area, stretcher, ice, and trained staff. These stations should have radio contact with the medical director.
- Safety vehicles should be stationed at check points (usually located at turns/areas of possible danger), in radio contact with race director/medical director.
- Dangerous areas or hazards should be avoided or modified (i.e. gravel on the road should be swept away, cattle grids on the road).
- A 'sag' vehicle should follow the latter athletes along the course to collect the injured, sick, or withdrawals.

Run leg

- Lanes should be clearly marked with witches hats and be wide enough to accommodate a large field of athletes. Marshals should be in assistance to indicate directions to athletes. This is especially important near the transition area and close to the finishing line.
- There should never be any crossover with traffic or with cyclists competing in the event. Preferably, the run leg should be on a different course to the cycling leg.
- Drink stations should be set up every 2km (1.25 miles). A first aid station should be set up with every second drink station. First aid stations should have a shaded area, stretcher, ice, and trained staff, and radio communication if possible. This is particularly important in the last 4km (2.5 miles) of the race.
- Personnel at the drink and first aid stations should be alerted to the symptoms of dehydration and hyperthermia, so that appropriate emergency first aid can be instituted.
- Trained spotters familiar with the symptoms of dehydration and hyperthermia should be distributed in large numbers, particularly over the second half of the course and around the finish line.

Table 25.1 Water temperature and distance guidelines for swimming

Maximum Distance	With wetsuit	Without wetsuit
1500m	16°C	18°C
1000m	15°C	17°C
500m	14°C	16°C

- A 'sag' vehicle should follow the latter athletes along the course to collect the injured, sick, or withdrawals.
- All athletes must be accounted for at the end of the event.
- If the event is likely to run into the night reflecting strips should be worn on the athletes' clothing. Alternatively, they can carry fluorescent torches.

Education

Many endurance events have large number of competitors in varying degrees of physical fitness and knowledge about the body's reactions to this level of physical stress. Participation in such an event is an opportunity to educate competitors in physical preparation, prevention of injuries, and recognition of conditions that may result in health risks unless precautions are taken (including withdrawal for the competition).

Registration in the race is the first chance to disseminate information to future entrants. Guidelines can contain information on the following items:[1]

- Perform adequate training
- Acclimatize to the expected environmental conditions
- Increase carbohydrate intake during the days prior to the competition
- Do not compete with a febrile illness, or in the 48h following a febrile illness, diarrhea
- Start the race at a comfortable pace
- If distressed, *stop and seek assistance*
- Adequate clothing (loose, light colored, cap or hat in hot or sunny conditions), footwear, eye goggles.
- Do not stand still at the finish (blood pooling)

Simple articles covering the above can be produced and published in the print media associated with the event.

Often, pre-event education sessions can be held. These provide another opportunity to inform competitors on specific aspects of preparation: fluid replacement; warm-up and stretching; clothing selection, heat acclimatization; signs and symptoms of heat/cold illness. These are to optimize performance and minimize health risks.

Communication

Good communications skills and electronic communication facilities are essential. The medical director of the race should be well known to all those involved in the organization of the event.

Liaison within the organizing committee

The medical director needs to liaise with the race director to ensure that all medical facilities required are in place prior to the race. The size of the facility required (at the finish line and/or in transition areas) must be determined by the medical director. The number of stretchers or beds required must also be specified.

Part of the planning stages is to determine who is responsible for supplying goods: stretchers, blankets, pillows, bed linen, water, water

1 R Richards *et al* 1979 *Med J Aust* **2** 470–4

containers and cups, food, tables, chairs, writing boards, paper and pens, adequate power supply, etc. for the medical facility at the finish line. The medical director needs to supervise and ensure that these goods are ready by race day.

The medical director must liaise with the directors of each of the three legs of the race to check that medical and first aid facilities are in place. Location of the drinks stations in the cycle and run legs must be known and such that first aid stations can be set up in the immediate vicinity, down course from the drinks stations. They must have safe access for both stretcher patients, walking athletes and ambulances. He/she must ensure that the first aid (and drinks) stations are adequately staffed by trained personnel, and that supplies are appropriate (ice, water cups, first aid supplies, shaded area, stretchers, access for athletes and ambulances, privacy).

Adequate numbers of trained personnel are required to operate water craft (rescue boats) in addition to any other marshaling or media (TV) craft on the water. It is helpful to have organizations, such as Surf Life Saving associations, to be involved in the swim leg, as they are familiar with water rescue procedures.

Communications on race day

The medical director must have one of the radio sets in the main race radio channel. There must be good (clear and fast) communication between the medical director and the various medical facilities. In large participation events, a separate medical channel is very useful. It should be mandatory in events with 1000 or more athletes. Every second first aid station, some 'spotters', the 'sag' medical vehicles, the medical facility at the finish line, and the station at the starting line and/or transition areas, and the medical director should all have sets on the medical channel, co-ordinated by a central base. The communication tent should be adjacent to the medical facility at the finish line.

It is very important to test the communication network prior to the race. As most staff will only be occasional users of these means it is important that they have adequate preparation to ensure smooth communications during race day.

The medical tent should have a direct radio link with the ambulance network or direct access to all ambulances involved in covering the race. In this way an ambulance can be directed to any part of the course, and the medical facility can be warned to prepare for specific casualties. In addition, the medical director will have a mobile phone. The number will be known to all personnel involved in the organization.

The medical and paramedical team

Setting up

The medical director bears the overall responsibility for the organization of medical personnel and facilities,[1] the operation of the medical back-up for the race, and the training of staff before the event. This section will concentrate on personnel and medical facilities. First aid and drink stations have already been covered, although they fall within the scope of medical attention.

1 M Moore 1983 *Physician Sports Med* **11** No.6

The medical director is also responsible to provide facilities for drug testing procedures to follow IOC guidelines. This will be done together with the race organizers.

Medical and paramedical personnel must be included in all waivers that athletes must sign. For medico-legal purposes, the categories of health professionals involved (doctors, nurses, trainers, first aiders, physiotherapists, masseurs, etc.) should be listed separately in the waiver. Professional indemnity that covers the event is necessary for all medical personnel.[1]

Medical staff

Although the function of the sports medicine team is one of support, the medical staff must be empowered to remove an athlete from the race if they fear for his/her health. Their decision should be final and binding.

Identification and access

Medical and paramedical staff should be easily identifiable (armbands, special T-shirts, bibs, etc.) to race marshals and competitors alike. They should be different from the rest of race marshals. Members of the sports medicine team should have access to all areas but should not abuse this privilege. Athletes should be familiar with the extent of medical back-up and access to it, before, during, and after the race. This can be achieved through the information provided with registration, and further publicity prior to the race.

Number of (para)medical personnel

The following information should be considered minimum guidelines, which need to be adapted to the distance, duration of the event, the number of competitors and their experience, the nature of the course, and the environmental conditions. Minimum numbers for a competition with 1000 athletes of varying degrees of fitness would be:

- 5 doctors and 10 nurses. 1 or 2 doctors should have accident and emergency background, and be familiar with intubation and resuscitation procedures. If wheelchair athletes take part, it is advisable to have 1 or 2 physicians and 2–4 nurses familiar with medical care of wheelchair athletes. (see Chapter 20)
- 1 or 2 first aiders or sports trainers at every first aid Station. They can treat minor injuries during the race. They can also double up as spotters. Should they observe any competitor in distress or who looks unwell, a radio message is forwarded to the mobile vehicle/ambulance for further medical assistance.
- 5–10 spotters. This number to double if conditions are expected to be hot and/or humid. The majority should be around the finish line and the transition zone
- Physiotherapists, massage therapists, and podiatrists should be in one section of the medical facility at the finish line to treat soft tissue injuries, and particularly foot problems at the end of the run leg.
- 2 doctors or trained paramedics in two mobile vehicles or ambulances on course when there is one cycle loop of 40km (25 miles), or when the run leg is a point to point race rather than a loop course.
- 1 doctor with experience in coverage of athletic events to triage

1 R Roos 1987 *Physician Sports Med* **15** No.11

patients and direct them to the appropriate medical area of the finish line medical facility.

Distribution of (para)medical personnel

- 60% at the finish line medical facility
- 10% at the finish line itself
- 20% at aid stations—non-medical staff
- 10% patroling the course in ambulances/bicycles/rubber duckies/ surf skis

Training

The majority of the members of the sports medicine team should be experienced in the coverage of this type of events. A pre-race seminar should be held to train those with little or no experience in the art of recognizing athletes in distress due to thermal illness or dehydration, treatment protocols, medical records, etc.

The medical facility

Will be set up in the immediate vicinity of the finish line. It should be adjacent to the race communications centre. A large enough tent may be used in the absence of an existing hall or other weather proof facility. It should be located within 50 meters of the finish line, and large enough to accommodate enough beds for 5–10% of the field. It must have good ventilation, adequate lighting, sufficient power and water supply and storage space for all emergency medical equipment and for the staff to move about. It should be at the same level as the finish line (no steps), accessible by wheelchair and to ambulances, with vehicular entrance independent of the race course. If there is more than one transition area, there should be an additional medical facility for each transition area.

The medical director is free to triage, direct athletes, organize staff, and handle communications. For a large part of the duration of the event he/she will control best his/her team from the medical facility or the race communications centre. In races with a large field (as the present case used as an example), the medical facility should be divided into three different sections, with independent entrance:

1 A massage area. Portable massage couches can be installed for this purpose.

2 A minor injury and treatment area. This section will house first aiders, podiatrists, nurses, and physiotherapists, with one or two sports physicians in attendance.

3 A 'field hospital' section for serious patients, where a degree of privacy is required. Emergency physicians, intensivists, and sports physicians are best suited. They should be familiar with intubation and resuscitation procedures. For every doctor there should be 2 nurses and 1 medical records clerk (i.e. medical student) per bed. Depending on weather conditions, up to 25 patients would be expected to be admitted to this section. Equipment required is outlined in *Appendix A*.

Single day mass participation event: triathlon (*cont*)

Race day coverage

On race day, the medical director's role is mainly one of supervision, with direct attention where required. To this end he/she should do a 'round' of all medical services related to the race. This includes contacting or visiting the following facilities connected to the race:

- Weather bureau latest forecast. Injuries forecast[1]
- State emergency services and local hospitals
- Briefing of all (para)medical personnel. Final instructions
- Radio posts/telephone numbers

Visit all posts, first aid stations, starting line, and main medical facility at the finish line. Set up permanent position in or near the main medical facility close to the communications center.

A briefing session should be held prior to the start of the race for all medical, paramedical, and first aid staff. They should be introduced to their respective supervisors and receive identification tags. The latest information on weather forecast, expected casualties, and other instructions for the day should be given at that time. A final check should be made on the adequate functioning of all equipment especially in the medical facility at the finish line. All personnel should be familiar with their respective functions. Treatment protocols for specific expected casualties (heat exhaustion,[2,3] hypothermia,[4] stings, abrasions, chaffing, etc.) should be clear to all involved, and spotters familiar with the signs of heat or cold distress.

The importance of keeping adequate medical records cannot be overemphasized, for clinical, research, and medico-legal reasons. Protocol forms for management of patients in the medical facility should be available in sufficient numbers.

In preparation of the briefing session mentioned above, the number of casualties should be predicted following consultation with the weather bureau, so that personnel and equipment can be deployed appropriately and without wastage.

The medical director or a representative should address the athletes should there be a pre-race briefing for them. Water temperature, possible hazards, location of first aid, and other medical services should be announced once more (information should be given to every athlete on registration). Drug testing facilities and procedures should also be explained briefly. It should be made clear to athletes that the medical personnel have the power to withdraw an athlete from the competition in the event of sickness or injury. During and after the race he/she should maintain direct or radio contact with all posts, receive and transmit updates of relevant information (from a 'pile-up' to unexpected problems, so that the appropriate personnel are made ready).

Debriefing, experiences, and follow-up

After the event all members of the medical team should be invited to attend a post race debriefing and education seminar to gather all records and discuss various aspects of the race. The purpose is to

1 R Richards *et al* 1984 *Med J Aust* 805–8 2 DM Lyle *et al.* 1994 *Med J Aust* 161 361–5 3 D Richards *et al* 1979 *Med J Aust* 2 457–61 4 American College of Sports Medicine 1996 *Med Sci Sports Exerc* 28 i–x

thank volunteers for their contribution and effort, to gather feedback from the field workers, to write down experiences, criticisms
and suggestions and to make recommendations for future events.

Appendix A Facilities for a sports medical room or a field tent (eg Olympic triathlon with 1000 participants)

Equipment	No. required
Couches, defibrillators, aerosols, fluids, IV, resuscitation	
Stretchers/beds	10
Cots	30
Wheelchairs	1
Wool blankets	1/bed/cot
Bath towels	30
High and low temperature thermometers	30
Elastic bandages (50, 100, 150mm; 2, 4, 6 inch)	6 each
Adhesive tape (35mm; 1.5 inch)	1 case
Skin prep	1 case
Surgical soap	1 case
Band-Aids	200
Moleskin	1 case
Petroleum jelly ointment	1 case
Latex gloves, disposable	3 cases (small, medium, large)
Stethoscopes	5 (preferably each physician brings his/her own)
Sphygmomanometers	6
IV giving sets	30
IV fluids (NS, D5%, D4%N1/5S)	30–50
Sharps containers	2
Biohazard disposal containers	2
Alcohol wipes	200
Small instruments kit	1
Athletic trainer's kit	1/athletic trainer
Podiatrist kit	1/podiatrist
Air splints (upper & lower limb)	2 each
Folding tables for medical supplies	5
Fans	2–4
Ice bags (in esky, small)	5–10
Sports drinks	100 liters
Disposable cups	2000
Nebulizer	1
Oxygen tanks	1
Oxygen masks and tubing	10
Urine dipsticks	20
Glucose monitoring kit	1
Oral and injectable drugs	See Appendix B
ECG monitor	1
Defibrillator	1
Water (drinking)	Unlimited supply
Power supply	(10–20) away from water/wet equipment
Toilet	1–2

Appendix B Medical kit for games

Dressings, Braces

blister kit 2nd skins
cotton buds × 1 pkt
cotton balls 2 × 5 (sterile pkts)
Adhesive dressing

non-adhesive dressing
finger splint
wrist splint

Adhesive dressing strips
steristrips
adhesive foam
ankle brace × 1
triangular bandage × 2
cohesive gauze bandage
dressing pack × 3
150mm (6 inch) crepe bandages × 4
  rolls
tubigrip sizes B, C, D, E
100mm (4inch) crepe bandages × 4
  rolls
sports tape × 2 rolls

Equipment

sterile suture sets × 3 comprising
scalpel blade, scissors, needle-holder
toothed forceps, mosquito forceps
syringes 5ml × 5
needles 23g × 5
needles 18g × 5
IV cannulae 15g × 2
sutures 5/0 Dermalon, 3/0 Dermalon
Guedel airway
alcohol swabs50 (1 box)
gauze swabs (sterile) × 5 packs of 5
scalpel blades × 3
oral/rectal thermometer
sphygmomanometer
stethoscope
laryngoscope
otoscope
toothed forceps
Swiss Army knife
plastic gloves
notebook/clipboard/pen
plastic bags × 5 (for ice)
pencil torch

Physiotherapy Kit for games

adhesive foam large roll
Adhesive dressing strip
Friars balsam
Cotton wool (large pkt)
sports tape: 38cm
underwrap
insect repellent
Chlorhexidine antiseptic

Medication
500 (paracetamol)

Salbutamol aerosol
Ibuprofen 400 × 4 bottles or other
  NSAIDs
Chlorhexidine antiseptic
Bupivicaine 0.5%, 5 × 10ml vials
Lidocaine 1% with Adrenaline, 5 ×
  10 ml vials
Lidocaine 1%, plain, 5 × 10ml vials
Antacid solution

'Sharps' container
iodine antiseptic solution
sterifoam
insect repellent
sunscreen
cotton buds
finger splints
bolt cutters
safety pins
cervical collars (soft and hard)
triangular bandages × 3
tongue depressors
airsplints
Dressing packs × 5
Eyestream—eye wash
kidney dish
Hartmann's solution.
nail clippers
small sharp scissors

Nonstick dressing 4 × 4cm × 3
Petroleum jelly
Eyestream
crepe bandages: 6 × 6cm; 6 × 4cm
disposable razors
2mm tape
scissors dressing
sunscreen

Comprehensive base medical kit

General
multipurpose Swiss army knife
torch (penlight) + batteries
pen
notebook/folder/clipboard
safety pins × 5
plastic bags (for rebreathing + ice)
fingernail and toenail clippers
hot air gun (for moulding formthotic material)

Bandages, tape, and dressings
ice packs (instant and reuseable gel)
crepe bandages 50mm × 6 rolls; 100mm × 6 rolls; 150mm × 6 rolls
aluminium finger splints × 5
sports tape: 25mm, 50m × 5 rolls; 38mm, 50m × 5 rolls
silk tape: 12m × 4 rolls
wrap (underwrap)
adhesive foam
skin adhesive spray
sterile cotton wool swabs—packs of 510 (J&J)
Adhesive dressing strips
dressing pads: small × 10
dressing pads: large × 10
antiseptic creme—Chlorhexidine
antiseptic solution—acriflavine or mercurochrome
Povidine iodine antiseptic 200ml
hand antiseptic—to prevent cross-infection
Friar's balsam solution or spray (tinc. benz. co.)
triangular bandages (slings) × 5
collar-and-cuff kit
Heat mouldable orthotics

Medical equipment
stethoscope
oral spatula
sphygmomanometer (aneroid type)
opthalmoscope/otoscope (diagnostic kit)
laryngoscope
alcohol swabs
disposable needles (18g, 21g, 23g) and syringes (2ml, 5ml, 20ml)
percussion hammer
tourniquet (rubber tubing)
sterile scalpel blades (for paring calluses, plantar warts)
scalpel handle
suture material and instruments (3/0 Dermalon, 5/0 Dermalon)
kidney dish × 2
sponge forceps
examination gloves (sterile)
sterile dressing packs
tape measure
thermometer—non-mercury (electronic or crystal)
tongue depressor × 20 (wooden spatulae)
bandage scissors × 2
Guedel airways (small, large)
splinter forceps or tweezers

Physiotherapy equipment
TENS unit
ultrasound unit

transformers/adaptors as appropriate
alkaline batteries (appropriate sizes) AA, AAA

Medications (*indicates script needed, supplied only by physician)
Check first for possible allergy

ANALGESICS (pain killers)

ANTIINFLAMMATORY MEDICATIONS (not if peptic ulcer)

ANTACIDS

ANTISPASMODIC (for colic, stomach cramps—**not in glaucoma**)

LAXATIVES

ANTIDIARRHEAS

NEVER USE MORE THAN DIRECTED.
CONSULT DOCTOR IF DIARRHOEA PERSISTS FOR 2–3 DAYS

SEDATIVE/HYPNOTICS (sleeping tablets for travel) (**Not recommended prior to competition**)

ANTINAUSEANTS (antimotion sickness)

COUNTER-IRRITANT AND ANTI-INFLAMMATORY CREAMS AND RUBS

TOPICAL VAGINAL MEDICATION (mixed tour parties)

ANTIBIOTICS **For more *severe* LOCAL INFECTIONS. Consult doctor always for more generalized infections with fever.**

ANTIFUNGAL (tinea, etc.)

OTHER LOCAL ANTI-INFECTIVE CREAMS

LOCAL SKIN AGENTS: ANTIITCH (insect bites, etc.), and antiallergy

DECONGESTANTS AND ANTIASTHMATIC BRONCHODILATORS

LOCAL EYE/EAR DROPS

HORMONAL (females, to modify menstruation)

Appendix C Principles and ethical guidelines of health care for sports medicine

(Medical Commission of the International Olympic Committee)

The Medical Commission of the International Olympic Committee recommends the following ethical guidelines for physicians who care for athletes and sportspersons (hereinafter termed athletes). These have been based on those drafted by the World Medical Association[1] and recognise the special circumstances in which medical care and guidance are provided for participants in sport(s).

1 All physicians who care for athletes have an ethical obligation to understand the specific physical and mental demands placed upon them during training for and participation in their sport(s).

2 It is recommended that undergraduate and postgraduate training in sports medicine be available to medical students and those doctors who desire or are required to provide health care for athletes.

3 When the sports participant is a child or an adolescent, the sports physician must ensure that the training and competition are appropriate for the stage of growth and development. Sports training and participation which may jeopardise the normal physical or mental development of the child or adolescent should not be permitted.

4 In sports medicine, as in all other branches of medicine, professional confidentiality must be observed. The right to privacy relating to medical advice or treatment the athlete has received, must be protected.

5 When serving as a team physician, it is acknowledged that the sports doctor assumes a responsibility to athletes as well as team administrators and coaches. It is essential that from the outset, each athlete is informed of that responsibility and authorises disclosure of otherwise confidential medical information but solely to specified and responsible persons and for the express purpose of determining the fitness or unfitness of that athlete to participate.

6 The sports physician must give an objective opinion on the ahtlete's fitness or unfitness as clearly and as precisely as possible. It is unethical for a physician with a financial investment or incentive in a team to act as a team physician.

7 At sports venues it is the responsibility of the team or contest physician to determine whether an injured athlete may continue in or return to the event or game. This decision should not be delegated to other professionals or personnel. In the physician's absence these individuals must adhere strictly to the guidelines established by the physician. In all cases, priority must be given in order to safeguard the athlete's health and safety. The outcome of the competition must never influence such decisions.

8 To enable him/her to undertake this ethical obligation, the sports physician must insist on professional autonomy over all medical decisions concerning the health, safety and legitimate interests of the athlete, none of which can be prejudiced to favor the interest of any third party whatsoever.

9 The sports physician should endeavour to keep the athlete's personal physician fully informed of relevant aspects of his or her health and treatment. When necessary, they should collaborate to ensure that the athlete does not exert himself or herself in a manner detrimental to their health and does not employ potentially harmful techniques to improve performance.

10 The sports physician should be cognizant of the contributions to athlete performance and health from other sports medicine professionals, including physical therapists, podiatrists, psychologists and sports scientists, including biochemists, biomechanists, physiologists, etc. As the person with the final responsibility for the health and the well-being of the athlete,

the physician should co-ordinate the respective roles of these professionals and those of appropriate medical specialists in the prevention and treatment of disease and injury from training and participation in sports.

11 The sports physician should publicly oppose and in practice refrain from using method which has been banned by the IOC Medical Commission, is not in accord with professional ethics or which might be harmful to the athlete especially: any

11.1 Procedures which artificially modify blood constituents or biochemistry.

11.2 The use of drugs or other substances whatever their nature and route of administration which artificially modify mental and physical ability to participate in sports.

11.3 Procedures used to mask pain or other protective symptoms for the express purpose of enabling the athlete to participate and thus risk aggravation of the condition, whereas in the absence of such procedures participation would be inadvisable or impossible.

11.4 Training and participating when to do so is incompatible with the preservation of the individual's fitness, health or safety.

12 The sports physician should inform the athlete, those responsible for him or her and other interested parties of the consequences of the procedures he or she is opposing, guard against their use, enlist the support of other physicians and other organisations with similar aims, protect the athlete against any pressures which might induce him or her to use these methods and help with supervision against these procedures.

13 Physicians who advocate or utilise any of the above mentioned unethical procedures are in breach of this code of ethics and are unsuited to act or be accredited as sports physicians.

14 The sports physician must never be party to any contract which obliges them to reserve any particular form of therapy solely and exclusively for any individual or group of athletes.

15 When sports physicians accompany national teams to international competitions in other countries, they should be accorded the rights and privileges necessary to undertake their professional responsibilities to their team members while abroad.

16 It is strongly recommended that a sports physician participates in the framing of sports regulations.

As an addition it can be stated that it is unwise for a team physician to hold a number of other offices in a club, for example President, Director or Selector as in so doing, he may be jeopardising a truly satisfactory confidential medical communication with team members.

Introduction

The illnesses encountered in diving medicine are related to the environment and/or the diving equipment. Thus it is conventional to subdivide the diving-related illnesses as to whether they occur during free diving, with open circuit diving, or with closed circuit diving equipment. The **free diving** hazards are due mostly to the aquatic environment, and therefore are common to all types of divers. Swimming and breathhold diving accidents include:

- drowning syndromes
- effects of cold and immersion
- marine animal injuries
- hyperventilation then breathholding hypoxia
- descent barotrauma

Apart from descent barotrauma, these disorders are well described in general medical texts and in the more comprehensive diving medical texts. The hazards associated with open circuit equipment are commonly encountered, as they include diving with **scuba**. The diseases are especially those of the extended environmental parameters, to which the equipment now allows the diver to explore. Thus, the illnesses of barotrauma, decompression sickness, bone necrosis and gas toxicities develop.

This chapter deals essentially with the dysbaric diseases (due to abnormal environmental pressures) as well as some of the common symptoms with which divers present (hearing loss, vertigo, headaches). The hazards with **rebreathing** equipment tend to be restricted to professional or technical divers, and their medical back-up. They are more related to the extremes of gas pressures (especially oxygen, carbon dioxide, nitrogen, and helium), and they develop because of the complexity of maintaining breathing gas pressures within an acceptable range for humans.

Despite the above, many of the accidents experienced by divers are initiated because of the medical illnesses and personal characteristics of the diver (inadequate physical fitness, psychological disturbances, inadequate training) and improper or unsafe diving techniques and practices. These are well covered in the conventional diving medical texts, and do not usually present as the problem in emergency medical situations. They are the provoking factors on which the medical disease will develop.

Diving with open circuit apparatus (scuba)

This equipment allows the inhalation of gases from a high pressure source, and the liberation of exhaled gas into the water. There is no rebreathing of exhaled gases involved. Open circuit diving may involve the use of:

- Self-contained underwater breathing apparatus (scuba). The breathing gas is compressed air and is carried in tanks on the diver's back.
- Surface supply breathing apparatus (SSBA). Air is carried to the diver via a hose from either storage cylinders or compressors ('hookah') on the surface.
- Standard diving equipment ('hard hat').

Gas mixtures (oxygen/nitrogen, oxygen/helium) may replace air for specific diving operations

The availability of non-expensive equipment has increased the popularity of this type of diving. Scuba and SSBA have largely replaced the old 'hard hat' or standard diving previously used in shell collecting and salvage. The **medical conditions** which can occur when diving with compressed gases include:

1 Barotrauma—ears, sinus, lung, dental, others
2 Decompression sickness
3 Dysbaric osteonecrosis
4 Salt water aspiration
5 Gas toxicities
6 Contamination of gas supply
7 Nitrogen narcosis
8 Syncope of ascent

Only the first four of these are likely to present to the emergency room clinician, and will be dealt with in this chapter. Common diving medical presentations have been included, with a checklist to aid in **differential diagnosis**:

- Disorientation and vertigo in diving
- Hearing loss
- Headaches

Physics review—1

To understand the physiological changes which occur, some knowledge of physics is needed. *Pascal's Principle* states that when pressure is applied to the surface of a fluid it is distributed equally and undiminished in all directions.

Since the pressure on sea water is atmospheric pressure, i.e. 100kPa , (1 Bar, 1 atmosphere absolute, or 1 ATA), then at a depth of 10 meters the pressure will be 1 ATA plus the pressure equal to 10m of sea water. In sea water, the pressure will increase by 100kPa (1 ATA) for every 10m depth. The pressure at 10m will then be as follows:

$$1 \text{ ATA} + 1 \text{ ATA} = 2 \text{ ATA}$$

Surface pressure = 1 ATA
At 10m = 2 ATA
At 20m = 3 ATA
At 30m = 4 ATA

Boyle's law states that at a given temperature, the volume of a given mass of gas will vary inversely with the pressure applied. $PV = K$ (where K is a constant)

This means that 1 liter (1L) of gas at the surface (where the pressure equals 1 ATA) will be reduced to 0.5L at 10m (2 ATA), or 0.33L at 20m depth (3 ATA), 0.25L at 30m depth (4 ATA), etc.

It can be seen that the volume change is proportionately greatest near the surface, and so it is in this zone that the effects of Boyle's law are most noticeable.

Barotrauma

Is the tissue damage resulting from the expansion or contraction of enclosed gas spaces, and is a direct effect of the gas volume changes causing tissue distortion. It is probably the most common occupational disease of divers. There are two types of barotrauma: descent and ascent. Both are caused by the effects of Boyle's law. The volume change is proportionally greatest near the surface, and so it is here that barotrauma is most noticeable.

Barotrauma of descent is that damage which occurs during descent in water (i.e. as a result of increasing pressures of the surrounding environment). Pressure imbalance is due to an inability to compensate for the reducing volumes within the body cavities as the depth increases. Because some cavities are surrounded by bone, no collapse can occur, and the space must be taken up by engorgement of the mucous membrane, edema, and hemorrhage. This, together with the compressed gas, assists in 'equalizing' the pressure balance. It is commonly called a 'squeeze'.

Barotrauma of ascent is the result of the distension of tissues around the expanding gas. This occurs when environmental pressures are reduced during ascent in water. Divers use the misnomer 'reverse squeeze' to describe it. The classification of barotrauma is as follows :

Ear barotrauma

- External ear barotrauma of descent
- Middle ear barotrauma of descent
- Middle ear barotrauma of ascent
- Inner ear barotrauma

Sinus barotrauma

- Sinus barotrauma of descent
- Sinus barotrauma of ascent

Dental barotrauma
Mask, suit, and helmet barotrauma

- Facial barotrauma of descent
- Skin barotrauma of descent
- Head and body barotrauma of descent
- Suit barotrauma of ascent

Gastrointestinal barotrauma
Other barotrauma and sequelae

- Localized surgical emphysema
- Bone cyst
- Pneumoperitoneum
- Pneumocephalus
- Cranial nerve palsies

Ear barotrauma

Is the commonest reason for divers to present to clinicians. Barotrauma is subdivided according to the anatomical sites. They may occur separately or in combination in the external ear, the middle ear, or the inner ear.

External ear barotrauma (external 'ear squeeze')

If the external meatus is blocked, water entry is prevented. Then contraction of the contained gas during descent is compensated for by tissue collapse, outward bulging of the tympanic membrane, congestion, and hemorrhage. These results are observed in as little as 2 meters (6 feet) of water. The common **causes** of blockage of the external auditory canal include: cerumen, exostoses, foreign bodies such as mechanical ear plugs, tight fitting hoods, and mask straps. **Clinical** symptoms are usually mild. Following ascent there may be an ache in the affected ear and/or a bloody discharge. **Examination** of the external auditory canal may reveal petechial hemorrhages and blood-filled cutaneous blebs which may extend on to the tympanic membrane.

Treatment for this condition includes maintaining a dry canal, removal of any occlusion, and prohibition of diving until epithelial surfaces appear normal. Secondary infection may result in a recurrence of the pain, and require antibiotics. This condition is easily **prevented** by ensuring patency of external auditory canals and avoidance of ear plugs or hoods which do not have apertures over the ear to permit water entry.

Middle ear barotrauma of descent ('middle ear squeeze')

Is the most common medical disorder experienced by divers, and it follows the failure to equalise middle ear and environmental pressures via the Eustachian tubes ('equalizing the ears'), during descent. Any condition which blocks the Eustachian tube, predisposes to middle ear barotrauma. Failure to voluntarily autoinflate the middle ears, usually by the Valsalva maneuver during descent, has the same effect. If the diver continues the descent without 'equalizing', mucosal congestion, edema, and hemorrhage within the middle ear cavity are associated with inward bulging of the tympanic membrane. This tends to compensate for the contraction of air within the otherwise rigid cavity. The tympanic membrane will become hemorrhagic (the 'traumatic tympanum' of older texts). Eventually it may rupture, although this is not common. Blockage of the Eustachian tubes may be due to mucosal congestion as a manifestation of upper respiratory tract infections, smoking, allergies, otitis media, mechanical obstructions such as mucosal polyps, or individual variations in size, shape, and patency.

Symptoms consist initially of discomfort followed by increasing pain in the ear if descent continues. This may be sufficiently severe to prevent further descent. Occasionally, a diver may have little or no symptomatology. Occasionally, there is a sensation of vertigo during the descent, but it is not as common as in middle ear barotrauma of ascent or inner ear barotrauma (see later), both of which can follow or be due to middle ear barotrauma of descent. Eventually, rupture of the drum may occur, usually after a descent of 1.5–10 meters (5–33 feet) from the surface. This causes instant equalization of pressures by allowing water entry into the middle ear cavity. If this occurs, pain is suddenly relieved. However, nausea and vertigo may follow the caloric stimulation by the cold water.

Following a dive which has resulted in descent barotrauma, there may be a mild residual pain in the affected ear. Blood or blood-stained fluid may be expelled from the middle ear during ascent, and be swallowed or produce epistaxis on the affected side. A full or blocked sensation may be experienced in the ear. This is sometimes associated with a mild conductive deafness especially involving low frequencies. It is usually temporary. Fluid may be felt within the middle ear for a week or so, before resolution. Middle ear barotrauma is classified into 6 grades based on the otoscopic appearance of the tympanic membrane (Table 26.1). Damage involves the whole of the middle ear space and not the tympanic membrane alone. The **clinical management** consists of:

- prohibition of all pressure changes such as diving and autoinflation techniques until resolution
- occasionally (very rarely) systemic or local decongestants
- antibiotics only where there is evidence of a pre-existing or developing infection, gross hemorrhage or perforation

Serial **audiometric examination** should be undertaken to exclude hearing loss, and to assist in further action if such loss is present. Diving can be resumed when resolution is complete, and voluntary autoinflation of the middle ear cleft has been demonstrated. If there is no perforation (grades 0–IV), recovery may take up to 2 weeks. With perforation (grade V) it may take 1–2 months, if uncomplicated and managed conservatively .

Note: it is important to identify clearly the contributing factors to the disease in each case, or it is likely to recur.

Middle ear barotrauma of ascent

This refers to the effects from distension by enclosed gases within the middle ear, expanding with ascent. Because it may prevent ascent, it is usually considered more serious than middle ear barotrauma of descent—which allows an unhindered return to safety.

Gas which has entered the middle ear by autoinflation at depth is at the surrounding environmental pressure, and on ascent it obeys Boyle's law. If the Eustachian tube restricts its release, the expansion of gas can cause **clinical manifestations** with sensations of pressure or pain in the affected ear, vertigo due to increased middle ear pressure difference (alternobaric vertigo), or tinnitus. The vertigo tends to develop when the middle ear's pressure differs by 60cm H_2O. Relief of the overpressure in the affected middle ear may be heard, with air felt hissing out the Eustachian tube.

Hearing loss in the affected ear, if present, may be either conductive or sensorineural and may follow damage to the tympanic membrane or the middle ear structures. Inner ear barotrauma is a possible complication. Seventh nerve palsy also is a complication (see later). Middle ear barotrauma of ascent usually follows recent, but sometimes mild, middle ear barotrauma of descent or the use of nasal decongestants. In each case, the common factor is probably a congestion and therefore blockage of the Eustachian tube. **Otoscopic examination** often reveals evidence of tympanic membrane injection or hemorrhage. **Treatment** is as for middle ear barotrauma of descent.

Prevention is achieved by avoiding nasal decongestants and by training the diver in correct middle ear equalisation techniques. Unless the descent barotrauma is prevented the ascent barotrauma is likely to recur.

Table 26.1 Middle ear barotrauma of descent grades.

Grade 0—Symptoms without signs

Grade I—Injection of the tympanic membrane, especially along the handle of the malleus

Grade II—Injection plus slight hemorrhage within the substance of the tympanic membrane

Grade III—Gross hemorrhage within the substance of the tympanic membrane

Grade IV—Free blood in the middle ear as evidenced by blueness and bulging

Grade V—Perforation of the tympanic membrane

Barotrauma (cont)

Inner ear barotrauma

There is always the possibility of a sensorineural hearing loss in divers who have experienced ear barotrauma of any type, or who have had difficulty in equalizing middle ear pressures by autoinflation or who subsequently apply force to achieve this. In these cases, the hearing loss may immediately follow the incident, or may develop over the next few days.

An inner ear (labyrinthine) window fistula is one pathological entity of inner ear barotrauma. Others include cochlear and vestibular hemorrhages, internal inner ear membrane ruptures, the entry of air into the cochlea, etc. It has been reported from dives as shallow as 2 meters (7 feet) and has been observed in a surfer who merely dived under a wave. **Symptoms** associated with inner ear barotrauma may include;

- a sensation of blockage in the affected ear
- tinnitus of variable duration
- high frequency hearing loss
- vestibular disturbances such as nausea, vomiting, vertigo, disorientation and ataxia
- clinical features of an associated middle ear barotrauma

Any combination of middle ear barotrauma symptoms, vertigo, tinnitus, and hearing loss should be immediately and fully investigated by serial measurements of clinical function, daily audiometry up to 8000Hz, and positional electronystagmography. Caloric testing is indicated only if the tympanic membrane is intact or if the technique guards against pressure or fluid transmission into the middle ear. **Other investigations** that may be of value include temporal bone polytomography, CT scans and other imaging techniques. Until now they have not been particularly helpful in diagnosis or treatment, but this should change with more experience. Cochlear injury is permanent in over half the cases, whereas vestibular injury is usually temporary. **Treatment**. Once damage has been confirmed, treatment should be initiated promptly. This includes:

1 Avoid straining, such as performing Valsalva maneuvers, sneezing, nose blowing, straining with defecation, sexual activity, coughing, lifting weights, or physical exertion. Any increase in cerebrospinal fluid pressure can be transmitted to the inner ear.

2 Immediate bedrest with the head elevated and careful monitoring of otological changes; this is given irrespective of which of the other treatment procedures are followed.

3 Bedrest should continue until all improvement has ceased and for up to a week thereafter, to allow the inner ear membranes to heal and the hemorrhages to resolve. Loud noises should be avoided.

4 If there is no improvement within 24–48h in cases of severe hearing loss, or if there is further deterioration in hearing, reconstructive microaural surgery must then be considered.

5 Prohibition of diving and flying. This is absolute for the first few weeks following a labyrinthine window fistula. If medical evacuation by air is required, an aircraft with the cabin pressurized to ground level is necessary.

Hyperbaric oxygen therapy has been used in some cases, but requires further confirmation before it can be generally recommended.

Sinus barotrauma

If a sinus ostium is blocked during descent, mucosal congestion and hemorrhage compensate for the contraction of the air within the sinus cavity. During ascent, expansion of the enclosed air expels blood and mucus from the sinus ostium. Ostia blockage may be the result of sinusitis with mucosal hypertrophy and congestion, rhinitis, redundant mucosal folds in the nose, nasal polyps, etc. Allergies and smoking may underly the pathology.

Sinus barotrauma of descent ('sinus squeeze')

Symptoms include pain over the sinus during descent. It may be preceded by a sensation of tightness or pressure. The pain usually subsides with ascent but may continue as a persistent dull ache for several hours. On ascent blood or mucus may appear in the nose or pharynx. The pain is usually over the frontal sinus, less frequently it is retroorbital, and maxillary pain is not common but may be referred to a number of upper teeth. Although they may feel hypersensitive, abnormal or loose, they are not painful on movement. Numbness over the maxillary division of the trigeminal nerve is possible. The superficial ethmoidal sinuses near the root of the nose occasionally rupture and cause a small hematoma or discoloration of the skin, between the eyes. Discomfort persisting after the dive may be due to fluid within the sinus (remaining from the dive), infection (usually starts a few hours post dive) or the development of chronic sinusitis or mucoceles.

Sinus x-ray examination, CT or MRI scan may disclose thickened mucosa, opacity or fluid levels. The opacities produced by the barotrauma may be serous or mucous cysts. The maxillary and frontal sinuses are commonly involved. The ethmoid and sphenoidal sinuses may also be affected. The new imaging techniques can clearly demonstrate these.

Treatment consists of temporary cessation of all diving and flying, with correction of any predisposing factors. Patients with a sinus or upper respiratory tract infection may require antibiotics and decongestants. Surgical drainage is rarely indicated. Even the mucoceles and chronic sinus pathology usually resolve without intervention, if diving is suspended.

Sinus barotrauma of ascent

This may follow the occlusion of sinus openings by mucosal folds or sinus polyps, preventing escape of expanding gases. The ostium or its mucosa will then blow out into the nasal cavity, with or without pain, and hemorrhage commonly follows. This disease is aggravated by rapid ascent.

If the expanding air cannot escape through the sinuses it may fracture the walls and track along the soft tissues. Rupture of air cells may cause sudden pain of a severe degree, often affecting the ethmoidal or mastoid sinuses, on ascent. Occasionally, the air may rupture into the cranial cavity and cause a pneumocephalus.

Dental barotrauma (aerodontalgia)

The tooth may cave in (implode) on descent, or explode on ascent. Gas spaces may exist in carious teeth, at the roots of infected teeth or within fillings which have undergone secondary erosion. During descent, the gas space contracts, filling with soft tissue or blood. Pain may prevent further descent. Gas expansion on ascent may be restricted by blood in these spaces, resulting in pain which may continue post dive. Pressure applied to individual teeth may cause pain and identify the affected tooth. **Treatment** consists of analgesia and dental repair. The **differential diagnosis** of sporadic or constant pain in the upper bicuspids or the first and second molars, but not localized in one tooth, must include referred pain from the maxillary sinus or the maxillary nerve. This may also present as a burning sensation along the mucobuccal fold.

Mask, suit, and helmet barotrauma

Facial barotrauma of descent ('mask squeeze')

A facemask creates an additional gas space external to, but in contact with, the face. Unless pressure is equalized by exhaling gas through the nose, facial tissues will be forced into this space, during descent. **Clinical** features include puffy edematous facial tissues especially under the eyelids, purpuric hemorrhages, conjunctival hemorrhages, and later, generalized bruising of the skin underlying the mask. *This condition is rarely serious*, and **prevention** involves exhaling into the facemask during descent. Diving should be avoided until all tissue damage is healed. Rare cases may involve the deeper orbital tissues and/or retina.

Skin barotrauma of descent ('suit squeeze')

This condition is encountered mainly with dry suits or poorly fitting wet suits. During descent the air spaces are reduced in volume and trapped in folds in the suit. The skin tends to be sucked into these folds, leaving linear weal marks or bruises. The condition is usually painless and clears within a few days.

Head and body barotrauma of descent ('diver's squeeze')

A rigid helmet, as used in standard and 'hard hat' diving, may cause this trauma. If extra gas is not added during descent to compensate for the effects of Boyle's law, or if pressure is lost for any reason, the suit and occupant may be forced into the helmet, causing fractured clavicles, bizarre injuries, or death.

Suit barotrauma of ascent ('blow up')

During ascent with a gas-filled diving suit (a 'dry suit'), the expanding gas must be able to escape. If it does not, then the whole suit will expand like a balloon and cause a rapid and uncontrolled ascent to the surface. This may result in barotrauma of ascent, decompression sickness, imprisonment of the diver and physical trauma.

Gastrointestinal barotrauma

Gas expansion occurs within the intestines on ascent, and may result in eructation, vomiting, flatus, abdominal discomfort and colicky pains. It is rarely severe, but has been known to cause syncopal and shock-like states. A small group of divers have experienced more serious symptoms, with gastric rupture on ascent.

Miscellaneous barotrauma

Localized surgical emphysema

This may result from the entry of gas into any area where the integument, skin, or mucosa is broken and in contact with a gas space. Although the classical site involves the supraclavicular areas in association with tracking mediastinal emphysema from pulmonary barotrauma, other sites are possible.

Orbital surgical emphysema, severe enough to completely occlude the palpebral fissure, may result from diving with facial skin, intra-nasal, or sinus injuries. The most common cause is a fracture of the nasoethmoid bones. The lamina papyracea, which separates the nasal cavity and the orbit, is of egg shell thickness. When these bones are fractured, any increase in pressure in the nasal cavity or ethmoidal sinus from ascent or Valsalva maneuver, may force air into the orbit.

Surgical emphysema over the mandibular area is common with buccal and dental lesions. The surgical emphysema, with its associated physical sign of crepitus and its radiological verification, tends to occur in loose subcutaneous tissue. **Treatment** is by administration of 100% oxygen by a non-pressurized technique, and complete resolution will occur within hours. Recompression is rarely indicated, but diving should be avoided until this resolution is complete and the damaged integument has completely healed.

Pneumoperitoneum

This has been observed following pulmonary barotrauma, gas dissecting along the mediastinum to the retroperitoneal area, into the peritoneum, and under the diaphragm. It is also possible that previous injury to the lung or diaphragm, producing adhesions, could permit the direct passage of air from the lung to the subdiaphragmatic area. Another possible cause of pneumoperitoneum is, as described above, from a rupture of a gastrointestinal viscus—from barotrauma of ascent. The **condition may be detected** by chest x-ray or positional abdominal x-ray (gas under the diaphragm). **Treatment** is by administration of 100% oxygen by a non-pressurized technique. Usually complete resolution will then occur within hours. Management of the cause (pulmonary or gastrointestinal) is required and surgical management of a ruptured gastrointestinal viscus may be needed.

Pneumocephalus

Occasionally, the cranial gas spaces (mastoid, paranasal sinuses) are affected by an ascent barotrauma, when the expanding gas ruptures into the cranial cavity. This may follow descent barotrauma, when hemorrhage occupies the gas space and its orifice is blocked. The **clinical presentation** may have all the features of a catastrophic intracerebral event. Excruciating headache immediately on ascent is probable, although the effects of a space occupying lesion may supervene. Neurological signs may follow brain injury or cranial nerve lesions. It is likely that the condition could be aggravated by excessive Valsalva maneuvers ('equalizing the ears') or ascent to altitude (air travel). Diagnosis can be verified by positional skull x-ray, or CT scan.

Treatment includes: bedrest, sitting upright; avoidance of Valsalva, sneezing, nose blowing, or other maneuvers that increase nasopharyngeal pressures; 100 % oxygen inhalation for many hours and follow-up x-rays to show a reduction of the air volume. **If untreated**, the disorder may last a week or so and subsequent infection is possible. Recompression or craniotomy could be considered in dire circumstances.

Bone cyst barotrauma

Occasionally pain may develop from an intraosseous bone cyst, probably with hemorrhage into the area, during descent or ascent, and may last for hours after the dive. The pelvic bones are most often involved, in the ilium and near the sacroiliac joints. An x-ray or CT scan may demonstrate the lesions.

Cranial nerve palsies

Cases occasionally present with cranial nerve lesions attributed to neurapraxis, due to the implosive tissue damaging effects during descent, the distension in enclosed gas spaces during ascent, or both. These presentations are usually associated with barotrauma symptoms and signs, as described earlier.

The **seventh or facial** cranial nerve may be affected, causing 'facial baroparesis', because of its passage through the middle ear space. Recorded in both aviators and divers, it is more frequent following ascent, presents as a unilateral facial weakness similar to Bell's palsy, and tends to recur in the same patient. A possible reason for an individual's susceptibility to this disorder is perhaps found in the anatomy of the facial canal. This opens into the middle ear in some people and shares its pathology.

The **fifth or trigeminal** nerve may be likewise influenced by gas pressure changes in the maxillary antrum and sinus barotrauma (see above). The most common presentation is with involvement of the maxillary division, especially the infraorbital nerve, which traverses the sinus. Hypoesthesia can be demonstrated for a variable time after the sinus barotrauma incident. It may involve the cheek, side of nose, lower eyelid, upper lip, maxillary teeth, and gums. It may also be a cause of pain from sinus barotrauma referred to the upper teeth on the same side.

Pulmonary barotrauma (PBT)

Of ascent is the most serious of the barotraumata, and causes concern in all types of compressed air diving. It is the clinical manifestation of Boyle's law as it affects the lungs and is the result of overdistension and rupture of the lungs by expanding gases during ascent. It is also called 'burst lung' or pulmonary overinflation. It is second only to drowning as a cause of death among young recreational scuba divers. Controversy surrounds the pathophysiology of PBT, but its cause, diagnosis, and treatment are well established.

Etiology. PBT may involve much of the lung, such as when the expanding lung gases are not exhaled during ascent. Alternatively, it may involve only small areas following obstructed air flow or altered compliance in some airways. With a breathhold ascent, the pressure change necessary to cause PBT is approximately 70mmHg near the surface (i.e. a force which could cause an increase in lung volume of about 10%, i.e. with an ascent from a depth of about 1 meter, to the surface).

Predisposing pathology causing local ruptures include previous spontaneous pneumothorax, asthma, sarcoidosis, cysts, tumors, pleural adhesions, intrapulmonary fibrosis, infection and inflammation, etc. These disorders may result in local compliance changes or airway obstructions.

There are four manifestations of PBT of ascent which may occur singly or in combination:
1 Pulmonary tissue damage
2 Mediastinal emphysema
3 Pneumothorax
4 Air embolism

Clinical features. *Pulmonary tissue damage*. Dyspnea, cough, and hemoptysis are symptoms of the lung damage, and widespread alveolar rupture may cause death from respiratory damage.

Mediastinal emphysema. **Symptoms** may appear rapidly in severe cases, or may be delayed several hours in lesser cases. They may include a voice change into a hoarseness or a brassy monotone, a feeling of fullness in the throat, dyspnea, dysphagia, retrosternal discomfort, syncope, shock, or unconsciousness. The voice changes are attributed to 'submucosal emphysema' of the upper airways and/or recurrent laryngeal nerve damage.

Clinical signs include: subcutaneous emphysema of neck and upper chest wall (i.e. crepitus under the skin, described as the sensation of egg shell cracking, by divers), decreased areas of cardiac dullness to percussion, faint heart sounds, left recurrent laryngeal nerve paresis, and cardiovascular effects of cyanosis, tachycardia, and hypotension.

Precordial emphysema may be palpable and give the pneumoprecordium or Hamman's sign—crepitus related to heart sounds. An extension of the mediastinal gas into the tissues between the pleura and the pericardium, rather than gas in the pericardial sac, has produced cardiac tamponade with its clinical signs. There may be radiological evidence of an enlarged mediastinum with air tracking along the cardiac border or in the neck.

Pneumothorax. If the visceral pleura ruptures, air enters the pleural cavity and expands during further ascent. It may be accompanied by hemorrhage, forming a hemopneumothorax. The pneumothorax may be unilateral or bilateral. **Symptoms** usually have a rapid onset and include sudden retrosternal or unilateral, sometimes pleuritic, pain with dyspnea, and an increased respiratory rate. **Clinical signs** may be absent, or may include: diminished chest wall movements, diminished breath sounds, and hyper-resonance on the affected side; movement of trachea and apex beat to the unaffected side with a tension pneumothorax; signs of shock; x-ray evidence of pneumothorax; arterial gas and lung volume changes.

A pneumothorax under pressure becomes a tension pneumothorax during ascent. Tension pneumothorax may also develop from coughing or exposure to altitude or aviation. Rarely a pneumoperitoneum may accompany the pneumothorax.

Air (gas) embolism. This is a dangerous condition and is the result of gas passing from the ruptured lung into the pulmonary veins and thence into the systemic circulation, where it can cause vascular damage or obstruction, hypoxia, and infarctions. **Serious effects may result** from blockage of cerebral (cerebral arterial gas embolism or CAGE) or coronary vessels by bubbles 25 microns–2 millimeters in diameter, or by otherwise interrupting blood flow (vascular endothelial and perfusion injury). Death may follow coronary or cerebrovascular embolism. Other tissues may be affected. The **manifestations** are usually acute and may include:

- Loss of consciousness; other neurological abnormalities such as confusion, aphasia, visual disturbances, paresthesiae or sensory abnormalities, vertigo, convulsions, varying degrees of paresis; gas bubbles in retinal vessels; abnormal electroencephalograms and brain scans, etc.
- Cardiac-type chest pain and/or abnormal electrocardiograms (ischemic myocardium, dysrhythmias or cardiac failure).
- Skin marbling; a sharply defined area of pallor on the tongue (Liebermeister's sign) is rare.

Of divers who experience symptoms of CAGE, many will show a partial, or even a complete, recovery within minutes or a few hours of the incident. This recovery presumably reflects a movement of the embolus through the cerebral vasculature. Even those who become comatose may improve to a variable degree after the initial episode. Unfortunately, the recovery is unreliable. It may not occur, or it may not be sustained. Recurrence of symptoms has an ominous prognostic significance.

Treatment. Once PBT has resulted in the distribution of gas within body tissues, it may be aggravated by other factors. Further ascent in a chamber or underwater, or ascent to altitude during air transport, will expand the enclosed gas and cause deterioration in the clinical state of the patient. Physical exertion, increased respiratory activity, breathing against a resistance, coughing, Valsalva maneuver, etc. may also result in further pulmonary damage, or in more extraneous gas passing through the lung tissues or into the pulmonary vessels. If the diver has exposed himself to depths and times resulting in tissue loading by inert gas, this gas will diffuse into the abnormal gas spaces. A situation develops which has aspects of both PBT and decompression sickness.

If the anesthetic, nitrous oxide, is used, this rapidly diffuses into tissues, causing expansion of bubbles.

Pulmonary tissue damage. The treatment is similar to that of near-drowning or the acute respiratory distress syndrome.

Mediastinal emphysema. The need for therapy may not be urgent. Exclusion of air embolism or pneumothorax is necessary and if in doubt, treatment for these should take precedence. Management of mediastinal emphysema varies according to the clinical severity. If the patient is asymptomatic, only observation and rest may be necessary. With mild symptoms, 100% oxygen administered by mask without positive pressure will increase the gradient for removal of nitrogen from the emphysematous areas. This may take 4–6h. **If symptoms are severe**, therapeutic recompression using oxygen is necessary.

Pneumothorax. Treatment depends on the clinical severity and the depth at which it is diagnosed. Any associated air embolism must be excluded. Mild cases require only administration of 100% oxygen, without positive pressure, bedrest, and analgesics. A pneumothorax may also respond rapidly to high oxygen pressures at depth, such as when it occurs in a compression chamber or when a patient is recompressed for other reasons, such as CAGE.

Serious cases, often with more than 20% lung collapse, may need to have the gas removed rapidly, by needle aspiration and/or intercostal cannulation and underwater drainage or a Heimlich valve, with or without low pressure suction. This may be needed while the patient is undergoing recompression therapy.

Air embolism. **Treatment of air embolism is urgent**, must be instituted immediately, and usually takes precedence over other manifestations of PBT. Immediate recompression is necessary, and a recompression chamber should always be available. To reduce the likelihood of further CAGE, the patient should be nursed horizontally, on his/her back or lying on his/her side in the 'coma' position.

Oxygen, 100% via a close fitting mask, should be administered in transit to the chamber. Oxygen may also be used intermittently following recompression therapy, for similar reasons and to reduce the growth of existing bubbles. Because a possible cause of death from air embolism is from a cardiac lesion, CPR before and during recompression may be necessary. Rehydration may be both important and needed. Intravenous fluids (saline, electrolytes) should correct hemoconcentration, and may contain glucose only if long-term infusion is needed. Drugs are not very valuable in most cases of CAGE, despite many attempts to affect the complications of blood bubble interactions. Heparin and aspirin are not indicated. The administration of steroids is sometimes used to reduce vasogenic cerebral and spinal edema.

Pulmonary barotrauma of descent

This is known by the divers as 'lung squeeze'. Descent barotrauma is not common in breathhold diving, and very rare with open circuit diving apparatus. In breathhold divers, the total lung volume contracts with descent, according to Boyle's law, until it approximates the residual volume. Further descent may be hazardous. The individual pulmonary vascular response determines the final volume limitation. The minimal residual volume, which if further reduced will result in pulmonary damage, is problematic.

Clinical features are poorly documented, but include chest pain, hemoptysis with hemorrhagic pulmonary edema, and death. **Treatment** is based on general principles. Intermittent positive pressure respiration may be needed. Initially, 100% oxygen should be used with replacement of fluids, treatment of shock, etc. The use of positive end expiratory pressure would seem hazardous and predispose to subsequent gas embolism, but may be necessary.

Physics review—2

Henry's Law

This law describes the dissolving of gas in a liquid and states that the quantity of gas which will dissolve in a liquid at a given temperature is proportional to the partial pressure of gas in contact with the liquid. This means that if the pressure of gas exposed to a liquid increases, then more gas will dissolve in the liquid. Thus, as the diver descends, more nitrogen is dissolved in his blood, and can produce 'nitrogen narcosis'.

An extension of this law can be seen whenever a soft drink bottle is opened. During the manufacture of these drinks, carbon dioxide is dissolved in the liquid under pressure and the pressure is maintained by the lid on the bottle. When the bottle is opened and the pressure released, the liquid will not allow as much gas to be dissolved and so the excess gas is released from solution in the form of bubbles.

Under certain circumstances, when the diver returns to the surface this nitrogen can come out of solution in the form of bubbles. These bubbles cause tissue injury which is the basis of decompression sickness ('bends').

Decompression sickness (DCS)

Is an illness caused by the effects of gas coming out of solution to form bubbles in the body after diving. It is due to the effect of Henry's law following diving exposures.

Etiology

In recreational divers the main gas bubble is nitrogen (N_2)—because these divers almost invariably breath air. However, the same principles apply to other inert gases, such as helium (He), which may be breathed by commercial divers at deeper depths. When a diver breaths air from scuba equipment at depth, N_2 is breathed at an increased partial pressure. Because gas diffuses from areas of high partial pressure, N_2 is taken up from the lungs by the blood and transported around the body and into the tissues. The greater the depth, the greater the partial pressure of N_2, and therefore the amount of N_2 absorbed.

The rate of uptake of N_2 in a tissue is exponential. The uptake of gas in any tissue is initially rapid but slows with time. Accordingly, it may take a long time for a tissue to become saturated with gas, but the more vascular tissues become saturated sooner than others.

N_2 is eliminated in a reverse of the uptake process. As the diver ascends there is a reduction in the partial pressure of N_2 in the air he breathes, allowing blood to release N_2 into the lungs. The decrease in the blood level of N_2 causes N_2 to diffuse into the blood from the tissues. The pressure of N_2 dissolved in the tissues may become greater than the environmental pressure. The tissue is then said to be supersaturated.

The tissues are able to tolerate a certain degree of supersaturation. Nevertheless, if the pressure of N_2 in the tissues exceeds the environmental pressure by a critical amount, bubble formation occurs. *Bubbles can form in any tissue in the body, including blood.*

At the onset of DCS, the pressure of N_2 in the tissues is supersaturated (greater than the environmental pressure) so there is an immediate diffusion (pressure) gradient of N_2 into any bubbles present, causing them to expand.

Once a bubble has formed its behavior depends on several factors. Any increase in pressure such as diving or recompression, will reduce its size while any decrease in pressure such as ascent in the water, over mountains or in aircraft will expand it. The bubble will continue to grow in any tissue until the N_2 excess in that tissue has been eliminated. Once this has occurred (which may take hours or days) the bubble will begin to decrease in size but it may take hours, days or weeks to disappear. In the meantime the bubble can damage the tissues which host it.

There is good evidence that subclinical bubbles frequently form in tissues and blood of recreational divers after routine non-decompression dives.

Tissue damage by a bubble results from several factors. Bubbles in the blood may damage vascular endothelium or even obstruct blood vessels in vital organs such as the brain. Bubbles forming in the tissues may impair blood flow. Bubble pressure in or on nerves may interfere with function. Bubbles in the blood can also stimulate the clotting mechanism. Blood/bubble and tissue/bubble interaction results in progressive pathology.

Classification

DCS is best classified according to the organ or tissue affected, and the development (worsening, stationary, or improving). If there is difficulty in the provisional diagnosis between cerebral DCS and CAGE, an umbrella term is used '*acute decompression illness*' as the treatment is similar.

Onset

DCS develops after the subject has commenced decompression or ascent. Most cases present within 6 hours of the dive. Over 50% of cases of DCS develop symptoms within 1h of the dive and 90% within 6h.

Generalized symptoms

Perhaps the commonest presentations of DCS are generalized symptoms described as weakness, apathy, weariness, tiredness, or malaise. Other less tangible presentations include deviations from normal personality and/or behavior.

Musculoskeletal

This is also termed 'joint bends'. First, there is an ill-defined discomfort or numbness poorly localized to a joint, periarticular, or muscular area. The subject may protect or guard the affected area, although in the early stages relief may be gained by moving the limb. Over the next hour or so the discomfort develops into a deep dull ache, then a pain with fluctuations in intensity, sometimes throbbing, and occasionally with sharp exacerbations. Limitation of movement is due to pain, and the limb is placed in a position which affords the most relief. The duration of pain is often related to the severity of symptoms.

The shoulder is the more common joint affected in recreational divers, in approximately one-third of cases. Other joints, about equally affected, are the elbows, wrists, hands, hips, knees, and ankles. Often, when two joints are involved, they are adjoining ones, and frequently the localisation of pain is between joints, over the scapula, on tendon insertions, etc. The involvement is rarely symmetrical. The **application of local pressure** by means of a sphygmomanometer cuff, may result in considerable relief and thus be of diagnostic value. The site of pain can sometimes be transferred by massage of the area.

In the mild cases, fleeting symptoms are referred to as 'niggles', and may only last a few hours. The pain of the more severe cases usually increases over 12–24h and, if untreated, abates over the next 3–7 days to a dull ache. Local skin reactions may occur over the affected joint.

Neurological

Newer brain imaging techniques suggest that multifocal, small vessel, cerebral involvement, especially in the frontal and parietal lobes, are demonstrable with most neurological DCS cases and with CAGE. The **clinical subdivisions** of neurological presentations are: cerebral, cerebellar, spinal, inner ear, vision, and peripheral nerve.

Cerebral. Any cerebral tissue may be damaged by gas bubbles, and causes a great variety of manifestations, analogous to those of the diffuse cerebrovascular disease of general medicine. Especially noted are the homonymous scotomata, unilateral or bilateral. Others include hemiplegia, monoplegia, focal or generalized convulsions, aphasia, alexia, agnosia, hemisensory or monosensory disturbances, and confusional states. Raised intracranial pressure has been observed, and may be associated with severe headache.

Cerebellar. These lesions produce ataxia, incoordination with typical neurological signs of hypotonia, diminished or pendular tension reflexes, asynergia with dysmetria, tremor, dysdiadokokinesis, rebound phenomenon, scanning speech, and nystagmus. The 'staggers' which is variously described as vestibular, posterior column, spinal cord, and cerebral DCS, is probably more often due to cerebellar lesions, without nystagmus.

Spinal. The spinal cord changes are predominantly in the white matter, and are most often observed in the midthoracic, upper lumbar, and lower cervical areas, with the lateral, posterior and anterior columns suffering in that order. Often, there is sparing of some long sensory tracts. Local spinal or girdle pains may precede other symptoms, developing into serious spinal cord disease. It is more common in patients who also have respiratory symptoms ('chokes'). The symptoms and signs vary from mild paresthesia to paraplegia or paraparesis, and include urinary retention with overflow incontinence. *Note*: the lower abdominal pain due to a distended bladder from spinal DCS, is frequently misdiagnosed.

Somatosensory evoked cortical responses and imaging techniques do not demonstrate the extent of the pathology.

Inner ear. In deep helium or hydrogen dives the most common serious problem is DCS affecting the inner ear. **Clinically**, it may be characterized by cochlear damage (tinnitus, sensorineural hearing loss) and/or vestibular disorder (prostrating vertigo, nausea, vomiting, syncope). In cases of generalized neurological DCS, vestibular symptoms are **misdiagnosed** and often confused with cerebellar disease. Investigations, including electronystagmography, clarify the peripheral (vestibular) or central (cerebellar) nature of the disease. In shallow scuba air diving, isolated inner ear DCS is not common. It is much more likely to be due to inner ear barotrauma.

Vision. Bubbles have been observed in the ocular fluids and in the lens. The latter are longer lasting, but both may cause blurring of vision in one or both eyes. Retinal lesions with intravascular bubbles and hemorrhages have been described. Vision is more commonly affected by interference with the neural pathways, with appropriate visual field defects. Long-term retinal lesions, with low retinal capillary density at the fovea, microaneurysms and small areas of capillary non-perfusion are said to be related to DCS incidence.

Peripheral nerve. Bubble formation in the myelin of peripheral nerves will result in a patchy sensory damage or motor impairment, predominantly involving the limbs. In severe cases there may be a glove-and-stocking distribution, but the usual presentation is with paresthesia, numbness, and weakness. Pain may be related to the major plexus, and may be long lasting.

Cutaneous

Skin manifestations range from being local and innocuous, to generalized and ominous, with a complete spectrum in between. If they develop with water exposure they are more likely to be serious than with chamber exposures, in which the inert gas can be absorbed through the skin. They include:

- **Pruritis.** It is often a transient effect, presenting very soon after decompression, and is not considered a systemic or serious manifestation of DCS. The symptoms are attributed to small gas bubbles in the superficial layers of the dermis, and especially near its entry via the epidermis and the sebaceous glands.
- **Scarlatiniform rash**. The distribution is predominantly over the chest, shoulders, back, upper abdomen, and thighs, in that order. The rash may last for several hours.
- **Erysipeloid rash.** This is a definite sign of systemic DCS. Some of the skin appearance is thought to be a reflex vascular reaction.
- **Cutis marmorata marblization**. This commences as a small pale area with cyanotic mottling. Swelling and edema result in a mottled appearance. Recompression gives dramatic relief. Marbling of the skin is a cutaneous manifestation of what is occurring elsewhere in the body, and is a serious sign of DCS.
- **Subcutaneous emphysema**. This has the typical crepitus sensation on palpation, either in localized areas or along the tendon sheaths. It can be verified radiologically and should not be confused with the supraclavicular subcutaneous emphysema extending from the mediastinum, due to pulmonary barotrauma.
- **Lymphatic obstruction**. This presents as a localized swelling which may be associated with an underlying DCS manifestation. If it involves hair follicles, a *peau d'orange* or pigskin appearance with brawny edema is characteristic. It is common over the trunk, but is also seen over the head and neck.
- **Formication** may be the presentation in any of the skin manifestations described above, or due to involvement of the peripheral nervous system or the spinal cord. The neural involvement may also result in numbness, hypoesthesia, paresthesia, or hyperesthesia of the skin.

Gastrointestinal

Mildly affected patients may present only with anorexia, nausea, vomiting or retching, abdominal cramps, and diarrhea. *When the condition is severe*, local ischemia and infarction of bowel, with secondary hemorrhages, may result. In such cases, the use of drugs which encourage hemorrhage, such as aspirin or heparin, could be detrimental. In some of the DCS fatalities, gastointestinal hemorrhage was the final cause of death.

Cardiorespiratory

Intravascular bubbles are more common in the venous system after diving. Although many of these bubbles may be trapped in the pulmonary capillaries, some may pass into the arterial circulation, either through the pulmonary plexus, a patent foramen ovale, or a septal defect. The presence of gas bubbles in the blood may hamper microcirculation and produce both local hypoxia and generalized hematological sequelae.

Local ischemic effect. This may follow cerebral, coronary, or other visceral effects from vascular damage or occlusion. The clinical manifestations will vary according to the organs involved.

Pulmonary involvement ('chokes'). After uneventful dives bubbles may be entrapped in the pulmonary circulation. **Clinical manifestations** develop when 10% or more of the pulmonary vascular bed is obstructed. The effect of gas in the pulmonary vessels is to displace blood and inflate the lungs intravascularly. This may reflexly produce a shallow rapid breathing, reduce alveolar ventilation, and compliance. *Note*: interference with the pulmonary circulation can result in a decrease in pulse rate and a reduction in left ventricular return, progressing to circulatory collapse in severe cases.

Post decompression shock. In very severe cases (e.g. in explosive—very rapid—decompression or following grossly inadequate decompression), there may be a generalized liberation of gas into all vessels, resulting in rapid death. The presence of gas bubbles in the circulating blood results in a bubble/blood interaction and if the fibrin clotting mechanism is activated, then all manifestations of disseminated intravascular coagulation may result.

Treatment

Therapeutic recompression is the most effective treatment for DCS. Delay increases the likelihood of a poor final result. The increase in pressure reduces the bubble size (Boyle's law) and usually relieves the clinical features. It also increases the surface area to volume ratio of the bubble, which may collapse the bubble. The increased pressure in the bubble also enhances the diffusion gradient, encouraging nitrogen to leave the bubble. Oxygen, sometimes at toxic levels, is used to hasten the process. This is a treatment performed by diving medical experts. **First aid management** includes 100% oxygen administration, fluid replacement and transfer to a recompression facility.

Mountainous roads should be avoided whenever an evacuation route by land is planned. Transportation in aircraft presents problems. Apart from movement which aggravates DCS, environmental pressure decreases with altitude, causing DCS bubbles to expand and more gas to pass from the tissues into any bubbles. Whenever possible, the aircraft cabin altitude should be maintained at 1 ATA. This is attainable by many modern commercial jet aircraft, and some military aircraft (Hercules C–130). This requirement is not popular with commercial airlines since it necessitates flying lower than the most efficient altitude, resulting in excessive fuel consumption. This requirement may also limit the range of certain aircraft.

Dysbaric osteonecrosis

The cause of the disorder is probably a delayed effect of damage caused by gas bubbles produced during a dive. In this sense it is a delayed form of decompression sickness. This was first described as being an area of localized bone death, predominantly occurring in the long bones of the arms and thigh.

X-ray changes have been seen as soon as 3 months after a dive and it has been reported following a single deep dive. When joint involvement does occur, the onset of symptoms is usually delayed for many years, reflecting the time required for joint destruction.

Type A lesions

With these, the joints may become involved as the overlying bone is destroyed and the joint surface collapses. This may produce symptoms which are potentially crippling. Hips and shoulders are more frequently affected.

Type B lesions

These rarely cause symptoms and are generally of little clinical importance, except to suggest more conservative diving procedures. The most common areas affected are the long bones of the thigh, leg, and upper arm. Occasional cases of neoplasia have developed in these lesions.

Investigations. X–rays have been the traditional investigative method but these will only reveal lesions once bone changes have developed. This may take months or years. Early lesions can now be identified with newer techniques. Injected radioactive Technetium (bone scans) will bind to an osteonecrotic area and can be detected within 2 weeks of the injury. The lesions can also be identified in excellent detail, using magnetic resonance imaging.

Treatment. The pain associated with movement can be reduced with an antiinflammatory drug such as NSAIDs. Severe cases may require the fusion of a joint or its replacement with a synthetic joint. While this procedure relieves the pain and increases mobility, a replacement joint is never as robust and its endurance is indefinite.

Salt water aspiration syndrome

This condition is due to the aspiration of small amounts of salt water, nebulized by the diver breathing through a leaking demand valve. Experienced divers used the term 'salt water fever'. Other marine sports persons to present with a similar disorder, but possibly not as frequently, are snorkellers, surfers, and rescuees picked up by helicopter.

Clinical

Immediate symptoms. A history of aspiration is given by most. Often this is not causally associated by the novice diver with the subsequent events. Most also have a post dive cough, with or without sputum. Only in the more serious cases is the sputum bloodstained, frothy, and copious.

Respiratory symptoms. There is often a delay of 1–2h before dyspnea, cough, sputum and retrosternal discomfort on inspiration are noted. In the mild cases, respiratory symptoms persist for only an hour or so, while in the more severe cases they continue for days. In about half the cases there are crepitations or occasional rhonchi, either generalized or local. Administration of 100% oxygen was reliably effective in relieving respiratory symptoms and removing cyanosis when present. Expiratory spirometry shows a drop in both FEV_1 and vital capacity measurements and can persist for up to 24h. Arterial blood gases revealed oxygen tensions of 40—75mmHg with low or normal carbon dioxide tensions.

Generalized symptoms. The patient complains of being feverish in most cases. Malaise, headaches, and generalized aches were important in some cases, but usually not dominant. In some, there is an impairment of consciousness, including a transitory mild confusion or syncope with loss of consciousness on standing. Pyrexia is often present, up to 40°C with tachycardia over the first 6h. These systemic signs and symptoms usually revert to normal within 6h, and rarely persist beyond 24h, unless the case is severe. Hemotological and electrolyte changes are unusual, although a mild leucocytosis is sometimes present. X-ray of the chest reveals areas of patchy consolidation, or an increase in respiratory markings, in about half the cases. These usually clear within 24h, but remain longer in severely affected cases.

There is a gradation of clinical manifestations between salt water aspiration and near drowning cases. The intensity of the symptoms and the degree of consciousness depend on various circumstances, the activity of the victim and the administration of oxygen.

Headaches after diving: differential diagnosis

Some causes of headache in diving:

- Anxiety
- Sinus barotrauma, sinusitis and other pathology
- Infections
- Cold exposure
- Exercise provocation
- Salt water aspiration
- Tight facemask straps
- Carbon dioxide and carbon monoxide toxicity
- Decompression sickness (DCS)
- Pulmonary barotrauma
- Migraine
- Cervical spondylosis
- Drugs

These causes are not all inclusive, and the clinical details of each type of headache are to be found in general medical texts. The differential diagnosis will depend on a detailed clinical and diving history, a physical examination, and laboratory investigation, and may even require the provoking of the symptoms by re-exposure of the diver to the specific diving condition.

Anxiety (tension). The psychological reaction induced in susceptible novice divers, exposed to a stressful underwater environment, may produce a typical tension headache.

Sinus barotrauma pain occurs during the diver's change of depth— reflecting the volume changes on the sinus gas spaces. Barotrauma of descent affecting the frontal sinus is the most common. It is **often relieved by ascent**. Ethmoidal sinus pain if referred to the intraorbital area and maxillary sinus pain may be referred to the teeth. Sphenoidal sinus pain may be referred to the parieto-occipital area.

Sinus pathology, such as mucocoele or mucosal congestion, can be produced by diving. Rupture of the air cells in the ethmoidal sinus air cells can cause a sudden and explosive headache and result in a small hematoma or bruising below the glabella, at the root of the nose. A similar explosive headache can develop, often during ascent and following middle ear barotrauma, with rupture of the mastoid air cells causing a generalized pain, localizing later to the mastoid region. Pneumocephalus can follow the sinus ruptures. **X-rays and diagnostic imaging** demonstrate these lesions with precision.

Infections in the mastoid cavities or sinuses usually cause pain 4–24h after the dive, and are commonly associated with a pre-existing upper respiratory tract infection and/or barotrauma. Other generalized infections, including *Nagleria*, are related to marine exposure.

Cold. In some susceptible subjects, exposure to cold water may induce a throbbing pain over the frontal area especially, but sometimes also including the occipital area. It is probably analogous to ice cream headaches. The onset may be rapid after cold water contact, or it may progressively increase in intensity with the duration of exposure. It usually remains after the diver has left the water.

Salt water aspiration. Headache following aspiration of sea water usually follows a latent period, and is usually associated with myalgia and is aggravated by exercise and cold.

Mask tension. Inexperienced divers tend to adjust the facemask straps far too tightly and this may result in a headache not dissimilar

Hearing loss in diving: Aetiological checklist

1 Conductive

- External ear obstruction
  - Cerumen
  - Otitis externa
  - Exostoses
- Tympanic membrane perforation
  - Middle ear barotrauma of descent
  - Forceful autoinflation
  - Shock wave
- Middle ear cleft disorder
  - Middle ear barotrauma of descent
  - Otitis media
  - Forceful autoinflation
  - Increased gas density in middle ear.
  - Ossicular disruptions

2 Sensorineural

- Noise induced
- Decompression sickness (DCS)
- Inner ear barotrauma

3 Others

- Dysacusis

to that of a tight hat, misfitting spectacle frames, etc. due to direct local pressure effects. It is related to the duration of the dive, and clears in an hour or so. It sometimes may be related to migraine.

Gas toxicity. Specific gas toxicities may sometimes cause a characteristic headache. The carbon dioxide-induced headache usually develops with a gradually increasing carbon dioxide tension, or follows a reduction in a sharply rising carbon dioxide tension (i.e. a carbon dioxide 'off effect'). It is throbbing in nature, lasts a few hours, and is not relieved by analgesics or antimigraine preparations. Headaches have also been described with oxygen toxicity, carbon monoxide toxicity and other gas contaminations.

DCS and *CAGE*. Headache is an ominous symptom in both neurological DCS and CAGE from pulmonary barotrauma. It is associated with intracerebral bubbles and/or raised intracranial pressure. Usually, it arises within minutes of ascent, and implies an intravascular origin. Other neurological manifestations and a disturbance of conscious state are often associated. The headache is likely to persist for a week or more, but is rapidly relieved by recompression therapy. Its recurrence is indicative of a deterioration in the patient's neurological state and is also amenable to recompression or oxygen therapy.

Migraine. Traditionally, migraine sufferers are often advised not to take up diving. Attacks are occasionally induced by the diving environment, and may be of greatly increased severity. The precipitation of the migraine attack may be due to any of the other headache-producing stimuli discussed in this section (e.g. cold, anxiety, oxygen or carbon dioxide tensions, intravascular bubbles, etc.).

Neuromuscular pain. Headaches produced by the environment or by locomotor stress may produce severe pains which are difficult to assess and diagnose. Many such patients give consistent accounts of headaches being induced by diving, and sometimes only by scuba diving, but with none of the specific features mentioned above.

One specific type is due to minor degrees of *cervical spondylosis*. In these there may be loss of lordotic curvature, narrowing of intervertebral spaces, and osteophytosis in the lateral x-ray views. Many divers who develop this disorder are older or have a history of head and neck trauma. They often swim underwater with flexion of the lower cervical spine (to avoid the tank) and their upper cervical spine hyperextended (to view where they are going). This produces C1, C2, and C3 compression and distortion of the cervicocranial relationships—an unnatural posture aggravating underlying disease.

The headache is usually occipital and may persist for many hours after the dive. The area is often tender on palpation. Persistent occipital neuralgia can have a similar etiology. Occasionally, the pain is referred to the top and front of the head, possibly due to the trigeminal nerve.

Others. Many other obvious reasons may be incriminated in the etiology of headache in divers. These include such diverse factors as alcohol overindulgence, head injury usually sustained during ascent, glare from the sun, drugs such as vasodilators, and calcium channel blockers.

Vertigo in diving: Aetiological checklist

DUE TO UNEQUAL VESTIBULAR STIMULATION

1 Caloric

- Unilateral external auditory canal obstruction
  - Cerumen
  Otitis externa
  Miscellaneous
- Tympanic membrane perforation
  - Shock wave
  - Middle ear barotrauma of descent
  - Forceful autoinflation

2 Barotrauma

- External ear barotrauma
- Middle ear barotrauma of descent
- Middle ear barotrauma of ascent
- Forceful autoinflation
- Inner ear barotrauma
- Fistula of the inner ear windows
- Other causes

3 Decompression sickness (DCS)

4 Miscellaneous

- Tullio Phenomenon

DUE TO UNEQUAL VESTIBULAR RESPONSES

1 Caloric
2 Barotrauma
3 Gas toxicity
4 Sensory deprivation

Recommended reading for Chapter 26

P Bennett, D Elliott 1993 *The physiology and medicine of diving* 4th edition. Saunders, London.

AA Bove, JC Davis 1997 *Diving medicine.* Saunders, Philadelphia.

Diving Accident Management 1990 *41st Undersea and Hyperbaric Medical Workshop*, Bennett, Moon (ed). Undersea and Hyperbaric Medical Society, National Oceanic and Atmospheric Administration, and the Divers Alert Network.

C Edmonds, B McKenzie, R Thomas 1997 *Diving medicine—for scuba divers.* JL Publications, Australia and DAN, USA.

C Edmonds 1989 *Dangerous marine creatures.* Best Publishing, Arizona.

C Edmonds, C Lowry, J Pennefather 1991 *Diving and subaquatic medicine*, 3rd edn. Butterworth-Heinemann, Oxford

CW Shilling, MF Werts, NR Schandolmeier 1976 *The underwater handbook, a guide to physiology and performance for the engineer*. Undersea and Hyperbaric Medical Society, Maryland. J Wiley, London.

CW Shilling, CB Carlston, RA Mathias 1984 *The physician's guide to diving medicine.* Plenum Press, New York.

Further reading

CL Baker (Ed) 1996 *The Hughston Clinic Sports Medicine Field Manual*. Williams and Wilkins, PA.

RB Birrer (Ed) 1994 *Sports medicine for the primary care Physician* 2nd Ed. Florida

J Bloomfield *et al*. 1992 *Science and medicine in sport.* Blackwell, Oxford.

A Dirix, HG Knuttgen, and K Tittel 1988 *The Olympic book of sports medicine.* Blackwell, Oxford.

LY Griffin (Ed) 1994 *Orthopaedic knowledge update sports medicine.* AAOS, IL

M Harries *et al*. (Eds) 1994 *The Oxford textbook of sports medicine.* OUP.

WL Kenney (Ed) 1995 *ACSM's guidelines for exercise testing and prescription.* Williams and Wilkins, Philadelphia

WB Kibler (Ed) 1996 *ACSM's Handbook for the Team Physician.* Williams and Wilkins, Philadelphia

MB Meillion (Ed) 1994 *Sports medicine secrets.* Hanley and Belfus, Inc, Philadelphia

E Sherry 1997 *Colour guide sports medicine.* Churchill Livingstone, Edinburgh

E Sherry, D Bokor (Ed) 1997 *Sports medicine problems and practical management.* GMM, London

Further contacts

The Internet

WorldOrtho—The World of Orthopaedics and Sports Medicine
Visit www.worldortho.com

Sports Medicine Centre

Australian Institute of Sport
Canberra, ACT 2601, Australia

Centre for Disease Control

Division of Injury, Epidemiology and Control
Atlanta, GA 30333
USA

Sports Council

16 Upper Woburn Place
London, WC1H OQP
UK

American College of Sports Medicine

PO Box 1440
Indianapolis, IN 46206–1440
USA

**National Injury Information Clearinghouse/National
Electronic Injury Surveillance System (NEISS)**

US Consumer Product Safety Commission
5401 Westbard Ave
Room 625
Washington DC, 20207
USA

Index

A